The Most Common Manual For Medical Students

Second Edition

*A reference manual for medical students
and house staff*

Steven M. Grosso, M.D.
Department of Surgery
Vanderbilt University School of Medicine
Nashville, Tennessee

TABLE OF CONTENTS

PREFACE

This medical reference manual is a compilation of many of the "**most commons**" of medicine. It is my intention in writing this manual to provide **second and third year medical students** with a resource which will be useful when studying for examinations and reviewing material. It is also designed to be a good size to carry in the white coat on the hospital wards; this should provide both students and residents with a good source with which to gear up for rounds. It is by no means an exhaustive compilation, and is not intended to be a complete listing. However, this edition contains over 3,500 entries, organized into 15 chapters, and is a handy source by which one can quickly access information.

The organization of the manual is **alphabetical**. Chapters are arranged this way, and listings within each chapter are also alphabetical. This provides the reader with a convenient system of identifying entries in the text. There are a few exceptions, however. For example, in the neoplasm chapter, neoplasms are identified as benign or malignant, and then miscellaneous listings follow.

An additional comment about the organization is in order. Some entries are more difficult to categorize than others, consisting of both adjectives and nouns. For example, the most common causes of metabolic acidosis could have been listed as "...metabolic acidosis" or "...acidosis, metabolic". In many cases *both* entries have been listed to eliminate confusion.

Answers listed under a heading are intended to be in order of **greatest to least frequency**. This means that the first entry is the most common, the next is the second most common, and so on. However some sources do not identify their entries (answers) in order of frequency, and group them collectively as the most common. This pattern is duplicated here as well. Answers either *are* in decreasing order, or they are the most common as a group. This still yields a collection of the "most commons" and not the "zebras".

It should be noted that **geographic differences** do exist in most commons. For example, the two most common causes of meningitis in neonates may be reversed in order on the coasts compared with the midwest. However, as noted above, the answers will still collectively be the most common causes, and should be viewed this way.

Finally, some chapters are quite extensive. Others have fewer listings. In compiling this edition, I have decided to include all chapters for which I have current entries. I encourage all readers to give me input regarding the content and organization of this text. This will only continue to be a valuable text if its readers can access the information that they need. If readers find themselves referring to chapters which are not extensive enough, I would like to hear those comments. In future editions, I can expand chapters commonly referred to and eliminate those which readers use less often. This will insure that the manual remains small, convenient, and valuable.

Please send any comments and suggestions to the address indicated on the copyright page (ii).

Good luck, and good reading!

October, 1991
Steven M. Grosso, M.D.

The Most Common

Causes Of...

The Most Common
CAUSES OF:

...ABNORMAL BLEEDING:
   thrombocytopenia
...ABNORMAL PLATELET FUNCTION:
   drug related platelet dysfunction (e.g., aspirin
   or other anti-inflammatory drug use)
...ABSCESSES:

Anorectal: a mixed infection usually occurs; *Escherichia coli, Proteus vulgaris,* streptococci, staphylococci, and bacteroides are predominant causes

Axillae: aerobes alone or a mixture of aerobes and anaerobes is usual. The most frequent anaerobic species are *Peptococcus* and *Propionibacterium*; the most common aerobic organisms are *Staphylococcus aureus* and *epidermidis.*

Brain: the bacteria isolated from these abscesses usually are anaerobic, not uncommonly mixed, and often include anaerobic *Streptococcus* or *Bacteroides.* Fungal abscesses occur as well.

in the Newborn and debilitated elderly patient:
   facultatively anaerobic enteric rods; *H. influenzae* essentially is found only in children in the 1- to 5-year old age group

Buttock: these abscesses contain organisms found in the stool, commonly anaerobes alone or a combination of aerobes and anaerobes. *Peptococcus,* Peptostreptococcus, *Lactobacillus, Bacteroides,* and *Fusobacterium* species are the predominant anaerobic isolates; α– and non-hemolytic streptococci are the most frequent aerobes

Cutaneous: these abscesses usually follow minor skin trauma

Axillae: aerobes alone or a mixture of aerobes and anaerobes is usual. The most frequent anaerobic

3

The Most Common
CAUSES OF:

species are *Peptococcus* and *Propionibacterium*; the most common aerobic organisms are *Staphylococcus aureus* and *epidermidis*.

Extremities:
aerobes alone or a mixture of aerobes and anaerobes is usual. The most frequent anaerobic species are *Peptococcus* and *Propionibacterium*; the most common aerobic organisms are *Staphylococcus aureus* and *epidermidis*.

Head and neck:
aerobes alone or a mixture of aerobes and anaerobes is usual. The most frequent anaerobic species are *Peptococcus* and *Propionibacterium*; the most common aerobic organisms are *Staphylococcus aureus* and *epidermidis*.

Perineal (inguinal, vaginal, buttock, and perirectal):
these abscesses contain organisms found in the stool, commonly anaerobes alone or a combination of aerobes and anaerobes. *Peptococcus, Peptostreptococcus, Lactobacillus, Bacteroides,* and *Fusobacterium* species are the predominant anaerobic isolates; $\alpha-$ and non-hemolytic streptococci are the most frequent aerobes

Trunk:
aerobes alone or a mixture of aerobes and anaerobes is usual. The most frequent anaerobic species are *Peptococcus* and *Propionibacterium*; the most common aerobic organisms are *Staphylococcus aureus* and *epidermidis*.

Dentoalveolar:the abscess is secondary to an infection of the dental pulp usually due to caries. However, it may occur after trauma to the teeth or from periapical localization of organisms, usually

4

The Most Common
CAUSES OF:

Extremities:
α− hemolytic streptococci or staphylococci aerobes alone or a mixture of aerobes and anaerobes is usual. The most frequent anaerobic species are *Peptococcus* and *Propionibacterium*; the most common aerobic organisms are *Staphylococcus aureus* and *epidermidis*.

Hand:
Felon (an infection of the pulp space of the finger pad): nearly always follows minor finger injury (e.g., a splinter or needle prick)

Head and neck:
aerobes alone or a mixture of aerobes and anaerobes is usual. The most frequent anaerobic species are *Peptococcus* and *Propionibacterium*; the most common aerobic organisms are *Staphylococcus aureus* and *epidermidis*.

Hepatic, in the Western World:
hepatic abscesses are usually amebic or bacterial (pyogenic)

Bacterial:
secondary to an infectious process in the abdomen, particularly appendicitis, diverticulitis, or purulent cholecystitis. Also may be the result of seeding from a distant infectious focus, such as subacute bacterial endocarditis. In some cases, no primary source can be identified. Streptococci or staphylococci are the most common bacteria when the infection results from systemic bacteremia. Abscesses originating from a biliary tract infection usually contain aerobic gram-negative rods - e.g., *E. coli* and *Klebsiella*, while those secondary to portal bacteremia from an intra-abdominal infection typically contain both aerobic gram-

The Most Common
CAUSES OF:

Inguinal:
negative bacilli and anaerobic bacteria
these abscesses contain organisms found in
the stool, commonly anaerobes alone or a
combination of aerobes and anaerobes. *Peptococcus, Peptostreptococcus, Lactobacillus, Bacteroides,* and *Fusobacterium* species are
the predominant anaerobic isolates; α- and
non-hemolytic streptococci are the most frequent aerobes

Intra-abdominal:
gastrointestinal perforations, operative complications, penetrating trauma, and genitourinary infections

Intraperitoneal:
Intrinsic causes:
perforation of a hollow viscus such as the appendix, duodenum, or colon, seeding of bacteria from a source outside the abdomen, or ischemia and infarction of tissue within the
abdomen, such as bowel ischemia

Extrinsic causes:
penetrating trauma and surgical procedures

Left lower-quadrant:
usually occur from perforation of a diverticulum in the descending or sigmoid colon, less
commonly from a perforated colonic carcinoma

Lung:
aspiration of infected material or foreign body
with subsequent pneumonia (50%). The aspiration is usually infected material from the
upper airway when a patient is unconscious or
obtunded from alcoholism, CNS disease, general anesthesia, or excessive sedation. Usually due to anaerobes, lung abscesses are often

associated with periodontal disease; sometimes multiple organisms act synergistically. Bacteria cultured from lung abscesses include common pyogenic bacteria and nasopharyngeal flora, particularly anaerobes, and less often aerobic bacteria or fungi. Other less common causes include: necrotizing pneumonia (20%); septic embolus or infection of a pulmonary infarct; bronchial obstruction due to any cause (e.g., tumor) may result in infection behind the obstruction and abscess formation (bronchogenic carcinoma is an occasional cause of lung abscess in persons over age 55); infection of a cyst or bulla; extension of bronchiectasis into the parenchyma; penetrating chest trauma; transdiaphragmatic extension of infection (e.g., from a subphrenic bacterial or amebic abscess). When a lung abscess develops in childhood, a foreign body should be suspected, whereas in older age groups, bronchial obstruction by cancer should be considered. In the Immunocompromised host, lung abscess is usually due to *Nocardia,* cryptococcus, *Aspergillus, Phycomyces*, or gram-negative bacilli

in the Immunocompromised host:

usually due to *Nocardia,* cryptococcus, *Aspergillus, Phycomyces*, or gram-negative bacilli. Other less common causes of lung abscess include septic pulmonary emboli, secondary infection of pulmonary infarcts, and direct extension of amebic or bacterial abscesses from the liver through the diaphragm into the lower lobe of the lung.

The Most Common
CAUSES OF:

Mid-abdominal:

    Left lower-quadrant:

        usually occur from perforation of a diverticulum in the descending or sigmoid colon, less commonly from a perforated colonic carcinoma

    Right lower-quadrant:

        develop most commonly as complications of acute appendicitis and less frequently from colonic diverticulitis, regional enteritis, or a perforated duodenal ulcer with drainage down the right paracolic gutter

Pancreatic: the usual organisms are bowel flora - aerobic gram-negative rods and anaerobes, but how they reach the pancreas is uncertain. Staphylococcus and candida are surprisingly frequent isolates, as well

Parapharyngeal: usually secondary to pharyngitis or tonsillitis and may occur at any age

Pelvic: usually are complications of acute appendicitis, pelvic inflammatory disease, or colonic diverticulitis

Perianal: infected anal glands that erode into underlying tissues

Periapical (dentoalveolar): the abscess is secondary to an infection of the dental pulp usually due to caries. However, it may occur after trauma to the teeth or from periapical localization of organisms, usually α- hemolytic streptococci or staphylococci

Perineal (inguinal, vaginal, buttock, and perirectal): these abscesses contain organisms found in the stool, commonly anaerobes alone or a combination of aerobes and anaerobes. *Pep-*

8

The Most Common
CAUSES OF:

tococcus, Peptostreptococcus, *Lactobacillus, Bacteroides*, and *Fusobacterium* species are the predominant anaerobic isolates; α– and non-hemolytic streptococci are the most frequent aerobes

Perinephric: abscess between the renal capsule and the perirenal fascia most often results from rupture of an intrarenal abscess into the perinephric space. The infecting bacteria are usually gram-negative enteric bacilli and occasionally gram-positive cocci when the infection is of hematogenous origin. *E. coli* is the most common, and *Proteus mirabilis* is also frequently cultured from these abscesses

Perirectal: these abscesses contain organisms found in the stool, commonly anaerobes alone or a combination of aerobes and anaerobes. *Peptococcus*, Peptostreptococcus, *Lactobacillus, Bacteroides*, and *Fusobacterium* species are the predominant anaerobic isolates; α– and non-hemolytic streptococci are the most frequent aerobes

Peritonsillar (Quinsy): a Group A β-hemolytic streptococcus. Anaerobic microorganisms such as bacteroides also cause peritonsillar infection

Pharyngomaxillary: usually arise from infections in the pharynx, including the nasopharynx, adenoids, and tonsils. Less common sources are dental infections, parotitis, and mastoiditis

Prostatic: aerobic gram-negative bacilli or, less frequently, *Staphylococcus aureus*

Psoas:

The Most Common
CAUSES OF:

Primary: these are caused by hematogenous spread of *Staphylococcus aureus* from an occult source

Secondary: these result from spread of infection from adjacent organs, principally from the intestine, and are therefore most often polymicrobial. The most common cause is Crohn's disease

Renal: while renal abscess (carbuncle) is occasionally due to hematogenous spread of a distant staphylococcal infection, most abscesses are secondary to chronic non-specific infection of the kidney, often complicated by stone formation

Retroperitoneal: pyogenic bacteria have replaced *Mycobacterium tuberculosis* as the major causative organisms. Retroperitoneal abscesses arise chiefly from injuries or infections in adjacent structures: gastrointestinal tract abscesses due to appendicitis, pancreatitis, penetrating posterior ulcers, regional enteritis, diverticulitis, or trauma; genitourinary tract abscesses due to pyelonephritis; and spinal column abscesses due to osteomyelitis or disk space infections

Retropharyngeal: usually a complication of suppurative retropharyngeal lymph nodes to which infection has spread from the pharynx, sinuses, adenoids, nose, or middle ear. Occasional causes in adults or children are TB or perforation of the posterior pharyngeal wall by foreign bodies or instrumentation (although these abscesses usually occur in infants or young children)

Right lower-quadrant: develop most commonly as complications of

10

acute appendicitis and less frequently from colonic diverticulitis, regional enteritis, or a perforated duodenal ulcer with drainage down the
right paracolic gutter

Spinal epidural:

Staphylococcus aureus is the most common
causative organism, followed by *Escherichia
coli* and mixed anaerobes. Rarely, a tuberculous abscess may develop in conjunction with
Pott's disease of the thoracic spine

Splenic:

most occur from uncontrolled infection else-
where and are small, multiple, and clinically
silent abnormalities found incidentally at autopsy. Clinically evident splenic abscesses
usually are solitary and arise from (1) systemic bacteremia (e.g., endocarditis or salmonellosis) that originated in another site and is
now causing infection in a previously normal
spleen; (2) infection, presumably of hematogenous origin, in a spleen damaged by blunt or
penetrating trauma (with superinfection of a
hematoma), bland infarction (such as occurs
in hemoglobinopathies, especially sickle trait
or hemoglobin SC disease), or other diseases
(malaria, hydatid cysts); or (3) extension from
a contiguous infection, such as a subphrenic
abscess. The most commonly infecting organisms are staphylococcus, streptococci, anaerobes, and anaerobic gram-negative rods, including salmonella

Subphrenic:

most subphrenic abscesses arise from direct
contamination of the area following local disease, injury, or most frequently, surgery.
They develop from peritonitis secondary to
another cause, such as perforated viscus; ex-

The Most Common
CAUSES OF:

Trunk:

Vaginal:

tension from an abscess in an adjacent organ; or, most commonly, as a postoperative complication of abdominal surgery, especially on the biliary tract, duodenum, or stomach aerobes alone or a mixture of aerobes and anaerobes is usual. The most frequent anaerobic species are *Peptococcus* and *Propionibacterium*; the most common aerobic organisms are *Staphylococcus aureus* and *epidermidis.*

these abscesses contain organisms found in the stool, commonly anaerobes alone or a combination of aerobes and anaerobes. *Peptococcus, Peptostreptococcus, Lactobacillus, Bacteroides,* and *Fusobacterium* species are the predominant anaerobic isolates; $\alpha-$ and non-hemolytic streptococci are the most frequent aerobes

...ABRUPTIO PLACENTA:

toxemia, diabetes, vascular disease, trauma, sudden decrease in uterine size (e.g. concealed hemorrhage), compression of inferior vena cava, folic acid deficiency, vitamin C deficiency, short umbilical cord, cigarette smoking, amniocentesis

...ACIDOSIS:

Metabolic:

with Elevated "anion gap":

the principle causes are renal failure, diabetic ketoacidosis, lactic acidosis, and exogenous poisons (ethylene glycol, salicylates, methanol, paraldehyde)

with Normal "anion gap":

the principle causes are GI alkali loss (diarrhea, ileostomy, colostomy), renal tubular aci-

12

The Most Common
CAUSES OF:

dosis, interstitial renal disease (e.g., "selective hypoaldosteronism"), ureterosigmoid loop, uncommonly ureteroileal conduit, ingestion of acetazolamide or ammonium chloride

Respiratory
Acute: obstruction of the airway, neuromuscular disorders and diseases of the central nervous system are common causes of acute respiratory acidosis, according to Devlin

Chronic: seen in patients with chronic obstructive lung disease, such as emphysema

...ACQUIRED ACUTE RENAL FAILURE IN INFANTS AND CHILDREN:

hemolytic-uremic syndrome

...ACUTE ABDOMEN:

gastrointestinal tract disorders (appendicitis, small and large bowel obstruction, strangulated hernia, perforated peptic ulcer, bowel perforation, Meckel's diverticulitis, Boerhaave's syndrome, diverticulitis, inflammatory bowel disorders, Mallory-Weiss syndrome, gastroenteritis, acute gastritis, mesenteric adenitis); liver, spleen, and biliary tract disorders (acute cholecystitis, acute cholangitis, hepatic abscess, ruptured hepatic tumor, spontaneous rupture of the spleen, splenic infarct, biliary colic, acute hepatitis); pancreatic disorders (acute pancreatitis); urinary tract disorders (ureteral or renal colic, acute pyelonephritis, acute cystitis, renal infarct); gynecologic disorders (ruptured ectopic pregnancy, twisted ovarian tumor, ruptured ovarian follicle cyst, acute salpingitis, dysmenorrhea, endometriosis); vascular disorders (ruptured aortic and visceral aneurysms, acute ischemic colitis,

The Most Common
CAUSES OF:

mesenteric thrombosis); peritoneal disorders (intra-abdominal abscesses, primary peritonitis, tuberculous peritonitis); retroperitoneal disorders (retroperitoneal hemorrhage)

Requiring surgical intervention:

acute appendicitis. Others include small and large bowel obstruction, strangulated hernia, perforated peptic ulcer, bowel perforation, Meckel's diverticulitis, Boerhaave's syndrome, acute cholecystitis, acute cholangitis, hepatic abscess, ruptured hepatic tumor, spontaneous rupture of the spleen, ruptured ectopic pregnancy, twisted ovarian tumor, ruptured ovarian follicle cyst, ruptured aortic and visceral aneurysms, acute ischemic colitis, mesenteric thrombosis, intra-abdominal abscesses

...ACUTE ARTERIAL OCCLUSION OF THE LOWER EXTREMITY:

an embolus or, frequently, multiple emboli

...ACUTE BACTERIAL GASTROENTERITIS:

The causative agent usually is not identified in most clinical situations, according to the Merck manual. However, the most common bacterial pathogens identified by stool culture are listed: *Campylobacter* species (causes 11% of infectious dysentery in U.S. hospitals - this is greater than *Salmonella* species), according to Rubin. Overall, those isolated most often include a variety of strains of *Escherichia coli*, *Shigella*, *Salmonella* (almost exclusively non-*S. typhi*), *Campylobacter jejuni*, and *Yersinia enterocolitica* in North America and *Vibrio cholera* in Asia.

...ACUTE BRONCHITIS:

14

The Most Common
CAUSES OF:

Hemophilus influenzae and Pneumococcus are
commonly encountered pathogens

...ACUTE CHOLECYSTITIS:

impacted stone in the gallbladder neck or the
cystic duct. Others include sepsis, trauma, or
collagen vascular disease

...ACUTE EPIDIDYMITIS:

in Older Males:

infection secondary to urinary tract obstruction or instrumentation

in Young Males:

bacterial infection ascending from the urethra
or prostate

...ACUTE EPIGLOTTITIS IN CHILDREN:

H. influenzae type b

...ACUTE GASTROENTERITIS:

The causative agent usually is not identified in
most clinical situations, according to the
Merck manual. However, the most common
bacterial pathogens identified by stool culture
are listed below:

Bacterial:

Campylobacter species (causes 11% of infectious dysentery in U.S. hospitals - this is greater than *Salmonella* species), according to Rubin. Overall, those isolated most often
include a variety of strains of *Escherichia
coli, Shigella, Salmonella* (almost exclusively
non-*S. typhi*), *Campylobacter jejuni,* and *Yersinia enterocolitica* in North America and *Vibrio cholera* in Asia.

Viral:

the most common viral agent is human rotavirus, causing 40-50% of acute diarrhea in children requiring hospitalization (usually those <
36 months old). Other viral agents implicated

15

The Most Common
CAUSES OF:

include enterovirus strains (echo-, polio-, coxsackie-), astroviruses, parvoviruses, adenoviruses, and picornaviruses

...ACUTE LARYNGITIS:

viruses. Viral causes include influenza virus, rhinovirus, and adenovirus. Bacterial causes (less common) include group A β-hemolytic streptococcus (*S. pyogenes*) in some cases and, rarely, *C. diphtheriae*

Bacterial: group A β-hemolytic streptococcus (*S. pyogenes*) in some cases and, rarely, *C. diphtheriae*

Viral: influenza virus, rhinovirus, and adenovirus

...ACUTE LARYNGOTRACHEOBRONCHITIS (Croup):

the parainfluenza viruses, especially Type 1, are the major pathogens. Less common causes are respiratory syncytial virus (RSV) and influenza A and B viruses, followed by adeno-, entero-, rhino-, and measles virus and *Mycoplasma pneumoniae*

...ACUTE OTITIS MEDIA in children:

Streptococcus pneumoniae, which accounts for 25% to 40% of cases. Next in order of frequency is *Haemophilus influenzae*, which causes 25% of cases. Group A streptococcus is somewhat less common, although it was a frequent cause of severe otitis media before the age of antibiotics. Recent studies indicate that *Branhamella (Moraxella) catarrhalis* is increasingly important in the etiology of acute otitis media. *Staphylococcus aureus* frequently is implicated in chronic otitis media; however, it rarely is a cause of acute infection

...ACUTE PANCREATITIS:

16

The Most Common
CAUSES OF:

Postoperative: the pathogenesis in most cases appears to be mechanical trauma to the pancreas or its blood supply

in the United States:

alcohol abuse or gallstones (about 70%). Less common causes include postoperative pancreatitis (10%) (may be quite severe and is especially common after hepatobiliary tract surgery), abdominal trauma, hyperlipidemia (an associated finding in 15% of cases but also may be causative since dietary and medical treatment of hypertriglyceridemia reduces recurrences), drugs (such as azathioprine, thiazides, sulfonamides, and corticosteroids), hypercalcemia, uremia, peptic ulcer disease (with penetration into the pancreas), cystic fibrosis (in rare cases), endoscopic retrograde cholangiopancreatography (ERCP), viral infections (especially mumps), vascular insufficiency, pancreatic cancer (probably by localized ductal obstruction), hereditary pancreatitis (which may be inherited in an autosomal dominant pattern and carries an increased risk for development of pancreatic carcinoma), ampullary lesions or duodenal disease involving the ampulla and periampullary regions, idiopathic causes

...ACUTE PHARYNGITIS:

viral. However, the clinically most significant cause of acute pharyngitis is the group A β-hemolytic streptococcus (*S. pyogenes*)

...ACUTE RENAL FAILURE:

acute tubular necrosis

Acquired, in infants and children:

hemolytic-uremic syndrome

The Most Common
CAUSES OF:
in Hospitalized patients:

prerenal azotemia (50% of cases). Common causes of prerenal azotemia include intravascular volume depletion (hemorrhage, gastrointestinal losses [e.g., diarrhea, vomiting, nasogastric suction], renal losses [e.g., osmotic diuresis, diuretics, adrenal insufficiency], skin losses [e.g., burns, excessive sweating], sequestration in third spaces [e.g., pancreatitis, peritonitis, massive trauma with crush injury]); reduced cardiac output (cardiogenic shock, congestive heart failure, pericardial tamponade, massive pulmonary embolism); systemic vasodilatation (anaphylaxis, antihypertensive drugs, sepsis, drug overdose); systemic or renal vasoconstriction (anesthesia, surgery, alpha adrenergic agonists or high dose dopamine, hepatorenal syndrome); impaired renal autoregulation (nonsteroidal antiinflammatory drugs, angiotensin-converting enzyme inhibitors); hyperviscosity syndromes (multiple myeloma or macroglobulinemia, polycythemia)

...ACUTE RESPIRATORY ACIDOSIS:

obstruction of the airway, neuromuscular disorders and diseases of the central nervous system are common causes of acute respiratory acidosis, according to Devlin

...ACUTE SINUSITIS, bacterial:

S. pneumoniae and *Staphylococcus aureus* are commonly encountered pathogens. *H. influenzae*, *Staphylococcus epidermidis* and β- hemolytic streptococcus are less commonly encountered pathogens

18

The Most Common
CAUSES OF:

...ACUTE SURGICAL CONDITION IN THE ABDOMEN:
>acute appendicitis

...ACUTE THYROIDITIS:
>*Staphylococcus aureus, Streptococcus hemolyticus,* and pneumococcus

...ACUTE TUBULAR NECROSIS:
>renal hypoperfusion leading to ischemia with inadequate restoration of renal perfusion accounts for 50% of cases. Ischemic damage may occur also in the absence of systemic hypotension, as is the case in more than 50% of patients with postsurgical ATN. The other major cause of ATN is nephrotoxic injury from either exogenous (25%) or endogenous (20%) toxins. Approximately 70% of patients with ATN will have more than one possible cause for their renal failure

...ACUTE TUBULOINTERSTITIAL NEPHRITIS:
>acute bacterial pyelonephritis and acute drug-induced hypersensitivity

...ACUTE URETHRITIS:
>the major single specific etiology of acute urethritis is *Neisseria gonorrhoeae.* Urethral inflammation of all other etiologies is referred to collectively as non-gonococcal urethritis (NGU). NGU is twice as common as gonorrhea in the United States and in much of the developed world as well. In some underdeveloped areas, however, gonorrhea accounts for 80 percent of the cases of acute urethritis.

Non-specific (NGU; non-gonococcal):
>*Chlamydia trachomatis* (30-50% of cases), serotypes D through K; *Ureaplasma urealyticum* (formerly the T strain of *Mycoplasma*)

19

The Most Common
CAUSES OF:

also fairly common, has been recovered from 81% of men with *Chlamydia*-negative NGU (Mandell), causing about 10% of cases (Braunstein); Herpes simplex virus; Nonspecific, various causes include chemical, physical, etc.; Reiter's syndrome. Rare causes include *Trichomonas vaginalis* (isolated from 3-15% of patients with NGU [Mandell]), tuberculosis, and syphilis

...ACUTE VIRAL GASTROENTERITIS:

The causative agent usually is not identified in most clinical situations, according to the Merck manual. However, the most common pathogens are listed: The most common viral agent is human rotavirus, causing 40-50% of acute diarrhea in children requiring hospitalization (usually those < 36 months old). Other viral agents implicated include enterovirus strains (echo-, polio-, coxsackie-), astroviruses, parvoviruses, adenoviruses, and picornaviruses

...ADENITIS, cervical:

in Childhood: *S. aureus* and group A streptococci. In addition, group B streptococci are common causes in neonates. Recent studies also have implicated anaerobic bacteria, which may cause cervical adenitis alone or in combination with other bacteria. Less common agents include cat-scratch disease, atypical mycobacteria (most commonly *Mycobacterium scrofulaceum* and *Mycobacterium avium-intracellulare*), Epstein-Barr virus, *Mycobacterium tuberculosis*, *Francisella tularensis*, *S. pneumoniae*, *Yersinia pestis*, *H. influenzae*

The Most Common
CAUSES OF:

type b, fungi, and *T. gondii*

...ADRENAL INSUFFICIENCY IN THE SURGICAL PATIENT:

ACTH suppression by corticosteroid drugs

...ADRENOCORTICAL INSUFFICIENCY, secondary:

ACTH suppression by corticosteroid drugs is the usual cause. Primary pituitary pathology is less common

...AIR IN THE SMALL INTESTINE:

secondary to obstruction of the intestine

...AIR WITHIN THE BILIARY TREE:

a surgical connection created to provide biliary drainage (e.g., choledochoduodenostomy), or a gas-forming infection within the biliary tree (cholangitis)

...ALKALOSIS:

Metabolic:

the principle causes are diuretic therapy (thiazides, ethacrynic acid, furosemide), vomiting or gastric drainage, hyperadrenocorticism (Cushing's syndrome, aldosteronism, exogenous corticosteroid administration). The most common clinical setting for chronic metabolic alkalosis may be extracellular fluid volume contraction and avid renal sodium reabsorption, according to the Merck manual

in Children:

the use of diuretics, which leads to volume contraction and potassium and chloride depletion. These in turn lead to increased bicarbonate reabsorption and aldosteronism with increased hydrogen ion secretion. Loss of acid due to recurrent vomiting is also a common cause. A gain of base can be the result of excessive alkali administration. Less common causes include Bartter syndrome, familial

21

The Most Common
CAUSES OF:

chloride diarrhea, and chronic steroid administration

Respiratory: hyperventilation due to anxiety
("hyperventilation syndrome") is probably the
most common cause, according to Devlin.
Other common causes include overventilation
of patients on assisted ventilation, primary
CNS disorders, salicylism, hepatic cirrhosis,
hepatic coma, hypoxemia, fever, and gram-
negative septicemia

...α (ALPHA)- THALASSEMIA:

gene deletion

...AMBIGUOUS GENITALIA in infants:

congenital adrenal hyperplasia

...AMENORRHEA in a young woman (of reproductive age):

pregnancy. Others include chronic endometritis or scarring of the endometrium (Asherman
syndrome), hypothyroidism, and premature
ovarian failure. Also emotional stress, extreme weight loss, and adrenal cortical insufficiency can bring about secondary amenorrhea.
According to Gregory, *mild to moderate so-
cial stress is the most common cause of secondary amenorrhea* in young women (excluding
pregnancy)

...AMNESTIC SYNDROME, organic:

thiamine deficiency associated with chronic
abuse of alcohol (Korsakoff's disease), but it
may also result from any pathologic process
that causes selective damage to diencephalic
and medial temporal structures (e.g., encephalitis, hypoxia, or head trauma)

...ANAL FISSURE:

persistent trauma in the anal canal

22

The Most Common
CAUSES OF:

...ANAPHYLAXIS:
> antibiotic (penicillin) injections and Hymenoptera (bee) stings, but nearly any foreign substance could cause anaphylaxis

...ANEMIA:
> iron deficiency. The second most common form of anemia in the world is iron-reutilization anemia (anemia of chronic disease)

in Children:
> iron deficiency anemia. The majority of cases result from inadequate intake of iron; however, loss of iron through hemorrhage must be considered in the differential diagnosis

Autoimmune, hemolytic:
> idiopathic

due to (vitamin) B_{12} deficiency:
> pernicious anemia (in which the gastric mucosa fails to secrete intrinsic factor). Other causes of deficient secretion of intrinsic factor include gastrectomy, chronic atrophic gastritis, myxedema, and, rarely, congenital. In addition to deficient intrinsic factor, decreased B_{12} absorption may be due to blind loop syndrome (competition for available B_{12} and cleavage of intrinsic factor by bacteria), fishtapeworm infestation, and decreased or absent ileal absorptive sites due to congenital causes, destruction by inflammatory regional enteritis, or surgical resection. Less common causes of decreased B_{12} absorption include chronic pancreatitis, malabsorption syndromes, and administration of certain drugs (e.g., oral calcium-chelating agents, aminosalicylic acid, biguanides). Inadequate B_{12} intake in ve-

23

The Most Common
CAUSES OF:

gans, or, very rarely, increased metabolism if B_{12} in longstanding hyperthyroidism may also be causes

Hemolytic, in the Black population:
> Hgb S hemoglobinopathy

Hypoproliferative anemia:
> parvovirus

Iron deficiency:
> hemorrhage must be the foremost consideration in any adult. Other bases for anemia may be decreased absorption of iron after gastrectomy, upper small-bowel malabsorption syndromes, and occasionally some forms of pica (primarily clay), but such mechanisms are rare compared to bleeding. Most forms of pica (starch, ice, etc) are associated with decreased intake due to caloric substitution rather than with decreased absorption. In circumstances of chronic intravascular hemolysis (e.g., paroxysmal nocturnal hemoglobinuria, chronic disseminated intravascular coagulation, etc.), RBC fragmentation (recognizable on a peripheral smear) may produce iron lack by chronic hemoglobinuria and hemosiderinuria

in the Adult male:
> chronic occult bleeding, usually from the gastrointestinal tract

in the Postmenopausal female:
> gastrointestinal blood loss

Megaloblastic anemia:
> mechanisms that cause megaloblastic states most often include deficiency or defective utilization of vitamin B_{12} *or* folic acid; cytotoxic agents (generally antineoplastics or im-

24

The Most Common
CAUSES OF:

munosuppressives) that interfere with DNA synthesis; and a rare autonomous form, the Di Guglielmo syndrome

Myelophthisic anemia:

carcinoma metastasizing to bone marrow from primary tumors, most often located in the breast, prostate, kidney, lung, or adrenal or thyroid gland. Another frequent cause is myelofibrosis, which may be of undetermined origin, or sometimes appears in a late stage of polycythemia vera or chronic granulocytic leukemia. In children a rare cause is marble-bone disease of Albers-Schonberg

in the Newborn:

hemolytic disease of the newborn (erythro-blastosis fetalis)

in Pregnancy: iron deficiency

due to Vitamin B_{12} deficiency:

pernicious anemia (in which the gastric muco-sa fails to secrete intrinsic factor). Other caus-es of deficient secretion of intrinsic factor in-clude gastrectomy, chronic atrophic gastritis, myxedema, and, rarely, congenital. In addi-tion to deficient intrinsic factor, decreased B_{12} absorption may be due to blind loop syn-drome (competition for available B_{12} and cleavage of intrinsic factor by bacteria), fish-tapeworm infestation, and decreased or absent ileal absorptive sites due to congenital causes, destruction by inflammatory regional enteritis, or surgical resection. Less common causes of decreased B_{12} absorption include chronic pancreatitis, malabsorption syndromes, and

The Most Common
CAUSES OF:

administration of certain drugs (e.g., oral cal-cium-chelating agents, aminosalicylic acid, biguanides). Inadequate B12 intake in ve-gans, or, very rarely, increased metabolism if B_{12} in longstanding hyperthyroidism may also be causes

...ANERGY:

in Surgical patients:

malnutrition and disorders of leukotaxis are among the most common causes of anergy

...ANEURYSM:

Mycotic (caused by infection):

embolization of thrombotic material; the source of infection remains unidentified in about 50% of cases. When identified, Staphy-lococcus, Streptococcus and Salmonella spe-cies are most commonly involved

Thoracic aorta:

atherosclerotic aneurysms are the most com-mon. Other causes include syphilis, trauma, bacterial infection, arteritis, neoplasm and connective tissue disorders

...ANTERIOR MEDIASTINAL MASS:

thymoma

...ANTEROSUPERIOR MEDIASTINAL MASS:

thyroid, thymus, teratoma, lymphoma, lipo-matosis

...AORTIC INSUFFICIENCY:

chronic rheumatic valvular disease or syphilit-ic heart disease are most often associated, ac-cording to Braunstein. Jarrell reports that myxomatous degeneration accounts for most cases. Less commonly SBE, valvular rupture, dissecting aneurysm, Marfan's disease, psori-

The Most Common
CAUSES OF:

atic and ankylosing spondylitis, interventricular septal defects, and annuloaortic ectasia

...AORTIC STENOSIS:

    acquired valvular disease (rheumatic, degenerative [senile]). Congenital aortic stenosis is much less common, and syphilis *never* causes stenosis

...ARTERIAL AIR EMBOLISM:

    tears in pulmonary parenchyma, opening venous channels

...ARTERIAL DISEASE, peripheral:

Pathologic (causes):

    atherosclerosis, trauma, and thromboemboli

...ARTHRITIS:

Infectious: any pathogenic microbe may infect a joint. Bacteria are most often the etiologic agents, typically producing an acute arthritis

Acute: bacteria are most often the etiologic agents, typically producing an acute arthritis. Acute arthritis at any age may be associated with viral infections (e.g., rubella, mumps, human parvovirus, or hepatitis B)

Chronic: may be caused by *Mycobacterium tuberculosis* and other mycobacteria or fungi such as *Sporothrix schenckii, Coccidioides immitis, Blastomyces dermatitidis,* and *Candida albicans*

in Young Children:

    the predominating pathogens are staphylococci, *Hemophilus influenzae*, and gram-negative bacilli

in Older Children and Adults:

    gonococci, staphylococci, streptococci, or pneumococci

The Most Common
CAUSES OF:

Rheumatoid: etiology is unknown. The immunologic changes may be initiated by multiple factors

Septic: *Staphylococcus aureus*

...ASTHMA:

(Precipitants): allergen exposure, by exercise in cold dry air, or by environmental pollutants

...ATRIAL FIBRILLATION:

coronary artery disease. Other etiologies include valvular heart disease (especially mitral valve disease), cardiomyopathy, hypertension, pericarditis, chronic obstructive pulmonary disease and hyperthyroidism

...ATROPHY (of muscles):

decrease of workload, loss of innervation and verve function of muscle fibers, diminished blood supply causing inadequate nutrition, loss of endocrine stimulation

...AUTOIMMUNE HEMOLYTIC ANEMIA IN CHILDHOOD:
idiopathic

...BACTEREMIA:
gram-negative bacteremia, staphylococcal bacteremia, gonococcal bacteremia, meningococcal bacteremia, typhoid fever, bacteremia due to bacteroides, clostridial bacteremia, bacteremias of miscellaneous etiology

Clostridial: *Clostridium perfringens*

Gonococcal: usually evolves from asymptomatic gonorrhea

Gram-negative:

Escherichia coli, Klebsiella, Enterobacter, Serratia, Pseudomonas aeruginosa, Proteus

in Hospitalized patients:

catheter-related urinary tract infection (UTI)

in Neonates and older infants:

Streptococcus agalactia

Staphylococcal:

28

coagulase-positive *Staphylococcus aureus.*
Also coagulase negative staphylococci, *S. epidermidis,* and *Staphylococcus saprophyticus*
occasionally cause bacteremia

Coagulase-negative staphylococcal:

contaminated intravenous catheters, cannulae,
hydrocephalic shunts, or the paraphernalia
used in intravenous drug abuse

Typhoid fever: *Salmonella typhi*

...BACTERIAL DIARRHEA:

in the United States:

Campylobacter infection

...BACTERIAL ENDOCARDITIS:

Acute: staphylococcus (fulminant). Others include
pneumococcus, gram-negative rods

Subacute (SBE):

α–Hemolytic streptococci. Others include enterococcus, other low-grade pathogens

...BACTERIAL GASTROENTERITIS, acute:

The causative agent usually is not identified in
most clinical situations, according to the
Merck manual. However, the most common
bacterial pathogens identified by stool culture
are listed: *Campylobacter* species (causes
11% of infectious dysentery in U.S. hospitals
- this is greater than *Salmonella* species), according to Rubin. Overall, those isolated
most often include a variety of strains of *Escherichia coli, Shigella, Salmonella* (almost
exclusively non-*S. typhi*), *Campylobacter jejuni,* and *Yersinia enterocolitica* in North America and *Vibrio cholera* in Asia.

...BACTERIAL MENINGITIS in the United States:

Haemophilus influenzae, type b. Over 80 per-

The Most Common
CAUSES OF:

cent of the cases are caused by three encapsulated organisms: *Haemophilus influenzae*, *Neisseria meningitidis*, and *Streptococcus pneumoniae*. The balance are caused by *Listeria monocytogenes*, gram-negative enteric rods, *Staphylococcus aureus*, *Streptococcus pyogenes*, *Staphylococcus epidermidis*, *Pasteurella multocida*, *Acinetobacter calcoaceticus*, *Mycobacterium tuberculosis*, and other pathogenic bacteria.

(by age)

in Neonates: *E. coli*, *Streptococcus agalactia* (Group B streptococci)

in Infants (2 months to 3 years) and children (to 6 years): *Hemophilus Influenza* type b, *Streptococcus pneumoniae*, *Neisseria meningitidis*

in Adolescents and young adults: *Neisseria meningitidis*

in Adults (over 25) and elderly: *Streptococcus pneumoniae*

in Cancer and Immunosuppressed individuals: *Listeria monocytogenes*

...BILIARY TREE INFECTIONS: *E. coli*, *Streptococcus faecalis* (the aerobic gram-positive enterococcus), *Salmonella*, anaerobic organisms, especially *C. perfringens*

...BIRTH DEFECTS in man: unknown; hereditary diseases; cytogenetic diseases; drugs, chemicals, radiation; maternal infection; maternal metabolic factors; birth trauma and uterine factors

Chemically induced: alcohol (Fetal Alcohol Syndrome)

The Most Common
CAUSES OF:

...BLADDER INFLAMMATION:

        infection

...BLEEDING:

  Abnormal: thrombocytopenia

  Gastrointestinal:

  (Upper or lower GI):

        neoplasms (carcinoma, leiomyoma, sarcoma, hemangioma, lymphoma, melanoma, polyps), arterial-enteric fistulas, vascular anomalies (Rendu-Osler-Weber syndrome, blue rubber bleb nevus syndrome, CRST syndrome, arteriovenous malformations, angiodysplasia [vascular ectasia]), hematologic diseases, elastic tissue disorders (pseudoxanthoma elasticum, Ehlers-Danlos syndrome), vasculitis syndromes, amyloidosis

    Lower GI:

        hemorrhoids, anal fissure, diverticulosis, Meckel's diverticulum, ischemic bowel disease, inflammatory bowel disease, solitary colonic ulcer, intussusception

    Upper GI:

        duodenal ulcer, gastric ulcer, marginal ulcer, esophageal varices, Mallory-Weiss tear, gastritis, esophagitis, hematobilia, Menetrier's disease

  Genitourinary:

    in Young women:

        menstrual. Also uterine tumors, pregnancy (most common type of anemia in pregnancy, caused by diversion to fetus, delivery, lactation), renal dialysis, intravascular hemolysis (Hgb loss through kidney)

  Hemorrhagic: trauma

    Intra-cerebral:

The Most Common
CAUSES OF:

hypertension, intrinsic vessel disease, arteriovenous malformations, blood dyscrasias, trauma

Gastrointestinal (massive hemorrhage):

Lower GI:

diverticulosis, or vascular ectasia

Upper GI:

peptic ulcer (duodenal ulcer [25-40%], gastric ulcer [10-20%]) is the most common cause, accounting for over half of all cases. Other causes include diffuse erosive gastritis (15-20%), esophageal varices (10-20%), Mallory-Weiss tear of the gastroesophageal junction (10%). Uncommon causes (5%) include gastric carcinoma (up to 5%), esophagitis, pancreatitis, hemobilia, duodenal diverticulum

in cirrhotic patients:

varices, erosive gastritis, peptic ulcer disease, and esophageal tears (Mallory-Weiss syndrome)

Obstetrics (serious bleeding):

postpartum hemorrhage

Postpartum:

uterine atony, precipitous or prolonged labor, multiparity, history of postpartum hemorrhage, overextended uterus (macrosomia, multiple gestation, hydramnios), drugs (general anesthesia, oxytocin [Pitocin, Syntocinon], magnesium sulfate), toxins (amnionitis, intrauterine fetal demise), genital tract disruption (ruptured uterus, inverted uterus, lacerations or hematomas), retained products of conception (often late hemorrhage), placental abnormalities (placenta accreta, placenta increta, placenta percreta), coagulation disorders (idio-

32

The Most Common
CAUSES OF:

pathic thrombocytopenic purpura, thrombotic thrombocytopenic purpura, hemophilia, Von Willebrand's disease, drugs [aspirin, other nonsteroidal anti-inflammatory drugs, antibiotics, thiazide diuretics, sedatives, tranquilizers]), miscellaneous obstetric complications (preeclampsia/eclampsia, abruptio placentae, saline abortion, sepsis, thromboembolic disease)

Subarachnoid:

aneurysm (rupture)

in the Surgical patient:

thrombocytopenia

...BLINDNESS, preventable:

in the World: infection with *Chlamydia trachomatis*, subgroups A, B, Ba, and C

...BLOODY NIPPLE DISCHARGE:

intraductal papilloma

...BOWEL OBSTRUCTION:

postoperative adhesions, carcinoma of the colon, and inguinal hernias

...BRAIN ABSCESS:

Bacterial causes:

indigenous anaerobic gram-positive *Streptococci* (may be in combination with other anaerobes [*Bacteroides* and *Propionibacterium*] or enterobacteriaceae [*E. coli* and *Proteus*]); capnophilic aerotolerant streptococci; *Staphylococci*

in Children: congenital heart disease (Tetralogy of Fallot)

in the Newborn and debilitated elderly patient:

facultatively anaerobic enteric rods; *H. influenzae* essentially is found only in children in the 1- to 5-year old age group

33

The Most Common
CAUSES OF:

...BRONCHIOLITIS, Acute:
>>> usually viral in origin (most commonly respiratory syncytial virus). Other causes include parainfluenza virus and adenovirus

> in Infants and young children:
>>> viral

...BRONCHITIS, acute:
>>> *Hemophilus influenzae* and Pneumococcus are commonly encountered pathogens

...BRONCHOCENTRIC PULMONARY GRANULOMATOSIS:
>>> allergic aspergillosis

...BRONCHOPNEUMONIA:
>>> *Streptococcus pneumoniae*

...BRONCHOPULMONARY INFECTIONS (recurrent bronchitis, bronchiectasis, and bronchopneumonia) IN PATIENTS WITH CYSTIC FIBROSIS:
>>> *Staphylococcus aureus* and a mucoid form of *Pseudomonas aeruginosa*

...BRUCELLOSIS:

> in much of the World:
>>> unpasteurized dairy products (in the United States brucellosis is an occupational disease of farmers, employees of abattoirs, and veterinarians; in the arctic and subarctic regions humans acquire brucellosis by eating raw bone marrow of infected reindeer)

> on a Worldwide basis:
>>> *B. melitensis*

...CANCER:
>>> dietary factors, smoking. Others include occupational exposure to carcinogens such as asbestos and radiation. Unknown causes may be due to viruses, genetic factors, and sponta-

The Most Common
CAUSES OF:

neous mutational events.

...CANCER DEATH:

in Cystic Fibrosis patients:

respiratory failure (95%); others die of liver failure or other complications

in the United States:

Bronchogenic carcinoma. Cancer of the pancreas #4

Men (years of age):

Less than 15:

leukemia, CNS, lymphoma, connective tissue, bone

15-34: leukemia, CNS, lymphoma, skin, Hodgkin's

33-54: lung, bowel, CNS, pancreatic adenocarcinoma, leukemia

55-74: lung, bowel, prostate, pancreas, stomach

More than 75:

lung, prostate, bowel, pancreas, bladder

All ages: lung, bowel, prostate, pancreas, leukemia

Women (years of age):

Less than 15:

leukemia, CNS, connective tissue, bone, kidney

15-34: breast, leukemia, uterus, CNS, Hodgkin's

35-54: breast, lung, bowel, ovary, uterus

55-74: lung, breast, bowel, ovary, pancreas

More than 75:

bowel, breast, lung, pancreas, uterus

All ages: lung, breast, bowel (colon), ovary, pancreas

(1988 data: lung ↑ to #1 in women)

...CANDIDIASIS, vaginal:

Candida albicans

35

The Most Common
CAUSES OF:

...CAPILLARY ENDOTHELIAL PERMEABILITY, localized:
  inflammation

...CARBUNCLES: *Staphylococcus aureus* is a commonly encountered pathogen. *Staphylococcus epidermidis* is a less commonly encountered pathogen

...CARCINOMA:
  In situ of vulva:
  human papilloma virus

...CARDIAC ARREST, sudden and unexpected, in persons not already hospitalized:
  coronary artery disease or trauma

...CARDIAC CONDUCTION DISTURBANCES:
  idiopathic degeneration of the specialized conductive tissue of the heart. Other causes are myocardial infarction or ischemia secondary to coronary atherosclerosis, cardiomyopathy, drug effects, operative injury, and congenital defects

...CARDIAC EDEMA:
  acute left heart failure

...CARDIAC FAILURE, postoperative:
  left ventricular failure and pulmonary edema appear in 4% of patients over age 40 undergoing general surgical procedures with general anesthesia. Fluid overload in patients with limited myocardial reserve is the most common cause. Postoperative myocardial infarction and dysrhythmias producing a high ventricular rate are other causes

...CARDIAC TAMPONADE:
  rapid, massive accumulations of blood in the pericardial cavity. Causes include ruptured aortic aneurysm, dissecting aneurysm, heart trauma, rupture of recent myocardial infarct,

anticoagulant therapy, bleeding caused by leukemia, thrombocytopenia, scurvy, heart tumors, infection

...CARDIOMYOPATHY

Congestive — unknown. Viral infection has been implicated in the pathogenesis of this disease, but proof of cause generally is lacking. In addition, the following conditions have been linked to cardiomyopathy: prolonged ethanol abuse (the most common known cause), doxorubicin therapy, exposure to toxins (e.g., cobalt, mercury, and lead and high-dose catecholamines), endocrinopathies (thyrotoxicosis, hypothyroidism, and acromegaly have been reported to cause congestive cardiomyopathy), metabolic disorders (e.g., hypophosphatemia, hypocalcemia, and thiamine deficiency), and hemoglobinopathies (e.g., sickle cell anemia and thalassemia).

...CARPAL TUNNEL SYNDROME:

non-specific tenosynovitis. Hyperthyroidism, and hypothyroidism, diabetes mellitus, pregnancy, and amyloidosis are sometimes associated with CTS, but the syndrome most often develops in the absence of disease or trauma

...CELL INJURY:

Persistent: chronic inflammation associated with prolonged viral or bacterial infections

Reversible (sub-lethal):
anoxia

...CELLULITIS: *Staphylococcus aureus* and β- hemolytic streptococcus are commonly encountered pathogens. *Staphylococcus epidermidis* is a less commonly encountered pathogen

The Most Common
CAUSES OF:

in Children: group A streptococcus or *Staphylococcus aureus*; *Haemophilus influenzae* type b is the cause in a few cases. Cellulitis that is characterized by a sharply demarcated, firm, raised border is called erysipelas; group A streptococcus is the predominant cause of this infection. Cellulitis that is associated with painful red streaks along the course of lymph vessels (lymphangitis) also is caused primarily by group A streptococcus. Cellulitis that occurs with fever and is characterized by violaceous (purple) discoloration of the skin is most likely due to *H. influenzae* type b.

Orbital: this may follow directly from a wound or bacteremia, but the most common path is by extension from the paranasal sinuses. The organisms most frequently involved as pathogens are *Haemophilus influenzae*, *Staphylococcus aureus*, group A β-hemolytic streptococci, and *Streptococcus pneumoniae*

...CEREBROVASCULAR ACCIDENT (CVA):

Postoperative: these are almost always the result of ischemic neural damage due to poor perfusion

...CEREBROVASCULAR INFARCTION:

thrombosis of an atherosclerotic plaque

...CERVICAL ADENITIS IN CHILDREN:

S. aureus and group A streptococci. In addition, group B streptococci are common causes in neonates. Recent studies also have implicated anaerobic bacteria, which may cause cervical adenitis alone or in combination with other bacteria. Less common agents include cat-scratch disease, atypical mycobacteria (most commonly *Mycobacterium scrofula-*

ceum and *Mycobacterium avium-intracellulare*), Epstein-Barr virus, *Mycobacterium tuberculosis*, *Francisella tularensis*, *S. pneumoniae*, *Yersinia pestis*, *H. influenzae* type b, fungi, and *T. gondii*

...CHILDHOOD DIARRHEA in developed countries: rotavirus

...CHOLANGITIS: *E. coli, Klebsiella, Pseudomonas,* enterococci, and *Proteus. Bacteroides fragilis* and other anaerobes (e.g., *Clostridium perfringens*) can be detected in about 25% of appropriately cultures specimens, and their presence correlates with multiple previous biliary operations (often including a biliary enteric anastomosis), severe symptoms, and a high incidence of postoperative suppurative complications. Anaerobes are nearly always seen in the company of aerobes. Two species of bacteria can be cultured in about 50% of cases

...CHOLECYSTITIS:

Acute: impacted stone in the gallbladder neck or the cystic duct. Others include sepsis, trauma, or collagen vascular disease

Emphysematous:

Clostridia species are those most commonly implicated, but other virulent gas-forming anaerobes such as coliforms (*E. coli*), or anaerobic streptococcal species may be found

...CHOLESTATIC SYNDROME IN NEONATES:
neonatal hepatitis and biliary atresia

...CHORIOAMNIONITIS:
ascending infection, hematogenous spread (e.g. with *Listeria monocytogenes*)

...CHRONIC ACTIVE HEPATITIS:

The Most Common
CAUSES OF:

viral infection or drugs. When associated
with neither of these etiologies, chronic active
hepatitis generally is thought to be immunologically mediated, although an immunologic
mechanism has not been proven. This form of
chronic active hepatitis sometimes is called lupoid hepatitis because the typical patient is a
young woman with elevated antinuclear antibody

...CHRONIC DISEASE:

in Children: chronic lung disease; asthma is the most common of the chronic lung diseases

...CHRONIC KIDNEY TRANSPLANT DYSFUNCTION:

chronic rejection and recurrent or *de novo* kidney disease

...CHRONIC OBSTRUCTIVE PULMONARY DISEASE
(COPD):

chronic bronchitis. (LiVolsi reports that emphysema is the most common cause, although
this source is not as recent as Braunstein, who
reports that chronic bronchitis causes most
cases)

...CHRONIC PANCREATITIS:

alcohol is the most common cause. Biliary
tract disease rarely progresses to this stage despite acute attacks

in Adults: alcoholism (90%)
in Children: cystic fibrosis

...CHRONIC RENAL FAILURE IN CHILDHOOD:

congenital nephropathies

...CIRRHOSIS AND LIVER FAILURE:

chronic alcoholism, followed by postnecrotic
cirrhosis and biliary cirrhosis

...CLOSTRIDIAL INFECTIONS, other than tetanus:

six species cause infection in humans. Sever-

The Most Common
CAUSES OF:

al species may be found in the same lesion. *Clostridium perfringens* (*Clostridium welchii*) is recovered in about 80%, *Clostridium novyi* (*Clostridium oedematiens*) in 40%, and *Clostridium septicum* in 20%

...COIN LESIONS (of the lung):

Benign:
: granuloma (35-40% histoplasmosis), hamartoma, bronchial adenomas (relatively uncommon), carcinoid tumors, cylindromas (adenoid cystic tumors), mucoepidermoid tumors

Malignant:
: primary lung carcinoma (all types), primary lymphoproliferative lesions, metastatic lesions

...THE "COMMON COLD":

rhinoviruses

...COMPLICATIONS AFTER MAJOR SURGICAL PROCEDURES:

respiratory complications

...COMPRESSION IF THE TRACHEA OR CARINA:

carcinoma of the lung, trachea, and esophagus

...CONDUCTION DISTURBANCES OF THE HEART:

idiopathic degeneration of the specialized conductive tissue of the heart; myocardial infarction or ischemia secondary to coronary atherosclerosis, cardiomyopathy, drug effects, operative injury, and congenital defects

...CONGENITAL ADRENAL HYPERPLASIA:

21-hydroxylase deficiency (90% of cases), 11-hydroxylase deficiency (5% of cases)

...CONGENITAL DEFECTS:

unknown; DNA perturbations (genetic); environmental: maternal metabolic disorders, environmental chemicals, intrauterine infections, ionizing radiation, drugs (teratogens) and medications, trauma

41

The Most Common
CAUSES OF:

...CONGENITAL HEART DISEASE:

in most cases the etiology is unknown. Rubella occurring in the first trimester of pregnancy is known to cause congenital heart disease (e.g., patent ductus arteriosus); Down's syndrome is associated with septal defects

...CONGESTION (vascular), systemic passive:

left ventricular failure and cor pulmonale

...CONGESTIVE HEART FAILURE:

coronary artery disease. Hypertension is also still a major cause

in Children: congenital heart disease

...CONJUNCTIVITIS, neonatal:

conjunctivitis in the newborn is secondary to inflammation caused by silver nitrate and to infection with *Neisseria gonorrhoeae* (gonococcal conjunctivitis), *Chlamydia trachomatis* (inclusion conjunctivitis caused by *C. trachomatis* serotypes D through K), and *Staphylococcus aureus*. Less common causes include infection with group A or B streptococcus, *Pseudomonas aeruginosa*, and other bacteria, or herpesvirus hominis type 2. *N. gonorrhoeae, C. trachomatis*, group B streptococcus, and herpesvirus hominis are acquired on passage through a colonized or infected birth canal; other bacteria are usually acquired after birth

...CONN'S SYNDROME (primary hyperaldosteronism):

a unilateral adenoma of the adrenal in 85% of cases, and to bilateral adenomas in fewer than 5%. Bilateral hyperplasia causes about 10% of the cases. Rarely, the syndrome is due to an adrenocortical carcinoma

The Most Common
CAUSES OF:

...COPD (Chronic Obstructive Pulmonary Disease):

> chronic bronchitis. (LiVolsi reports that emphysema is the most common cause, although this source is not as recent as Braunstein, who reports that chronic bronchitis causes most cases)

...CORONARY ARTERY DISEASE:

> atherosclerosis with and without thrombosis. Other causes include vasculitis (occurring with collagen vascular disorders); inflammatory occlusion caused by rheumatic fever, polyarteritis, thromboangiitis obliterans, tuberculosis, syphilis, bacterial infection, Kawasaki disease; embolism and/or thrombotic; radiation injury; trauma; rare causes (neoplasms, trauma, aneurysm, anomalies, calcification)

...CORONARY EMBOLISM:

> nonbacterial thrombotic endocarditis (marantic endocardiosis)

...CORYZA (common cold):

> rhinoviruses

...COURVOISIER GALLBLADDER:

> an obstructing pancreatic neoplasm

...CROUP (Acute Laryngotracheobronchitis):

> the parainfluenza viruses, especially Type 1, are the major pathogens. Less common causes are respiratory syncytial virus (RSV) and influenza A and B viruses, followed by adeno-, entero-, rhino-, and measles virus and *Mycoplasma pneumoniae*

...CUSHING'S SYNDROME (Hyperadrenocorticalism):

> Hsu reports that the most common cause is iatrogenic, and that the most common non-

The Most Common
CAUSES OF:

iatrogenic cause is Cushing's disease (hypersecretion of ACTH from the pituitary). Jarrell does not mention iatrogenic causes, and lists the most common as Cushing's disease, or pituitary Cushing's syndrome (about 70% of cases). The other causes are adrenal Cushing's syndrome (excess cortisol produced autonomously by the adrenal cortex due to adenoma, carcinoma, or bilateral nodular dysplasia) - (15%); ectopic Cushing's syndrome (ACTH produced by an extra-adrenal, extrapituitary neoplasm (most commonly oat cell carcinoma of the lung, but also with bronchial carcinoids, thymomas, and pancreatic and liver tumors) - (15%). Tisher cites the same numbers as Jarrell

in Children older than age 7 years:
bilateral adrenal hyperplasia due to chronic pituitary ACTH secretion (Cushing's disease)

...CYSTITIS: *Escherichia coli* (>80%), *Enterobacter* spp., *Klebsiella* spp., and *Proteus* spp. are commonly encountered pathogens. Enterococcus and *Pseudomonas aeruginosa* are less commonly encountered pathogens

in Men: usually occurs in association with urethral or prostatic obstruction, prostatitis, foreign bodies, or tumors

in Women: usually due to an ascending infection

...CYSTS, vaginal:
in Infants: ectopic ureter

...DKA (DIABETIC KETOACIDOSIS) IN A KNOWN DIABETIC:
omission of insulin doses

44

The Most Common
CAUSES OF:

...DEATH:

Accidental:
> in Adolescents:
>> motor vehicle accidents, drowning
> in Children:
>> see listings by age. Drowning #3

in Acute Renal Failure patients:
> infections, particularly sepsis, pneumonia, and urinary tract. Other causes include progression of the underlying disease, gastrointestinal hemorrhage, and fluid and electrolyte disturbances

in Adolescents and young adults:
> accidents, homicide, suicide
> Females: suicide #4
> Males: suicide #3 (according to Dworkin), (#2 according to Tomb)

in AIDS patients:
> sepsis

Ages 1 to 6 months old:
> sudden infant death syndrome (SIDS), child abuse

Ages 6 months to 1 year:
> mechanical suffocation

under Age 1 year:
> Injury-related:
>> choking

under Age 4 years:
> in Underdeveloped and developing countries:
>> acute infectious gastroenteritis

Ages 6 months to 19 years:
> trauma to child passengers in motor vehicles

Ages 1 to 5 years old:
> accidents, child abuse

Ages 1 to 15: accidents, cancer

The Most Common
CAUSES OF:

Ages 5 to 18: accidents

Ages 15 to 24: accidents, suicide

Ages 5 to 32: traffic crashes

Age under 40 years:
: trauma; violence (accidents, suicide and homicide)

Ages 1 to 45: trauma, especially head injury

Ages 35-55: not available. Alcoholic liver disease #4

Ages over 55:
: Men: not available. Aortic aneurysm is the tenth leading cause in this group

Anesthetic, in obstetrics:
: pneumonitis from inhalation of gastric contents

in Arnold-Chiari malformation (type 2):
: cardiopulmonary arrest

after Billroth II gastrectomy:
: blowout of the duodenal stump

due to Cancer: cancer of the lung (bronchogenic carcinoma). Cancer of the pancreas #4

Gastrointestinal:
: colon carcinoma, adenocarcinoma of the pancreas

in Men:
: in 1930:
: stomach, colon and rectum, prostate, liver, bladder, lung, pancreas, esophagus, leukemia
: in 1940:
: stomach, colon and rectum, prostate, lung, liver, bladder, pancreas, leukemia, esophagus
: in 1950:
: colon and rectum, stomach, lung, prostate, pancreas, liver, bladder, leukemia, esophagus
: in 1960:
: lung, colon and rectum, prostate, stomach,

46

pancreas, leukemia, bladder, liver, esophagus

in 1970:

lung, colon and rectum, prostate, pancreas, stomach, leukemia, bladder, esophagus, liver

in 1980:

lung, colon and rectum, prostate, pancreas, leukemia, stomach, bladder, esophagus, lever

in 1986:

(years of Age):

Less than 15:

leukemia, CNS, lymphoma, connective tissue, bone

15-34:

leukemia, CNS, lymphoma, skin, Hodgkin's

33-54:

lung, bowel, CNS, pancreatic adenocarcinoma, leukemia

55-74:

lung, bowel, prostate, pancreas, stomach

More than 75:

lung, prostate, bowel, pancreas, bladder

All ages:

lung, colorectal, prostate, pancreas, leukemia

in Women:

in 1930:

uterus, stomach, breast, colon and rectum, liver, ovary, pancreas, lung, leukemia

in 1940:

uterus, colon and rectum, breast, stomach, liver, ovary, pancreas, lung, leukemia

in 1950:

breast, colon and rectum, uterus, stomach, ovary, liver, pancreas, lung, leukemia

in 1960:

breast, colon and rectum, uterus, ovary, stom-

The Most Common
CAUSES OF:
ach, pancreas, liver, lung, leukemia

in 1970:
breast, colon and rectum, lung, uterus, ovary, pancreas, leukemia, stomach, liver

in 1980:
breast, colon and rectum, lung, ovary, uterus, pancreas, leukemia, stomach, liver

in 1986:
(years of Age):
  Less than 15:
  leukemia, CNS, connective tissue, bone, kidney

  15-34:
  breast, leukemia, uterus, CNS, Hodgkin's

  35-54:
  breast, lung, bowel, ovary, uterus

  55-74:
  lung, breast, bowel, ovary, pancreas

  More than 75:
  bowel, breast, lung, pancreas, uterus

  All ages:
  breast, lung, bowel (colon), ovary, pancreas

in 1988:
lung, breast, bowel (colon), ovary, pancreas
(1988 data: lung ↑ to #1 in women)

Genital tract cancers:
ovary (50%), cervix (invasive carcinoma) (32%), endometrium (14%), other sites (4%)

resulting from Cardiac Disease of all types:
ischemic heart disease

in Childhood: injuries
  prior to the 1940's:
  respiratory disease

48

The Most Common
CAUSES OF:

in Down's syndrome patients:
>> infections, congenital heart defects, and leukemia

from Drug abuse:
>> the intravenous injection of excessive amounts of heroin and other "street drugs"

in fatal Epstein-Barr virus infections:
>> meningoencephalitis

in Familial Dysautonomia (Riley-Day syndrome):
>> chronic pulmonary failure

Fetal (recognizable):
>> abruptio placenta

due to Gynecologic Cancers in the United States:
>> ovarian cancer

in Hypertensive Heart Disease:
>> congestive heart failure or cerebrovascular accident, especially hemorrhage (most frequent major complication). Impaired renal function also important

in Industrialized societies:
>> coronary artery disease

Infectious, worldwide:
>> tuberculosis

from Injuries in children:
>> foreign body injury #1. Falls #4

in Juvenile diabetics:
>> MI (myocardial infarction) due to coronary artery atherosclerosis

during Labor and delivery:
>> hemorrhage

in Marfan syndrome:
>> cardiovascular disorders

Maternal: postpartum hemorrhage

  During pregnancy:
>> preexisting heart disease (most commonly

The Most Common
CAUSES OF:
rheumatic heart disease)

Men over age 55:
aortic aneurysm is the tenth leading cause in
this group

associated with Myocardial Infarction:
congestive heart failure. Others include pulmonary embolus, rupture of heart, or cardiogenic shock, especially with large infarcts
(more than one third of the left ventricle)

Neonatal:
Endocrine cause:
the adrenogenital syndrome due to 21-
hydroxylase deficiency

Perinatal: secondary to complications arising from a preterm birth

Postoperative, in patients older than 60 years:
respiratory complications are #2

Post-partum, non-OB:
pulmonary embolism

in Preterm Infants:
respiratory distress syndrome

Preventable: smoking

in Rheumatic Fever:
Acute: congestive heart failure or embolism
Chronic: valvular deformity or subacute bacterial endocarditis with subsequent congestive heart failure

in Riley-Day syndrome (Familial Dysautonomia):
chronic pulmonary failure

in Sarcoidosis: cardiac failure

Sudden: coronary artery disease

in Teenagers: accidents (most commonly motor vehicle accidents), suicide (Sierles reports that #2 & 3
are homicide and suicide)

50

The Most Common
CAUSES OF:

in Toxic Shock Syndrome (TSS):
>   shock

in fatal cases of Toxoplasmosis:
>   encephalitis

due to Transfusion:
>   Immediate death:
>>   acute hemolysis due to transfusion of the wring unit of blood to the wrong patient
>
>   Late death:
>>   hepatitis

in Ulcerative Colitis patients with complications:
>   perforation of the colon, which occurs in about 3-5% of hospitalized patients, is responsible for more deaths than any other complication of ulcerative colitis

in United States:
>   diseases of heart and blood vessels (atherosclerotic heart disease; cardiovascular disease and stroke), cancer, cerebrovascular disease (CVA), accidents. Infection #4 (Rubin). Suicide #9 (Gregory & Woods); (#10 [Sierles]).
>
>   Homicide # 11 (Sierles)

in 1979:
>   heart disease, cancer, stroke (cerebral vascular accident), accidents, chronic obstructive pulmonary disease, influenza, pneumonia (infection of the lung), diabetes mellitus (#6 in 1981), cirrhosis (degeneration and deformity) of the liver, suicide, and perinatal (before, during and after childbirth) conditions.

...DEATH AND DISEASE:
>   in Childhood: infections, behavioral and educational problems, accidents

...DECUBITUS ULCERS:
>   Hospital acquired:

51

The Most Common
CAUSES OF:

these are nearly always the result of inadequate nursing care

...DEHISCENCE (of wounds):

Technical causes (in surgery):

infection and excessively tight sutures

...DELAYED PUBERTY IN BOYS:

constitutional delay of puberty

...DELAYED WOUND HEALING :

local sepsis

...DEMENTIA: Alzheimer's disease, multi-infarct dementia (lacunar formation), Hutchinson's chorea, Creutzfeldt-Jakob disease, Pick's disease (more common in Europe than US)

in Elderly population:

although estimates vary, it is currently believed that 50% of demented elderly suffer from senile dementia of the Alzheimer type (Alzheimer's disease). Approximately 20% of demented elderly suffer from cerebral arteriosclerosis (previously described as hardening of the cerebral arteries). Cerebral arteriosclerosis produces dementia by causing multiple cerebral infarcts. Normal pressure hydrocephalus and Huntington's disease are rare causes of dementia

Irreversible (probably):

Alzheimer's type, alcoholism, multiple infarct, Huntington's chorea

Reversible (potentially):

pseudodementia, normal pressure hydrocephalus, resectable mass lesions, drug toxicities

...DIABETES INSIPIDUS, nephrogenic:

lithium carbonate. Acquired > congenital. Acquired causes include chronic renal disease (medullary cystic disease, polycystic kidney disease, obstructive uropathy, pyelonephritis, severe chronic renal failure), pharmacologic agents (demeclocycline, lithium, glyburide, tolazamide, propoxyphene, methoxyflurane, amphotericin B, vinblastine, colchicine), electrolyte disorders (hypercalcemia, hypokalemia), dietary abnormalities (poor protein intake, excessive water intake, poor salt intake), and miscellaneous (amyloidosis, sarcoidosis, multiple myeloma, Sjogren's syndrome, sickle cell disease)

...DIABETIC KETOACIDOSIS (DKA) IN A KNOWN DIABETIC:

omission of insulin doses

...DIARRHEA:

Bacterial:

in the United States:

Campylobacter infection

Childhood in developed countries:

rotavirus

Chronic:

in otherwise healthy Children:

chronic nonspecific diarrhea or irritable bowel syndrome

Traveler's:

E. coli. Species of *Shigella*, *Salmonella*, and *Campylobacter* as well as *E. histolytica* and *Giardia lamblia* are other known causes of traveler's diarrhea

Water-borne, infectious:

G. lamblia, a flagellate protozoan

Watery:

in the Elderly:

The Most Common
CAUSES OF:

fecal impaction (as very liquid fecal matter passes around the obstruction)

...DISEASE:
    Chronic:
        in Children:

           chronic lung disease; asthma is the most common of the chronic lung diseases

        Human: *Pseudomonas aeruginosa*
        Systemic:
        in Children under 5 years of age:
           N. meningitidis, group B
        in Children 4 to 14 years of age:
           N. meningitidis, group C

...DIC (disseminated intravascular coagulation), in OB:

abruptive placenta, retained dead fetus, amniotic fluid embolism, saline induced abortion, blood dilution, sepsis, hydatidiform mole, eclampsia, liver disease

...DOWN'S SYNDROME:

trisomy of chromosome 21 in group G. The remaining cases are due to translocation (D/D or D/G, with 46 chromosomes), or to mosaicism (some cells containing 46 and some 47 chromosomes)

...DRUG POISONING IN CHILDREN:

aspirin poisoning

...DUODENAL VARICES:

in a recent review, intrahepatic portal hypertension as a result of cirrhosis accounted for 30% of the cases, splenic vein obstruction secondary to pancreatitis, tumor, or thrombosis accounted for 25%, and an additional 25% were caused by portal vein obstruction as a result of thrombosis, infection, or tumor. Rarer causes included veno-occlusive disease, inferior vena cava obstruction, arteriovenous aneurysm involving the hepatic artery and portal vein, and postoperative shunt thrombosis

...DYSFUNCTIONAL UTERINE BLEEDING (DUB):

abnormalities of endocrine origin; anovulation occurring during the extremes of menstrual life, just after menarche and before menopause

...ECHINOCOCCOSIS (Hydatid disease):

this is a zoonotic infection caused by larval cestodes (tapeworms) of the genus *Echinococcus*. The most common offender is *E. granulosus* (cystic hydatid disease). Rarely, *E. multilocularis* (alveolar hydatid disease) and *E. vogeli* (polycystic hydatid disease) infect humans

...EDEMA:

Cerebral: hypoxia due to heart or lung failure
Localized: increased vascular permeability
Pulmonary: heart failure

...ELECTRICAL BURNS:

injuries are principally caused by a child sucking on the plug-receptor connection of an extension wire, a child chewing on poorly insulated wire, a child inserting conducting objects into live wall sockets

...ELEVATED LEVEL OF MATERNAL SERUM ALPHA-FETOPROTEIN (assuming the dates are correct):

an open defect of the neural tube such as open spina bifida or anencephaly

...EMBOLI:

Cardiac: atrial fibrillation, mural thrombus, subacute

The Most Common
CAUSES OF:

	bacterial endocarditis, valvular heart disease
Coronary:	nonbacterial thrombotic endocarditis (marantic endocardiosis)
Non-cardiac:	artery to artery embolus

...EMPHYSEMATOUS CHOLECYSTITIS:

Clostridia species are those most commonly implicated, but other virulent gas-forming anaerobes such as coliforms (*E. coli*), or anaerobic streptococcal species may be found

...EMPHYSEMATOUS PYELONEPHRITIS:

this is secondary to a gas-producing bacteria (most often *E. coli*)

...EMPYEMA: spread of infection from the lung from bacterial or tuberculous pneumonia, necrotic infected tumor, lung abscess, bronchopleural fistula, or trauma

Bacterial causes:

streptococci, pneumococci, and staphylococci

...ENCEPHALITIS:

Acute: viruses.

Sporadic: herpes simplex virus is the most common cause of sporadic acute encephalitis in the United States, according to Dworkin. However, as noted under the "viral" sub-heading, other viral causes are more frequently isolated. Diagnosis of herpes encephalitis is certain only upon demonstration of the virus (by recovery of the virus or immunologic technics) in cerebral tissue obtained by brain biopsy or at post-mortem examination

Viral: enterovirus (i.e., echovirus, coxsackie [A and B] and non-paralytic poliomyelitis), and mumps virus are <u>the most frequently isolated agents</u>. Herpes virus (see "sporadic acute en-

56

cephalitis" sub-heading, above), rubella, vaccinia, cytomegalovirus (CMV), rabies virus, the arboviruses, and many other viral agents also may cause encephalitis

due to Herpes simplex virus

in Neonates:

HSV type 2

in Older children:

HSV type 1

...ENCEPHALOPATHY, Hepatic:

Precipitants in Chronic Liver Disease:

sedative or analgesic drugs, upper gastrointestinal hemorrhage, systemic infection, diuretic-induced electrolyte disturbances, constipation, uremia, acute decompensation of stable liver disease, extrahepatic biliary obstruction

...END-STAGE RENAL DISEASE:

in Adults: #1 not available. Polycystic kidneys (adult form, autosomal dominant) is the third leading cause

in Children and Adolescents:

Medullary cystic disease (nephronophthisis)

...ENDOCARDITIS:

Bacterial: viridans streptococci (an α- hemolytic streptococcus). *Staphylococcus aureus* is also a commonly encountered pathogen. Enterococcus, *Staphylococcus epidermidis*, and β- hemolytic streptococci are less commonly encountered pathogens

Acute: staphylococcus (fulminant). Others include pneumococcus, gram-negative rods

Right sided:

Staphylococcus aureus, Diplococcus pneumoniae

The Most Common
CAUSES OF:

Subacute (SBE):

> α- Hemolytic streptococci. Others include enterococcus, other low-grade pathogens

Infective, in children:

> viridans streptococcus (α- hemolytic streptococcus). *S. aureus* and *S. epidermidis* have become progressively more important causes since the introduction of antimicrobial therapy. Enterococcus, which is a common cause of infective endocarditis, rarely is implicated in childhood disease

Right sided:
> *Staphylococcus aureus*, *Diplococcus pneumoniae*

...ENLARGED, NON-TENDER GALLBLADDER:

> an obstructing pancreatic neoplasm

...ENLARGED HEAD IN NEONATES:

> hydrocephalus

...ENTERITIS, acute:

Bacterial:
> *Campylobacter* species (causes 11% of infectious dysentery in U.S. hospitals - this is greater than *Salmonella* species)

...ENURESIS, functional:

Primary (predating age 5):

> maturational lag of bladder development or neurophysiologic dysfunction

Secondary (usually between ages 5 and 8):

> more likely to be psychogenic, though such problems as infection, seizures, or onset of diabetes need to be ruled out

...EPIDIDYMITIS, Acute:

in Older Males:

> infection secondary to urinary tract obstruction or instrumentation

in Young Males:

bacterial infection ascending from the urethra or prostate

...EPIDIDYMITIS in sexually active men:

under 30 years of age:

Gonorrhea and *Chlamydia*

30 to 35 years of age:

Chlamydia

under 35 years of age:

Chlamydia trachomatis

over 35 years of age:

Escherichia coli

...EPIGLOTTITIS, acute:

in Children: *H. influenzae* type b

...ERYTHROCYTOSIS IN CHILDHOOD:

cyanotic cardiac disease

...ESOPHAGEAL VARICES:

alcoholic cirrhosis, although any condition producing portal hypertension, even in the absence of hepatic disease (i.e., portal vein thrombosis or idiopathic portal hypertension), may result in variceal bleeding

...FACIAL NERVE PALSY:

Bell's palsy

...FAILURE TO RESPOND TO A HAND-HELD NEBULIZER IN ASTHMA THERAPY:

improper technique

...FELON (an infection of the pulp space of the finger pad):

nearly always follows minor finger injury (e.g., a splinter or needle prick)

...FEVER:

Non-infectious causes:

neoplasms, central nervous system (CNS) disease, rheumatic diseases, hypersensitivity reactions, metabolic derangements

The Most Common
CAUSES OF:

Postoperative (by # of days post-op):

    in the First 48 hours:

        pulmonary complications; atelectasis is responsible for over 90% of febrile episodes during this period. Phlebitis is one of the most common causes of fever after the third postoperative day

    after the Second postoperative day:

        catheter related phlebitis, pneumonia, and urinary tract infection

    after the Third postoperative day:

        phlebitis is one of the most common causes of fever after the third postoperative day

    after the Fifth postoperative day:

        patients without infection are rarely febrile after the fifth postoperative day; therefore, fever developing this late in recovery suggests wound infection. Less common problems in this period are anastomotic breakdown and intra-abdominal abscesses

    after the First Week:

        fever is rare after the first week in patients who had a normal convalescence. Allergy to drugs, transfusion-related fever, septic pelvic vein thrombosis, and intra-abdominal abscesses are some causes

...FEVER OF UNKNOWN ORIGIN:

        malignant neoplasms, occult infections, and connective tissue disorders each account for about one-third of eventual diagnoses

    in Children: infectious diseases. Others include collagen vascular diseases, malignancies, and inflammatory bowel disease

    Infectious causes:

        tuberculosis, brucellosis, tularemia, salmonel-

losis, diseases due to rickettsiae or spiro-
chetes, infectious mononucleosis, cytomegalic
inclusion disease, and hepatitis

Infectious disease:

tuberculosis and hepatobiliary infection are
the most common types of infectious disease
associated with fever of unknown cause

Malignant neoplasms:

lymphoproliferative neoplasms and obscure
adenocarcinomas (biliary tree, pancreas, kidney) are the most common types of malignant
disease associated with fever of unknown
cause

...FIBRILLATION, atrial:

coronary artery disease. Other etiologies include valvular heart disease (especially mitral
valve disease), cardiomyopathy, hypertension,
pericarditis, chronic obstructive pulmonary
disease and hyperthyroidism

...FISTULAS:

Vesicointestinal:

inflammatory bowel disease: Crohn's disease,
diverticulitis, appendicitis

Vesicovaginal: these are commonly secondary to gynecologic
trauma, rarely as a complication of infiltrating
cervical carcinoma

...FLUID AND ELECTROLYTE DISTURBANCES IN CHIL-
DREN:

gastrointestinal illness (diarrhea, vomiting)
and some degree of dehydration

...FOOD POISONING:

in the United States:

Clostridia perfringens and *Staph. aureus*

In Japan: *Vibrio parahaemolyticus*

...FUNGAL INFECTIONS OF THE SKIN IN ADOLESCENTS:

61

The Most Common
CAUSES OF:

Microsporum, Trichophyton, Epidermophyton, and Pityrosporum

...FURUNCLES: staphylococci and anaerobic diphtheroids are the commonest organisms. *Staphylococcus aureus* is a commonly encountered pathogen. *Staphylococcus epidermidis* is a less commonly encountered pathogen

...GAS GANGRENE:

Clostridium perfringens (Clostridium welchii)

...GENITAL ULCERS:
in the United States:

genital herpes, followed by syphilis. Other causes include lymphogranuloma venereum (LGV), chancroid, and granuloma inguinale (donavanosis) - all of which are uncommon in the United States. (Gonorrhea is one sexually transmitted disease that does not cause genital ulcer syndromes.)

...GINGIVITIS: the greatest single cause is poor hygiene, characterized by bacterial plaque (microbial colonies growing in carbohydrate residues tenaciously attached to the tooth surfaces). Other local factors such as malocclusion, dental calculus (calcified plaque, called tartar), food impaction, faulty dental restorations, and mouth breathing play important secondary roles

...GRAFT LOSS in pancreatic transplant patient:
rejection of the graft

...GRANULOMA: tuberculosis, sarcoidosis, coccidioidomycosis

...GRANULOMATOSIS: pulmonary, bronchocentric:
allergic aspergillosis

...GRANULOMATOUS HEPATITIS:
systemic infections (e.g., tuberculosis and sarcoidosis), fungal infections, syphilis, and viral

62

infections(e.g., infectious mononucleosis, cytomegalovirus infection, and varicella). Q fever, parasitic diseases, Hodgkin's disease, and beryllium toxicity also may cause granulomatous hepatitis. In addition, granulomatous hepatitis may be a manifestation of drug reactions involving phenylbutazone, sulfa drugs, hydralazine, or allopurinol. Occasionally, no cause can be found

...GROWTH HORMONE DEFICIENCY:

idiopathic

...HEMATEMESIS:

in most recent patient series, ulcer disease, gastritis, esophageal varices, and Mallory-Weiss tears account for 90-95% of episodes of hematemesis

...HEMATOMA, Subdural:

a moving head striking a fixed object

Chronic: approximately 60% follow head trauma. Other causes include ruptured aneurysms and rapid deceleration injuries

...HEMATURIA, recurrent:

of Glomerular origin:

Berger's disease

...HEMOLYTIC ANEMIA:

in the Black population:

Hgb S hemoglobinopathy

Autoimmune:

in Childhood:

idiopathic

...HEMORRHAGE:

trauma

Intra-cerebral: hypertension, intrinsic vessel disease, arteriovenous malformations, blood dyscrasias, trauma

63

The Most Common
CAUSES OF:
Gastrointestinal (massive hemorrhage):

    Lower GI:

        diverticulosis, or vascular ectasia

    Upper GI:

        peptic ulcer (duodenal ulcer [25-40%], gastric ulcer [10-20%]) is the most common cause, accounting for over half of all cases. Other causes include diffuse erosive gastritis (15-20%), esophageal varices (10-20%), Mallory-Weiss tear of the gastroesophageal junction (10%). Uncommon causes (5%) include gastric carcinoma (up to 5%), esophagitis, pancreatitis, hemobilia, duodenal diverticulum

    in Cirrhotic patients:

        varices, erosive gastritis, peptic ulcer disease, and esophageal tears (Mallory-Weiss syndrome)

Postpartum: uterine atony, precipitous or prolonged labor, multiparity, history of postpartum hemorrhage, overextended uterus (macrosomia, multiple gestation, hydramnios), drugs (general anesthesia, oxytocin [Pitocin, Syntocinon], magnesium sulfate), toxins (amnionitis, intrauterine fetal demise), genital tract disruption (ruptured uterus, inverted uterus, lacerations or hematomas), retained products of conception (often late hemorrhage), placental abnormalities (placenta accreta, placenta increta, placenta percreta), coagulation disorders (idiopathic thrombocytopenic purpura, thrombotic thrombocytopenic purpura, hemophilia, Von Willebrand's disease, drugs [aspirin, other nonsteroidal anti-inflammatory drugs, antibiotics, thiazide diuretics, sedatives, tranquilizers]), miscellaneous obstetric complications

64

(preeclampsia/eclampsia, abruptio placentae, saline abortion, sepsis, thromboembolic disease)

Subarachnoid: aneurysm (rupture)

...HEMORRHAGIC PERICARDIAL EFFUSION:

tumors

...HEMORRHAGIC PERICARDITIS:

neoplasms. Also tuberculosis or severe acute bacterial infections

...HEPATIC ABSCESS (bacterial) in the Western World:

secondary to an infectious process in the abdomen, particularly appendicitis, diverticulitis, or purulent cholecystitis. Also may be the result of seeding from a distant infectious focus, such as subacute bacterial endocarditis. In some cases, no primary source can be identified.

...HEPATIC ENCEPHALOPATHY:

Precipitants in Chronic Liver Disease:

sedative or analgesic drugs, upper gastrointestinal hemorrhage, systemic infection, diuretic-induced electrolyte disturbances, constipation, uremia, acute decompensation of stable liver disease, extrahepatic biliary obstruction

...HEPATITIS:

Chronic active:

viral infection or drugs. When associated with neither of these etiologies, chronic active hepatitis generally is thought to be immunologically mediated, although an immunologic mechanism has not been proven. This form of chronic active hepatitis sometimes is called lupoid hepatitis because the typical patient is a young woman with elevated antinuclear antibody

65

The Most Common
CAUSES OF:

Granulomatous:
systemic infections (e.g., tuberculosis and sarcoidosis), fungal infections, syphilis, and viral infections(e.g., infectious mononucleosis, cytomegalovirus infection, and varicella). Q fever, parasitic diseases, Hodgkin's disease, and beryllium toxicity also may cause granulomatous hepatitis. In addition, granulomatous hepatitis may be a manifestation of drug reactions involving phenylbutazone, sulfa drugs, hydralazine, or allopurinol. Occasionally, no cause can be found

..."HONEYMOON CYSTITIS":
excessive sexual activity. Other causes include chlamydial disease, chemical (cyclophosphamide), radiation

...HOUSE FIRES: smoking, heating equipment and electrical malfunction (including faulty extension cords and frayed wires), matches and fire-setting

...HYDROCEPHALUS:

Congenital:
aqueductal stenosis, Arnold Chiari malformation with myelomeningocele, communicating hydrocephalus, Dandy Walker malformation, intrauterine infection, intraventricular bleeds, tumor, malformation of the vein of Galen

in Infants:
intraventricular hemorrhage, infection, and congenital malformations such as aqueductal stenosis and Arnold-Chiari deformity. Brain tumors rarely occur in the first year of life, and, if present at this age, they are most likely to be supratentorial

...HYPERADRENOCORTICALISM (Cushing's syndrome):
Hsu reports that the most common cause is

iatrogenic, and that the most common non-iatrogenic cause is Cushing's disease (hypersecretion of ACTH from the pituitary). Jarrell does not mention iatrogenic causes, and lists the most common as Cushing's disease, or pituitary Cushing's syndrome (about 70% of cases). The other causes are adrenal Cushing's syndrome (excess cortisol produced autonomously by the adrenal cortex due to adenoma, carcinoma, or bilateral nodular dysplasia) - (15%); ectopic Cushing's syndrome (ACTH produced by an extra-adrenal, extrapituitary neoplasm [most commonly oat cell carcinoma of the lung, but also with bronchial carcinoids, thymomas, and pancreatic and liver tumors]) - (15%). Tisher sites the same numbers as Jarrell

...HYPERALDOSTERONISM:

Primary (Conn's syndrome):

a unilateral adenoma of the adrenal in 85% of cases, and to bilateral adenomas in fewer than 5%. Bilateral hyperplasia causes about 10% of the cases. Rarely, the syndrome is due to an adrenocortical carcinoma

...HYPERBILIRUBINEMIA IN THE NEONATAL PERIOD:

Direct hyperbilirubinemia:

neonatal hepatitis and biliary atresia

Unconjugated hyperbilirubinemia:

a physiologic delay in the ability of the liver to clear, metabolize, and excrete the relatively large bilirubin burden at birth; hemolytic causes

...HYPERCALCEMIA:

The Most Common
CAUSES OF:

90% of cases are due to primary hyperparath-yroidism (most common cause), malignancy, or granulomatous diseases.In malignancy, hy-percalcemia, a paraneoplastic complication that afflicts 10-20% of all cancer patients, is usually caused by metastatic disease of bone. However, in about one tenth of cases it occurs in the absence of bony metastases (the tumor may produce parathormone, prostaglandins, osteoclast activating factor, and possibly other osteolytic agents). Hypercalcemia from bony involvement is most common with cancer of the breast and multiple myeloma; in the ab-sence of metastases lung cancer is the usual culprit

...HYPERCALCIURIA:
idiopathic

...HYPERKINETIC PULMONARY HYPERTENSION:
left-to right shunt of circulation

...HYPERNATREMIA:
loss of water in excess of salt (pure water or hypotonic fluid), and it may result from nonre-nal or renal sources

...HYPERPARATHYROIDISM, primary:
single adenoma (87%), primary parathyroid hyperplasia (8%), multiple parathyroid adeno-mas (4%), and parathyroid carcinoma (1%) (according to one study at the University of California Medical Center in San Francisco) (Way)

...HYPERSPLENISM, secondary:
portal hypertension. Others include inflam-matory diseases including malaria, tuberculo-sis, brucellosis, mononucleosis, and hepatitis; Boeck's sarcoid; collagen vascular diseases

68

The Most Common
CAUSES OF:

(Felty's syndrome, systemic lupus erythematosus [SLE]); neoplastic diseases

...HYPERTENSION:

primary (idiopathic, essential) (90-98%).
Then secondary causes (see below). Malignant hypertension accounts for less than 1%
of all hypertension

Pulmonary hyperkinetic:

left-to-right shunt of circulation

Secondary: renal parenchymal disease (3-5%), renal vascular disease (1-4%), Cushing syndrome
0.5%), primary aldosteronism (0.3%), pheochromocytoma (0.1%), drug related (0.5-1%).
Other causes include perinephric disease, obstructive uropathies, cerebral pressure, anxiety, tumors, heart failure, AV fistula, shock, coarctation of the aorta. Other endocrine causes
include adrenal cortical tumors, pituitary
adenomas, arrhenoblastoma, eclampsia

in Children:

renal disease. Virtually any renal disease, glomerular or interstitial, may be the
cause.Vascular causes are uncommon. Exam-
ples include coarctation of the aorta, renal artery stenosis, and renal artery occlusion. Endocrine causes of hypertension are very
uncommon and are conditions associated with
excess catecholamines or aldosterone. These
include pheochromocytoma, primary or secondary aldosteronism, and congenital adrenal
hyperplasia with 11-hydroxylase or 17-
hydroxylase deficiency. Neurologic disease
as a cause of hypertension is often hard to
document

...HYPERTHYROIDISM:

The Most Common
CAUSES OF:

Grave's disease (thyrotoxicosis), or hyperthyroidism secondary to diffuse thyroid hyperplasia (diffuse toxic goiter); Toxic multinodular goiter, toxic adenoma de Quervain's thyroiditis, silent thyroiditis, postpartum hyperthyroidism, disseminated thyroid autonomy, Jodbasedow syndrome, thyrotoxicosis factitia, hydatidiform mole and choriocarcinoma, struma ovarii, thyroid carcinoma, iatrogenic hyperthyroidism (overtreatment of hypothyroidism)

...HYPERVITAMINOSIS D (excess vitamin D):

the inordinate consumption of vitamin preparations

...HYPERVOLEMIA:

renal failure, congestive heart failure, and cirrhosis.

...HYPOCALCEMIA:

operative injury or excision of the parathyroids during either a thyroidectomy or parathyroid exploration. Also neonatal hypoparathyroidism associated with maternal hypercalcemia, renal insufficiency, intestinal malabsorption of calcium (gut disease or vitamin D deficiency), pseudohypoparathyroidism, drugs (phosphates, barbiturates), acute pancreatitis, hypoalbuminemia, hypomagnesemia

...HYPOGLYCEMIA:

in Children 1 to 4 years:

ketotic hypoglycemia

...HYPOKALEMIA:

chronic use of diuretics. Also gastrointestinal losses, as from vomiting or diarrhea, and renal losses, as from renal tubular acidosis.

70

...HYPOMAGNESEMIA:

> chronic alcoholism. Acute intake of alcohol increases urinary excretion of magnesium and when this is compounded by poor dietary intake of magnesium-containing foods (green, leafy vegetables), hypomagnesemia results

...HYPONATREMIA accompanied by hypervolemia:

> SIADH (syndrome of inappropriate ADH secretion)

...HYPOPROLIFERATIVE ANEMIA:

> parvovirus

...HYPOTHYROIDISM, juvenile:

> autoimmune destruction of the thyroid secondary to chronic lymphocytic thyroiditis (Hashimoto's thyroiditis). Other causes include ectopic thyroid dysgenesis, goitrogens (e.g., iodide cough syrup, antithyroid drugs), and surgical or radioactive ablation for treatment of hyperthyroidism

...HYPOTONIA:

in Floppy Infant Syndrome:

> CNS disease or lesion

of Neuromuscular origin:

> spinal muscular atrophy, congenital myopathy, congenital myotonic dystrophy, glycogen and lipid storage myopathies, neonatal and congenital myasthenia gravis, motor neuropathies (hereditary, Guillain-Barre syndrome)

...HYPOXIA: abnormalities of ventilation: perfusion ratio

...ILLNESS AFTER SURGERY FOR PEPTIC ULCER:

Late illness: marginal ulcer, dumping syndrome, anemia, malnutrition, and diarrhea

The Most Common
CAUSES OF:

...IMMUNE-MEDIATED THROMBOCYTOPENIA IN CHILD-
HOOD:
idiopathic

...IMPETIGO: group A streptococcus (β- hemolytic streptococcus) and *Staphylococcus aureus* are commonly encountered organisms. *Staphylococcus epidermidis* is a less commonly
encountered pathogen. Mixed *Staphylococcus*
and *Streptococcus* are also causes (both Staph
and Staph/Strep mix account for an equal percentage of cases)

...IMPOTENCE (Male):
(Impotence is the inability to achieve or main-
tain an erection sufficient to accomplish coital
connection. Therefore, this is a male phenomenon. In females, inhibited sexual excitement
is frigidity.) Causes are performance anxiety
due to fatigue or stress. Also early undiag-
nosed diabetes, low androgen level, estrogenic
medication, hepatic problems, abuse of alco-
hol/narcotics, neurological diseases, MS, tumors, operations (e.g., prostatectomy)

Primary: negative parental influences, religious scrupu-
losity, homosexual involvement, disturbing
experiences with prostitutes, and physiologic
disorders

Secondary: the same factors as above (for primary impotence); also episodes of alcohol or drug abuse,
and inept or negative input from professional
authority

...INADEQUATE VENTILATION in the trauma patient:
Inadequate placement of the endotracheal tube
into either the esophagus or the right main

The Most Common
CAUSES OF:
stem bronchus, the presence of a pneumothorax

...INCOMPETENT CERVIX:

idiopathic, congenital DES exposure, traumatic (amputation, conization, lacerations [for-
ceps, precipitate labors, therapeutic abortions?, dilatation and curettage?])

...INCREASED PRESSURE IN THE HEMORRHOIDAL
VEINS:

straining at stool, hereditary varicose tenden-
cies, pregnancy, prolonged upright position,
abdominal or pelvic tumors, and portal hypertension

...INFECTION: *Haemophilus influenza* type b

in Adolescents:

Fungal infections of the skin:

*Microsporum, Trichophyton, Epidermophy-
ton, and Pityrosporum*

of Arteriovenous fistulas, prosthetic:

endogenous *S. aureus*, although *P. aeruginosa*
is also a frequent isolate

after Aspiration under general anesthesia:

anaerobes

in B-cell deficiency disorders:

extracellular organisms, namely pyogenic and
enteric bacteria. Patients with X-linked (Bru-
ton's) agammaglobulinemia may also have
problems with certain enteric viruses (e.g., po-
lio virus, echo virus, and coxsackie virus).
Giardia lamblia, a gastrointestinal parasite,
affects patients with IgA deficiency or with
common variable hypogammaglobulinemia

Bacterial, and Neonatal Sepsis:

Gram-positive cocci, especially group B β–

The Most Common
CAUSES OF:

hemolytic streptococcus, but also *S. aureus* and *S. epidermidis*, Gram-negative rods, especially *E. coli* and *K. pneumoniae*, Gram-positive rods (e.g., *L. monocytogenes*)

of the Biliary tree:

E. coli, Streptococcus faecalis (the aerobic gram-positive enterococcus), *Salmonella*, anaerobic organisms, especially *C. perfringens*

Bronchopulmonary (recurrent bronchitis, bronchiectasis, and bronchopneumonia):

in Patients with Cystic fibrosis:

Staphylococcus aureus and a mucoid form of *Pseudomonas aeruginosa*

in Cancer patients:

endogenous flora

in Children: *Haemophilus influenza* type b

Following vascular surgery:

S. aureus, followed by coagulase-negative *S. epidermidis*. Coliform organisms are becoming more common.

Fungal infections of the skin in adolescents:

Microsporum, Trichophyton, Epidermophyton, and *Pityrosporum*

Intrauterine: cytomegalovirus

Incisional wound infection:

Staphylococcus aureus, affecting as many as 10 percent of all surgical incisions and resulting in purulent discharge. *Staphylococcus epidermidis*, once considered nonpathogenic, and coagulase-negative *S. aureus* are found with increasing frequency as etiologic agents

Mastitis, puerperal:

Staphylococcus aureus from the infant's nose

74

The Most Common
CAUSES OF:

and throat

Meningeal, in neonates and older infants:

> *Streptococcus agalactia*

Necrotizing subcutaneous (necrotizing fasciitis; synergistic necrotizing cellulitis):

> while *Streptococcus pyogenes* (Group A streptococcus) alone may occasionally cause these infections, usually they are caused by a mixture of aerobic and anaerobic bacteria, the most common isolates being aerobic streptococci other than Group A, aerobic gram-negative bacilli, anaerobic gram-positive cocci, and *Bacteroides* species

Nosocomial: invasive diagnostic, corrective, and maintenance procedures are leading causes of infection. The patient's indigenous flora, other patients, environmental contaminants, and hospital personnel are sources of etiologic agents of nosocomial infections

in Patients with:

Alcoholism:

> *Streptococcus pneumoniae, Klebsiella pneumoniae, Listeria monocytogenes*

Burns:

> *Pseudomonas aeruginosa*

Cortisone therapy:

> *Staphylococcus epidermidis, Staphylococcus aureus, Mycobacterium tuberculosis*, fungi, viruses

Diabetes:

> *Staphylococcus aureus, Candida albicans, Pseudomonas aeruginosa*, Phycomycetes

Foreign bodies (e.g., intravenous [IV] cannulas, catheters, and prostheses):

75

The Most Common
CAUSES OF:

Staphylococcus epidermidis, Staphylococcus aureus, Propionibacterium acnes, Candida species, *Aspergillus* species

Hematoproliferative disorders:

Cryptococcus neoformans, Varicella zoster virus, Cytomegalovirus (CMV), *Listeria monocytogenes*

Splenectomy:

Streptococcus pneumoniae

Surgery:

Staphylococcus epidermidis, Staphylococcus aureus, Bacteroides species, *Clostridium perfringens, Pseudomonas aeruginosa*, other aerobic, facultative, and anaerobic bacteria

Urinary catheter:

Serratia marcescens, Pseudomonas aeruginosa, Proteus species

Perinatal:

Group B β–hemolytic streptococcus, *Escherichia coli, Klebsiella* species, *Streptococcus pneumoniae*, herpes simplex virus, *Chlamydia trachomatis, Neisseria gonorrhoeae, Neisseria meningitidis*

Postnatal:

Staphylococcus aureus, Staphylococcus epidermidis, Pseudomonas aeruginosa, Candida albicans, E. coli, Klebsiella pneumoniae, Clostridia species, *Bacteroides* species, Enterococcus

of Prosthetic arteriovenous fistulas:

endogenous *S. aureus*, although *P. aeruginosa* is also a frequent isolate

Puerperal Mastitis:

Staphylococcus aureus from the infant's nose and throat

76

of the Skin in adolescents:
> Fungal infections:
>> *Microsporum*, *Trichophyton*, *Epidermophyton*, and *Pityrosporum*

Subcutaneous, necrotizing (necrotizing fasciitis; synergistic necrotizing cellulitis):
> while *Streptococcus pyogenes* (Group A streptococcus) alone may occasionally cause these infections, usually they are caused by a mixture of aerobic and anaerobic bacteria, the most common isolates being aerobic streptococci other than Group A, aerobic gram-negative bacilli, anaerobic gram-positive cocci, and *Bacteroides* species

Submandibular space (Ludwig's Angina):
> usually develops from dental or peridontal infection, especially of the 2nd and 3rd mandibular molars. It may occur in association with problems caused by poor dental hygiene (e.g., gingivitis and dental sepsis), tooth extractions, or trauma (e.g., fractures of the mandible, lacerations of the floor of the mouth, peritonsillar abscess)

Surgical:
> *Escherichia coli, Staphylococcus aureus, Pseudomonas aeruginosa, Proteus mirabilis, Bacteroides* species, *Proteus* species, hemolytic streptococci, Group A streptococci, *Clostridium perfringens*

> in Gynecology patients:
>> hemolytic streptococci, *Proteus* species, *Bacteroides* species, *Escherichia coli, Proteus mirabilis*, Group A streptococci, *Staphylococcus aureus, Pseudomonas aeruginosa, Clostridium perfringens*

The Most Common
CAUSES OF:

in Medicine patients:

Group A streptococci, *Pseudomonas aeruginosa, Staphylococcus aureus, Proteus* species, *Clostridium perfringens,* hemolytic streptococci, *Proteus mirabilis, Escherichia coli, Bacteroides* species

in Newborn patients:

Staphylococcus aureus, hemolytic streptococci, *Escherichia coli, Proteus* species, *Pseudomonas aeruginosa* and *Proteus mirabilis*

in Obstetric patients:

hemolytic streptococci, *Bacteroides* species, *Proteus* species, *Proteus mirabilis, Escherichia coli,* Group A streptococci, *Clostridium perfringens, Staphylococcus aureus, Pseudomonas aeruginosa*

in Pediatric patients:

Group A streptococci, *Pseudomonas aeruginosa, Staphylococcus aureus, Escherichia coli,* Hemolytic streptococci, *Proteus* species and *Clostridium perfringens, Proteus mirabilis and Bacteroides* species

in Surgery patients:

Clostridium perfringens, Pseudomonas aeruginosa, Staphylococcus aureus, Group A streptococci, *Escherichia coli, Proteus mirabilis, Bacteroides* species, *Proteus* species, hemolytic streptococci

in Wound infections after surgery on the colon:

E. coli

Transplacental, prior to birth:

cytomegalovirus, *Treponema pallidum* (the agent of syphilis), human immunodeficiency

The Most Common
CAUSES OF:

virus [HIV; the agent of acquired immune deficiency syndrome (AIDS)], rubella virus, *Toxoplasma gondii*, echovirus, *Listeria monocytogenes*

Urinary tract: the most common causes are gram-negative bacteria, particularly *Escherichia coli*. *E. coli* accounts for 80-90% of uncomplicated acute UTI in the ambulatory patient. Less common are *Enterobacter aerogenes*, *Proteus vulgaris*, *Proteus mirabilis*, *Pseudomonas aeruginosa*, and *Streptococcus faecalis*. Organisms such as Proteus, Klebsiella, Enterobacter, Pseudomonas, Enterococci, Serratia, and Staphylococcus assume more importance in hospitalized patients with recurrent infection, obstruction, calculi, immunosuppression, or following urinary tract instrumentation. *Staphylococcus saprophyticus* is responsible for 10-15% of acute UTI in young women. *Staphylococcus aureus* bacteriuria is uncommon and usually indicates the presence of an extrarenal source of infection (endocarditis, osteomyelitis, skin abscess) leading to hematogenous renal involvement. *Mycobacterium tuberculosis* and *Candida albicans* are other uncommon causes of hematogenous UTI

Viral:

Perinatal: herpes simplex virus, herpes zoster virus, hepatitis A and B viruses, respiratory syncytial virus, echovirus, coxsackie virus, cytomegalovirus (via blood transfusion)

Postnatal: herpes simplex virus, herpes zoster virus, hepatitis A and B viruses, respiratory syncytial virus, echovirus, coxsackie virus, cytomegalovi-

The Most Common
CAUSES OF:

rus (via blood transfusion)

Prenatal: rubella virus, cytomegalovirus, echovirus, herpes zoster virus

Wound infection, incisional:

Staphylococcus aureus, affecting as many as 10 percent of all surgical incisions and resulting in purulent discharge. *Staphylococcus epidermidis*, once considered nonpathogenic, and coagulase-negative *S. aureus* are found with increasing frequency as etiologic agents

in Wound infections after surgery on the colon:

E. coli

...INFECTIVE ENDOCARDITIS IN CHILDREN:

viridans streptococcus (α–hemolytic streptococcus). *S. aureus* and *S. epidermidis* have become progressively more important causes since the introduction of antimicrobial therapy. Enterococcus, which is a common cause of infective endocarditis, rarely is implicated in childhood disease

...INFERTILITY IN WOMEN:

Chlamydial infection

...INFLAMMATION OF THE BLADDER:

infection

...INJURY TO:

the Bladder: an external blow over a full bladder

Children: motor vehicle accidents, drownings, burns

the Kidney: athletic, industrial, or automobile accidents

the Vagina:

in Adult Women:

a "lost" tampon

...INSOMNIA: chronic depression and/or anxiety

...INTESTINAL OBSTRUCTION:

intestinal (postoperative) adhesions, then her-

80

The Most Common
CAUSES OF:

nias (may be internal or mesenteric), then malignant neoplasms. Other intrinsic lesions include congenital lesions (webs, malrotations, atresias), inflammatory lesions (Crohn's disease, diverticulitis, ulcerative colitis, infections such as tuberculosis), luminal foreign bodies (bezoars, parasites, gallstones), radiation injury, other trauma, or endometriosis. Other extrinsic lesions include large intra-abdominal tumors or abscesses

in acute Appendicitis:

fecaliths (inspissated stool). Less common causes include lymphoid hypertrophy, barium, intestinal worms.

in Crohn's disease:

stricture and inflammation

Large intestine:

carcinoma of colon (65%), diverticulitis (20%), volvulus (5%), miscellaneous (inflammatory bowel disease, benign tumors, ischemic stricture, fecal impaction, adhesions, hernia, intussusception - 10%). Diverticulitis seldom obstructs the colon completely; volvulus is the second most common cause of complete colonic obstruction

Small Intestine:

adhesions (60) (Stillman cites 75%), external hernia (15%), neoplasm (15%), miscellaneous (intussusception, internal hernia, volvulus, foreign body, gallstone, inflammatory lesions - particularly those due to untreated appendicitis or Crohn's disease, and stricture from ischemia or radiation injury - 10%)

with history of previous Abdominal operation:
adhesions

81

The Most Common
CAUSES OF:

without history of previous Abdominal operation:

a visible external hernia

Distal small bowel:

torsion of a loop of bowel around a fixed point resulting from a band between the diverticulum and the inferior surface of the umbilicus. Also kinking of the bowel caused by inflammation or from intussusception, volvulus of a segment of intestine around a remnant of the omphalomesenteric vessels and entrapment of a portion of bowel beneath a band extending from the mesentery to the diverticulum

during Pregnancy:

adhesive bands are the most common cause of intestinal obstruction, and displacement of the intestine is most likely to occur when uterine growth carries the pregnancy into the abdomen around the fourth or fifth month of gestation; near term, when lightening occurs; or postpartum, with sudden reduction in the size of the uterus. The most frequent causes of postoperative adhesions are appendectomies and gynecologic operations. Other causes of intestinal obstruction during pregnancy are volvulus, intussusception, and large bowel cancer

in the Early 1900's:

hernias

...INTRAUTERINE INFECTION:

cytomegalovirus

...JAUNDICE: drug toxicity. In most cases, this jaundice is cholestatic - that is, the type resembling biliary obstruction

Extrahepatic: biliary obstruction by a malignant tumor, cho-

82

ledocholithiasis, or biliary stricture. Pancreatic pseudocyst, chronic pancreatitis, sclerosing cholangitis, metastatic cancer, and duodenal diverticulitis are less common causes

Postoperative: hepatocellular insufficiency > pre- or posthepatic causes

Hepatocellular insufficiency:

viral hepatitis, drug-induced (anesthesia, others), ischemia (shock, hypoxemia, low-output states), sepsis, others (total parenteral nutrition, malnutrition), liver resection (loss of parenchyma)

Prehepatic jaundice (bilirubin overload):

hemolysis (drugs, transfusions, sickle cell crisis), reabsorption of hematomas

Posthepatic obstruction (to bile flow):

retained stones, injury to ducts, tumor (unrecognized or untreated), cholecystitis, pancreatitis

Prehepatic: hemolysis. Less common causes are Gilbert's disease and the Crigler-Najjar syndrome

...JUVENILE HYPOTHYROIDISM:

autoimmune destruction of the thyroid secondary to chronic lymphocytic thyroiditis (Hashimoto's thyroiditis). Other causes include ectopic thyroid dysgenesis, goitrogens (e.g., iodide cough syrup, antithyroid drugs), and surgical or radioactive ablation for treatment of hyperthyroidism

...KIDNEY TRANSPLANT DYSFUNCTION, chronic:

chronic rejection and recurrent or *de novo* kidney disease

...KYPHOSIS: postural problems

...LACTIC ACIDOSIS:

shock

The Most Common
CAUSES OF:
...LARGE BOWEL OBSTRUCTION:
carcinoma. Others include volvulus, adhesions, diverticulitis, hernia, and intussusception

...LARYNGITIS, acute:
viruses. Also bacterial, including group A β–hemolytic streptococcus (*S. pyogenes*) in some cases and, rarely, by *C. diphtheriae*. Also *Haemophilus influenzae* (epiglottitis) in some cases in infants

Viral: influenza virus, rhinovirus, and adenovirus

...LARYNGOTRACHEOBRONCHITIS, acute (Croup):
the parainfluenza viruses, especially Type 1, are the major pathogens. Less common causes are respiratory syncytial virus (RSV) and influenza A and B viruses, followed by adeno-, entero-, rhino-, and measles virus and *Mycoplasma pneumoniae*

...LEUKODYSTROPHY:
metachromatic leukodystrophy, Krabbe's disease

...LEUKORRHEA (vaginal discharge):
infections of the lower reproductive tract. Estrogen depletion (senile or atrophic vaginitis) and estrogen or psychic stimulation are other causes

...LOBAR PNEUMONIA:
Streptococcus pneumoniae. Also *Klebsiella*, others uncommon

...LOSS OF GAG REFLEX:
in the Younger population:
epilepsy and drug abuse

...LOWER GASTROINTESTINAL HEMORRHAGE (massive):
diverticulosis

The Most Common
CAUSES OF:

...LOWERING THE THYROIDAL RADIOISOTOPE UPTAKE EXOGENOUSLY:

    expansion of the body stores of iodine

...LUDWIG'S ANGINA (Submandibular space infection):

    usually develops from dental or peridontal infection, especially of the 2nd and 3rd mandibular molars. It may occur in association with problems caused by poor dental hygiene (e.g., gingivitis and dental sepsis), tooth extractions, or trauma (e.g., fractures of the mandible, lacerations of the floor of the mouth, peritonsillar abscess)

...LUNG ABSCESS:

    aspiration with subsequent pneumonia (50%). They aspiration is usually infected material from the upper airway when a patient is unconscious or obtunded from alcoholism, CNS disease, general anesthesia, or excessive sedation. Usually due to anaerobes, lung abscesses are often associated with periodontal disease; sometimes multiple organisms act syndrgistically. Bacteria cultured from lung abscesses include common pyogenic bacteria and nasopharyngeal flora, particularly anaerobes, and less often aerobic bacteria or fungi. Bronchial obstruction due to any cause may result in infection behind the obstruction and abscess formation. (Bronchogenic carcinoma is an occasional cause of lung abscess in persons over age 55.) In the Immunocompromised host, lung abscess is usually due to *Nocardia,* cryptococcus, *Aspergillus, Phycomyces*, or gram-negative bacilli. Other less common causes of lung abscess include septic pulmonary emboli, secondary infection

The Most Common
CAUSES OF:

of pulmonary infarcts, and direct extension of amebic or bacterial abscesses from the liver through the diaphragm into the lower lobe of the lung

...LUNG FLUKE: *Paragonimus westermani*

...LYMPHADENITIS AND LYMPHANGITIS:

staphylococci or β−hemolytic streptococci

...LYMPHANGITIS AND LYMPHADENITIS:

staphylococci or β−hemolytic streptococci

...LYMPHATIC FILARIASIS:

Wuchereria bancrofti and *Brugia malayi*

...LYMPHEDEMA, secondary:

in Developed countries:

obstruction by malignancies, postsurgical lymphedema, lymphatic destruction from therapeutic radiation

in Less well-developed countries:

Wuchereria bancrofti

...MACROCEPHALY IN INFANTS:

hydrocephalus. Macrocephaly can also be caused by several inherited metabolic or chromosomal anomalies and several leukodystrophies. Arachnoid cysts can also cause an enlarging head circumference

...MALARIA:

inTemperate climates:

Plasmodium vivax, Plasmodium malariae

in the Tropics: *Plasmodium falciparum*

...MALNUTRITION:

decreased intake

...MALPRACTICE LITIGATION:

a breakdown in communication

...MASSES:

of the Brain, in AIDS:

86

masses due to *Toxoplasma gondii*. The second most common is primary CNS lymphoma. Rare causes of mass lesions in AIDS patients include pyogenic and fungal abscesses, tuberculomas, and metastatic Kaposi's sarcoma

Intracranial, in AIDS:

masses due to *Toxoplasma gondii*

of the Kidney: simple benign cyst

of the Neck:

Nonthyroid:

lymphadenopathy due to inflammatory disease, lymphoma, or metastatic tumor (usually from head or neck primaries) comprise the majority of nonthyroid neck masses. Carotid aneurysms, pseudoaneurysms, neural tumors, carotid body tumors, and branchial cleft cysts are other major differential considerations.
Neck abscess secondary to "mainlining" heroin and other drugs has become an increasingly common diagnostic and therapeutic problem

Pulsatile: a coiled or redundant carotid or subclavian artery

...MASSIVE LOWER GASTROINTESTINAL HEMORRHAGE:

diverticulosis

...MASTITIS, puerperal:

Staphylococcus aureus from the infant's nose and throat

...MATERNAL DEATH:

postpartum hemorrhage, hypertension, infection, pulmonary embolism

...MEDIASTINAL MASS:

Anterior: thymoma

Anterosuperior mediastinum:

The Most Common
CAUSES OF:

thyroid, thymus, teratoma, lymphoma, lipomatosis

Middle mediastinum:

aneurysm, lymphoma, metastases, esophageal tumor, duplication cysts

Posterior mediastinum:

neurogenic tumor, aneurysm, duplication cysts, metastases, infection

...MENINGITIS:

Bacterial: *Haemophilus influenzae*, type b. Over 80 percent of the cases are caused by three encapsulated organisms: *Haemophilus influenzae, Neisseria meningitidis,* and*Streptococcus pneumoniae.* The balance are caused by *Listeria monocytogenes*, gram-negative enteric rods (e.g., *Escherichia coli*),*Staphylococcus aureus, Streptococcus pyogenes, Staphylococcus epidermidis, Pasteurella multocida, Acinetobacter calcoaceticus, Mycobacterium tuberculosis,* and other pathogenic bacteria.

(by age)

in Neonates: *E. coli, Streptococcus agalactia* (Group B streptococci)

in Infants (2 months to 3 years) and children (to 6 years):

Hemophilus Influenza type b, *Streptococcus pneumoniae, Neisseria meningitidis*

in Adolescents and young adults:

Neisseria meningitidis

in Adults (over 25) and elderly:

Streptococcus pneumoniae

in Cancer and Immunosuppressed individuals:

Listeria monocytogenes

Chronic: tuberculosis, cryptococcal disease, malignan-

The Most Common
CAUSES OF:

cy, and sarcoidosis

Epidemic: *N. meningitidis*, group A

Tuberculous: *Mycobacterium tuberculosis*

Viral: enterovirus (i.e., echovirus, coxsackie and non-paralytic poliomyelitis), and mumps virus. Herpes virus, rubella, vaccinia, cytomegalovirus (CMV), rabies virus, the arboviruses, and many other viral agents also may cause meningitis

Infants and children:

enterovirus (i.e., echovirus, coxsackie and non-paralytic poliomyelitis), and mumps virus

...MENTAL RETARDATION:

trisomy 21 (Down's syndrome)

associated with Natal and Prenatal infections:

cytomegalic inclusion body disease (CID)

in Seattle, Washington:

not available. Fetal alcohol syndrome #3

Teratogenic cause:

alcohol consumption in pregnancy

...METABOLIC ACIDOSIS:

with Elevated "anion gap":

the principle causes are renal failure, diabetic ketoacidosis, lactic acidosis, and exogenous poisons (ethylene glycol, salicylates, methanol, paraldehyde)

with Normal "anion gap":

the principle causes are GI alkali loss (diarrhea, ileostomy, colostomy), renal tubular acidosis, interstitial renal disease (e.g., "selective hypoaldosteronism"), ureterosigmoid loop, uncommonly ureteroileal conduit, ingestion of acetazolamide or ammonium chloride

in Surgical patients:

vomiting, dehydration, starvation, diabetes, or

The Most Common
CAUSES OF:

renal failure

...METABOLIC ALKALOSIS:

the principle causes are diuretic therapy (thiazides, ethacrynic acid, furosemide), vomiting or gastric drainage, hyperadrenocorticism (Cushing's syndrome, aldosteronism, exogenous corticosteroid administration). The most common clinical setting for chronic metabolic alkalosis may be extracellular fluid volume contraction and avid renal sodium reabsorption, according to the Merck manual

in Children: the use of diuretics, which leads to volume contraction and potassium and chloride depletion. These in turn lead to increased bicarbonate reabsorption and aldosteronism with increased hydrogen ion secretion. Loss of acid due to recurrent vomiting is also a common cause. A gain of base can be the result of excessive alkali administration. Less common causes include Bartter syndrome, familial chloride diarrhea, and chronic steroid administration

...MICROCEPHALY:

occurs as a result of a small brain (micrencephaly), since the skull generally grows in response to brain growth

...MIDDLE EAR INFECTION (otitis media):

S. pneumoniae (25% to 40%) and unencapsulated *H. influenzae* (25%). In addition, gram-negative bacilli cause about 20% of otitis media in neonates; however, these bacteria rarely are found in older children with otitis media. Less common causes include group A streptococcus, *Branhamella (Moraxella) catarrhalis*

90

(acute form), and *S. aureus* and *P. aeruginosa*
(chronic form)

...MIDDLE MEDIASTINAL MASS:

aneurysm, lymphoma, metastases, esophageal
tumor, duplication cysts

...MISCARRIAGE:
in First Trimester:

blighted ovum

...MITRAL INSUFFICIENCY:

rheumatic endocarditis. Less common causes
include bacterial endocarditis, Libman-Sacks
endocarditis (rare), endocardial fibroelastosis,
congenital anomalies (uncommon)

...MITRAL STENOSIS:

rheumatic endocarditis. Less common causes
include bacterial endocarditis, Libman-Sacks
endocarditis (rare), endocardial fibroelastosis,
congenital anomalies

in Adults: rheumatic heart disease

...MORBIDITY:
in the United States:

upper respiratory infections (i.e., infections involving the nose, throat, larynx, airways, and
adjacent structures). Viruses cause the over-
whelming majority of upper respiratory infections, although bacterial complications may
ensue.

in Infants and Children:

infectious diseases

...MORBIDITY AND MORTALITY IN THE BURN PATIENT:
sepsis, particularly pneumonia

...MYCETOMA: *Madurella mycetomatis, M. grisea, Leptosphaeria senegalensis, Petriellidium boydii, Aspergillus nidulans*, and *Acremonium*, and *Cur-*

91

The Most Common
CAUSES OF:
vularia species

...MYELOMENINGOCELE:

environmental or genetic factors

...MYOCARDIAL INFARCTION:

atherosclerosis with or without intramural hemorrhage or thrombosis. Uncommonly caused by aortic stenosis or insufficiency, CO poisoning, spasm, platelet aggregation

...MYOCARDITIS:
infection

in Children: enteroviruses, predominantly coxsackie B virus and echovirus. Important bacterial causes include *C. diphtheriae* and *Salmonella typhi*

...MYOPATHY: inflammatory myopathy (polymyositis and dermatomyositis), endocrine myopathy, metabolic myopathies, periodic paralysis, muscular dystrophy, congenital myopathies, drug-induced muscle weakness

...NECK MASSES:

Nonthyroid: lymphadenopathy due to inflammatory disease, lymphoma, or metastatic tumor (usually from head or neck primaries) comprise the majority of nonthyroid neck masses. Carotid aneurysms, pseudoaneurysms, neural tumors, carotid body tumors, and branchial cleft cysts are other major differential considerations. Neck abscess secondary to "mainlining" heroin and other drugs has become an increasingly common diagnostic and therapeutic problem

Pulsatile: a coiled or redundant carotid or subclavian artery

...NECROTIZING SUBCUTANEOUS INFECTIONS (necrotizing fasciitis; synergistic necrotizing cellulitis):

92

The Most Common
CAUSES OF:

while *Streptococcus pyogenes* (Group A streptococcus) alone may occasionally cause these infections, usually they are caused by a mixture of aerobic and anaerobic bacteria, the most common isolates being aerobic streptococci other than Group A, aerobic gram-negative bacilli, anaerobic gram-positive cocci, and *Bacteroides* species

...NECROTIZING FASCIITIS:

while *Streptococcus pyogenes* (Group A streptococcus) alone may occasionally cause these infections, usually they are caused by a mixture of aerobic and anaerobic bacteria, the most common isolates being aerobic streptococci other than Group A, aerobic gram-negative bacilli, anaerobic gram-positive cocci, and *Bacteroides* species

...NEONATAL CONJUNCTIVITIS:

conjunctivitis in the newborn is secondary to inflammation caused by silver nitrate and to infection with *Neisseria gonorrhoeae* (gonococcal conjunctivitis), *Chlamydia trachomatis* (inclusion conjunctivitis caused by *C. trachomatis* serotypes D through K), and *Staphylococcus aureus*. Less common causes include infection with group A or B streptococcus, *Pseudomonas aeruginosa*, and other bacteria, or herpesvirus hominis type 2. *N. gonorrhoeae, C. trachomatis*, group B streptococcus, and herpesvirus hominis are acquired on passage through a colonized or infected birth canal; other bacteria are usually acquired after birth

...NEONATAL DEATH:

The Most Common
CAUSES OF:
Endocrine cause:
>
> the adrenogenital syndrome due to 21-hydroxylase deficiency

...NEONATAL SEPSIS:
>
> Gram-positive cocci, especially group B β–hemolytic streptococcus, but also *S. aureus* and *S. epidermidis*, Gram-negative rods, especially *E. coli* and *K. pneumoniae*, Gram-positive rods (e.g., *L. monocytogenes*)

...NEPHRITIS:

Acute, Tubulointerstitial:
>
> acute bacterial pyelonephritis and acute drug-induced hypersensitivity

...NEPHROGENIC DIABETES INSIPIDUS:
>
> lithium carbonate. Acquired > congenital. Acquired causes include chronic renal disease (medullary cystic disease, polycystic kidney disease, obstructive uropathy, pyelonephritis, severe chronic renal failure), pharmacologic agents (demeclocycline, lithium, glyburide, tolazamide, propoxyphene, methoxyflurane, amphotericin B, vinblastine, colchicine), electrolyte disorders (hypercalcemia, hypokalemia), dietary abnormalities (poor protein intake, excessive water intake, poor salt intake), and miscellaneous (amyloidosis, sarcoidosis, multiple myeloma, Sjogren's syndrome, sickle cell disease)

...NEPHROTIC SYNDROME:

in Children: lipoid nephrosis

in Adults: membranous glomerulonephropathy

...NEPHROTOXICITY:

Drug-induced: methicillin

...NERVE PALSY:

94

The Most Common
CAUSES OF:

Facial (VII) nerve:

> Bell's palsy

Third (III) nerve, isolated palsy:

> in one recent neurological survey, the most common cause was aneurysm

...NEUROGENIC (Neuropathic) BLADDER:

in Children: a spinal cord disorder, including meningomye-locele, trauma, and tumors

due to Lower Motor Neuron Lesions (flaccid):

> trauma is the most common cause, but tumors, ruptured intervertebral disks, and meningom-yelocele may also cause this type of neuro-pathic bladder

due to Upper Motor Neuron Lesions (spastic):

> lesions above the voiding reflex arc are most commonly due to trauma

...NEUROPATHIC (Neurogenic) BLADDER:

in Children: a spinal cord disorder, including meningomye-locele, trauma, and tumors

due to Lower Motor Neuron Lesions (flaccid):

> trauma is the most common cause, but tumors, ruptured intervertebral disks, and meningom-yelocele may also cause this type of neuro-pathic bladder

due to Upper Motor Neuron Lesions (spastic):

> lesions above the voiding reflex arc are most commonly due to trauma

...NEUROPATHY:

Worldwide: leprosy

United States: diabetes mellitus

...NIPPLE DISCHARGE, bloody:

> intraductal papilloma

...NON-GONOCOCCAL URETHRITIS:

> *Chlamydia trachomatis* (30-50% of cases), serotypes D through K; *Ureaplasma urealyti-*

95

The Most Common
CAUSES OF:

cum (formerly the T strain of *Mycoplasma*) also fairly common, has been recovered from 81% of men with *Chlamydia*-negative NGU (Mandell), causing about 10% of cases (Braunstein); Herpes simplex virus; Nonspecific, various causes include chemical, physical, etc.; Reiter's syndrome. Rare causes include *Trichomonas vaginalis* (isolated from 3-15% of patients with NGU [Mandell]), tuberculosis, and syphilis

...NOSEBLEEDS:

Anterior (originating in Kiesselbach's plexus [Little's area]): these occur most frequently in children and are usually the result of local trauma caused by rubbing, picking (septal spurs), or the insertion of foreign objects. Anterior nosebleeds also may arise secondary to respiratory ailments that cause blood-vessel dilatation and congestion. In northern climates, nosebleeds occur with greater frequency in winter months because lack of moisture in the air tends to dry the nasal mucosa

Posterior: these bleeds usually are thought to result from arteriosclerotic disease or hypertension

...OBSTRUCTION:

Biliary, which predispose to cholangitis: choledocholithiasis, biliary stricture, and neoplasm. Less common causes are chronic pancreatitis, ampullary stenosis, pancreatic pseudocyst, duodenal diverticulum, congenital cyst, and parasitic invasion. Iatrogenic cholangitis may complicate transhepatic or T tube cholangiography

Intestinal: intestinal (postoperative) adhesions, then her-

96

nias (may be internal or mesenteric), then malignant neoplasms. Other intrinsic lesions include congenital lesions (webs, malrotations, atresias), inflammatory lesions (Crohn's disease, diverticulitis, ulcerative colitis, infections such as tuberculosis), luminal foreign bodies (bezoars, parasites, gallstones), radiation injury, other trauma, or endometriosis. Other extrinsic lesions include large intra-abdominal tumors or abscesses

in acute Appendicitis:

fecaliths (inspissated stool). Less common causes include lymphoid hypertrophy, barium, intestinal worms.

in Crohn's disease:

stricture and inflammation

Large intestine:

carcinoma of colon (65%), diverticulitis (20%), volvulus (5%), miscellaneous (inflammatory bowel disease, benign tumors, ischemic stricture, fecal impaction, adhesions, hernia, intussusception - 10%). Diverticulitis seldom obstructs the colon completely; volvulus is the second most common cause of complete colonic obstruction

Small Intestine:

adhesions (60) (Stillman cites 75%), external hernia (15%), neoplasm (15%), miscellaneous (intussusception, internal hernia, volvulus, foreign body, gallstone, inflammatory lesions - particularly those due to untreated appendicitis or Crohn's disease, and stricture from ischemia or radiation injury - 10%)

with history of previous Abdominal operation:
adhesions

The Most Common
CAUSES OF:

without history of previous Abdominal operation:
> a visible external hernia

Distal small bowel:
> torsion of a loop of bowel around a fixed point resulting from a band between the diverticulum and the inferior surface of the umbilicus. Also kinking of the bowel caused by inflammation or from intussusception, volvulus of a segment of intestine around a remnant of the omphalomesenteric vessels and entrapment of a portion of bowel beneath a band extending from the mesentery to the diverticulum

during Pregnancy:
> adhesive bands are the most common cause of intestinal obstruction, and displacement of the intestine is most likely to occur when uterine growth carries the pregnancy into the abdomen around the fourth or fifth month of gestation; near term, when lightening occurs; or postpartum, with sudden reduction in the size of the uterus. The most frequent causes of postoperative adhesions are appendectomies and gynecologic operations. Other causes of intestinal obstruction during pregnancy are volvulus, intussusception, and large bowel cancer

in the Early 1900's:
> hernias

Urethral, in infants and newborns:
> posterior urethral valves

...OCCLUSION, arterial (acute) of the lower extremity:
> an embolus or, frequently, multiple emboli

...OLIGURIA: hypovolemia (prerenal)
Acute:

The Most Common
CAUSES OF:

Extrinsic causes:

    Postrenal:

        Postrenal extrinsic causes of oliguria include prostatic hypertrophy, retroperitoneal tumor, and unilateral stone or tumor in a solitary kidney

    Prerenal:

        reduced effective blood volume, which may be due to external fluid loss (e.g., hemorrhage, dehydration, diarrhea) or to internal, third-space accumulation of fluid (e.g., bowel obstruction, pancreatitis, extensive soft tissue trauma)

Intrinsic causes:

    oliguria due to intrinsic renal damage is called acute renal failure. Renal failure may be due to acute glomerulonephritis complicating abdominal sepsis. Acute pancreatitis is also frequently a cause of acute renal failure, but the mechanism is unclear

Postoperative: decreased glomerular filtration rate owing to hypovolemia or sepsis

...ORBITAL CELLULITIS:

    this may follow directly from a wound or bacteremia, but the most common path is by extension from the paranasal sinuses. The organisms most frequently involved as pathogens are *Haemophilus influenzae*, *Staphylococcus aureus*, group A β-hemolytic streptococci, and *Streptococcus pneumoniae*

...ORCHITIS, chronic infectious granulomatous:

  in Tuberculosis:

    descending > hematogenous

...ORGANIC AMNESTIC SYNDROME:

    Korsakoff's disease (due to thiamine deficien-

The Most Common
CAUSES OF:
cy)
...ORGANIC BRAIN SYNDROME:
  Metabolic cause:
  uremia (probably)
...ORGANIC DELUSIONAL SYNDROME:
  amphetamine abuse. It may also be due to
  abuse of other drugs (e.g., cocaine, cannabis),
  encephalitis, psychomotor epilepsy, and occasionally other CNS pathology
...ORGANIC HALLUCINOSIS:
  drug abuse (usually hallucinogens) or sensory
  deprivation (e.g., deafness)
...OSMOTIC DIURESIS:
  in Surgical patients:
  glycosuria. Also previous administration of
  osmotic diuretics, such as mannitol, and the
  previous administration of intravenous contrast agents.
...OSTEOMYELITIS:
  Staphylococcus aureus is a commonly encountered pathogen. β− hemolytic streptococcus is less commonly encountered
  in Children: Staphylococci and streptococci. *H. influenzae*
  type b is a frequent cause in infants younger
  than 3 years. *Salmonella* is a common pathogen in patients with sickle cell anemia. *P. aeruginosa* is a common pathogen in patients
  with puncture wounds of the foot
  Chronic: *Staph. aureus*
...OTITIS MEDIA: *S. pneumoniae* (25% to 40%) and unencapsulated *H. influenzae* (25%). In addition, gram-
  negative bacilli cause about 20% of otitis media in neonates; however, these bacteria rarely
  are found in older children with otitis media.

100

The Most Common
CAUSES OF:

Less common causes include *Proteus* spp.; group A streptococcus, *Branhamella (Moraxella) catarrhalis* (acute form); and *S. aureus* and *P. aeruginosa* (chronic form)

...OVARIAN ENLARGEMENT DURING PREGNANCY:

a cystic corpus luteum

...OVARIAN FAILURE:

Primary: Turner syndrome

...PANCREATIC INSUFFICIENCY IN CHILDREN:

in the United States:

cystic fibrosis. Other conditions associated with insufficiency include malnutrition, Schwachman-Diamond syndrome (pancreatic insufficiency and bone marrow dysfunction), isolated enzyme defects

Worldwide: malnutrition

...PANCREATITIS:

biliary tract disease or alcohol abuse

Acute:

in the United States:

alcohol abuse or gallstones (about 70%). Less common causes include postoperative pancreatitis (may be quite severe and is especially common after hepatobiliary tract surgery) (10%), abdominal trauma, hyperlipidemia (an associated finding in 15% of cases but also may be causative since dietary and medical treatment of hypertriglyceridemia reduces recurrences), drugs (such as azathioprine, thiazides, sulfonamides, and corticosteroids), hypercalcemia, uremia, peptic ulcer disease (with penetration into the pancreas), cystic fibrosis (in rare cases), endoscopic retrograde cholangiopancreatography (ERCP), viral in-

101

The Most Common
CAUSES OF:

fections (especially mumps), vascular insufficiency, pancreatic cancer (probably by localized ductal obstruction), hereditary pancreatitis (which may be inherited in an autosomal dominant pattern and carries an increased risk for development of pancreatic carcinoma), ampullary lesions or duodenal disease involving the ampulla and periampullary regions, idiopathic causes

Postoperative:

the pathogenesis in most cases appears to be mechanical trauma to the pancreas or its blood supply

Chronic: alcohol is the most common cause. Biliary tract disease rarely progresses to this stage despite acute attacks

in Adults: alcoholism (90%)

in Children:

cystic fibrosis

...PAPILLEDEMA:

brain tumors, pituitary tumors, infections (meningitis, encephalitis), ischemia and infarcts, metabolic disorders, Giant cell arteritis

...PARAGONIMIASIS:

Paragonimus westermani

...PAROXYSMAL SUPRAVENTRICULAR TACHYCARDIA (PSVT):

AV nodal reentry (responsible for approximately 60% of cases)

...PELVIC INFLAMMATORY DISEASE (PID):

N. gonorrhoeae, *C. trachomatis*, and *Mycoplasma hominis*. Other organisms causing this infection include *S. aureus*, *Streptococcus*, *Escherichia coli*, and anaerobic bacteria

102

such as *Bacteroides*. PID is often caused by multiple organisms

...PERICARDIAL EFFUSION, hemorrhagic:
tumors

...PERICARDITIS: uremia and causes associated with extension of myocardial infarction are most common according to Braunstein. Way indicates that the most common variety is idiopathic - probably viral- occurring in young adults. Other causes include infectious (bacterial, fungal, viral; e.g., tuberculosis, direct bacterial contamination), neoplastic, post-pericardiotomy syndrome, causes associated with systemic disease, causes associated with rheumatic fever

in Children: bacteria, especially *S. aureus* and *H. influenzae* type b, and viruses, especially coxsackie B virus, echovirus, influenza virus, and adenovirus. Other causes include fungi and *M. tuberculosis*

Hemorrhagic: neoplasms. Also tuberculosis or severe acute bacterial infections

Purulent or fibrinopurulent:
staphylococci, streptococci, or pneumococci

...PERINATAL INFECTIONS:
Group B β–hemolytic streptococcus, *Escherichia coli*, *Klebsiella* species, *Streptococcus pneumoniae*, herpes simplex virus, *Chlamydia trachomatis*, *Neisseria gonorrhoeae*, *Neisseria meningitidis*

...PERINATAL MORTALITY:
preterm labor

...PERIOPERATIVE DEATHS in emergency portacaval shunts:
an acute reduction of portal blood flow to the liver following shunting, which leads to hepat-

103

The Most Common
CAUSES OF:
ic failure

...PERITONITIS:

Primary ("spontaneous"):
bacteria are seen on gram-stained smears in only 25% of cases. Culture usually reveals a single enteric organism, most commonly *E. coli*

Secondary: most often follows disruption of a hollow viscus

Mild: appendicitis, perforated gastroduodenal ulcers, acute salpingitis

Moderate:
diverticulitis (localized perforations), nonvascular small bowel perforation, gangrenous cholecystitis, multiple trauma

Severe: large bowel perforations, ischemic small bowel injuries, acute necrotizing pancreatitis, postoperative complications

...PHARYNGITIS: viral, group A strep

Acute: viruses (40% of cases): rhinovirus, adenovirus, parainfluenza virus, coxsackievirus, coronavirus, echovirus, herpes simplex virus, Epstein-Barr virus, cytomegalovirus; primary pathogens (bacterial; 30% of cases): group A β–hemolytic streptococcus (*S. pyogenes*) (common; the clinically most significant cause of acute pharyngitis), group C streptococci (uncommon), group G streptococci (uncommon), *Neisseria gonorrhoeae* (uncommon), *Corynebacterium haemolyticum* (rare); no pathogens are isolated in 30% of cases. Probable copathogens include *Staphylococcus aureus, Haemophilus influenzae, Moraxella (Branhamella) catarrhalis, Bacteroides mela-*

ninogenicus, *Bacteroides oralis, Bacteroides fragilis,* Fusobacterium species, peptostreptococci. Unlikely pathogens include *Chlamydia trachomatis* and *Mycoplasma pneumoniae*

Bacterial:

Group A β - hemolytic streptococcus is a commonly encountered pathogen and considered the most likely bacterial pathogen in symptomatic pharyngitis. Others include group C streptococci (uncommon), group G streptococci (uncommon), *Neisseria gonorrhoeae* (uncommon), *Corynebacterium haemolyticum* (rare) *Klebsiella* spp. is less commonly encountered. An increasing number of cases may reflect synergistic infection with *Staphylococcus aureus, Moraxella (Branhamella) catarrhalis, Haemophilus influenzae* or anaerobic organisms. This "copathogenicity" may create the most common clinical setting for recurrent group A streptococcal pharyngitis. Copathogens include *Staphylococcus aureus, Haemophilus influenzae, Moraxella (Branhamella) catarrhalis, Bacteroides melaninogenicus, Bacteroides oralis, Bacteroides fragilis,* Fusobacterium species, peptostreptococci

Recurrent:

An increasing number of cases may reflect synergistic infection with (Group A β-hemolytic streptococci and) *Staphylococcus aureus, Moraxella (Branhamella) catarrhalis, Haemophilus influenzae* or anaerobic organisms. This "copathogenicity" may create the most common clinical setting for recurrent group A streptococcal pharyngitis

The Most Common
CAUSES OF:

Viral: rhinovirus, adenovirus, parainfluenza virus, coxsackievirus, coronavirus, echovirus, herpes simplex virus, Epstein-Barr virus, cytomegalovirus

...PHARYNGOTONSILITIS (acute): influenza, parainfluenza, myxoviruses, adenoviruses

...PHLEBITIS: the causative organisms vary, although staphylococci are most common

...PID (Pelvic Inflammatory Disease): *N. gonorrhoeae, C. trachomatis*, and *Mycoplasma hominis*. Other organisms causing this infection include *S. aureus, Streptococcus, Escherichia coli*, and anaerobic bacteria such as *Bacteroides*. PID is often caused by multiple organisms

...PLATELET DYSFUNCTION: drug-induced (specifically aspirin-induced) thrombocytopathia

...PLEURAL EFFUSION: congestive heart failure, infection, and neoplasm

...PNEUMONIA:

in Adults: influenza A virus

Bacterial: *Streptococcus pneumoniae* is most common. Less commonly encountered pathogens include *Escherichia coli, Hemophilus influenzae, Klebsiella* spp., *Staphylococcus aureus*, and β-hemolytic streptococcus

in older Children: *S. pneumoniae, H. influenzae* type b, and group A streptococcus. Group B streptococcus is a common pathogen in neonates. Other

106

bacterial causes of pneumonia in children include *S. aureus*, gram-negative enteric organisms, anaerobes, and *M. tuberculosis*

Gram-negative, bacillary:

Klebsiella pneumoniae, Escherichia coli, and *Pseudomonas aeruginosa*

Childhood: viral (respiratory syncytial virus). Other common causes include parainfluenza virus, adenovirus, and enterovirus. Less common causes of pneumonia in children include rhinovirus, influenza virus, and herpesvirus). *Mycoplasma. pneumoniae* is the most common nonviral cause of pneumonia in children older than 5 years. Bacterial causes include *S. pneumoniae*, *H. influenzae* type b, and group A streptococcus. Group B streptococcus is a common pathogen in neonates. Other bacterial causes of pneumonia in children include *S. aureus*, gram-negative enteric organisms, anaerobes, and *M. tuberculosis*

Community-acquired:

S. pneumoniae

Elderly: *Streptococcus pneumoniae*

Lobar: *Streptococcus pneumoniae*, then *Klebsiella*. Others uncommon

Neonatal: *Streptococcus agalactiae* (Group B)

Secondary to influenza infection:

secondary bacterial infection of an already weakened individual

Viral: influenza, adenoviruses

in Adults: influenza A virus

in Children:

Under 2 years of age:

The Most Common
CAUSES OF:

respiratory syncytial virus. Other common causes include parainfluenza virus, adenovirus, and enterovirus. Less common causes of pneumonia in children include rhinovirus, influenza virus, and herpesvirus

Under 5 years of age:

respiratory syncytial virus. Influenza A and B viruses, parainfluenza virus, and adenovirus are other common causes of viral pneumonia

...PNEUMOTHORAX, spontaneous:

rupture of subpleural bleb

...POLYURIA:

disorders of renal concentrating ability, although it occasionally results from an abnormal desire for fluids (psychogenic polydipsia)

in the Surgical patient:

overhydration due to overzealous oral intake of fluids, of excessive parenteral administration of fluids or of mobilization of the third space. Also due to osmotic diuresis, drug-induced diuresis, postobstructive diuresis, diabetes insipidus (DI), and high-output renal failure, chronic renal failure, or the resolution phase of oliguric renal failure.

...PORTAL HYPERTENSION:

intrahepatic causes (i.e. cirrhosis of the liver, schistosomiasis [worldwide cause], acute alcoholic hepatitis, Wilson's disease, hepatic fibrosis, hemochromatosis, and idiopathic diseases), prehepatic causes (rare), postsinusoidal resistance to hepatic flow [(also rare) e.g. Budd-Chiari syndrome, constrictive pericarditis], increased portal venous flow, splenic vein thrombosis

...POSTERIOR MEDIASTINAL MASS:

neurogenic tumor, aneurysm, duplication

108

The Most Common
CAUSES OF:

cysts, metastases, infection

...POSTNATAL INFECTIONS:

Staphylococcus aureus, *Staphylococcus epidermidis*, *Pseudomonas aeruginosa*, Candida albicans, *E. coli*, *Klebsiella pneumoniae*, Clostridia species, *Bacteroides* species, Enterococcus

...POSTPARTUM HEMORRHAGE:

uterine atony, precipitous or prolonged labor, multiparity, history of postpartum hemorrhage, overextended uterus (macrosomia, multiple gestation, hydramnios), drugs (general anesthesia, oxytocin [Pitocin, Syntocinon], magnesium sulfate), toxins (amnionitis, intrauterine fetal demise), genital tract disruption (ruptured uterus, inverted uterus, lacerations or hematomas), retained products of conception (often late hemorrhage), placental abnormalities (placenta accreta, placenta increta, placenta percreta), coagulation disorders (idiopathic thrombocytopenic purpura, thrombotic thrombocytopenic purpura, hemophilia, Von Willebrand's disease, drugs [aspirin, other nonsteroidal anti-inflammatory drugs, antibiotics, thiazide diuretics, sedatives, tranquilizers]), miscellaneous obstetric complications (preeclampsia/eclampsia, abruptio placentae, saline abortion, sepsis, thromboembolic disease)

...POSTRENAL OBSTRUCTION:

bladder neck or urethral obstruction, frequently due to prostatic hypertrophy or blood clots in the bladder in surgical patients. Also bilateral ureteral or ureteropelvic obstruction and

The Most Common
CAUSES OF:

unilateral ureteral or ureteropelvic obstruction in patients with only one kidney.

...POSTSPLENECTOMY SEPSIS:
pneumococcus

...PRECOCIOUS PUBERTY:

in Girls: idiopathic. Only 1 to 2 percent of patients with precocious puberty have an estrogen-producing ovarian tumor as the causative factor. Albright syndrome (polyostotic fibrous dysplasia) is also relatively rare. Also hypothyroidism and tumors of the central nervous system

Isosexual: idiopathic

...PREMATURE RUPTURE OF MEMBRANES (PROM, placental):
idiopathic, amniocentesis, local defects or area of weakness, genital pathogens which can cause infection, previous PROM, polyhydramnios, abruptio placenta, smoking, coitus, bleeding, multiple induced abortions, incompetent cervix, preterm labor (recognized or unrecognized)

...PRIAPISM: about 25% of cases are associated with leukemia, metastatic carcinoma, sickle cell anemia, or trauma. In most cases, the cause is uncertain, according to Way

...PRIMARY HYPERALDOSTERONISM (Conn's syndrome):
a unilateral adenoma of the adrenal in 85% of cases, and to bilateral adenomas in fewer than 5%. Bilateral hyperplasia causes about 10% of the cases. Rarely, the syndrome is due to an adrenocortical carcinoma

...PRIMARY LUNG DISEASES CAUSING PULMONARY VASCULAR OBLITERATION:
silicosis, alveolar destruction caused by em-

110

physema, and pulmonary histiocytosis

...PRIMARY OVARIAN FAILURE:

Turner syndrome

...PROCTITIS, Nongonococcal:

in Homosexual men:

herpes simplex virus. *Chlamydia trachomatis* infections are also common in this group

...PROGRESSIVE RENAL INSUFFICIENCY IN THE FIRST DECADE OF LIFE:

renal dysplasia

...PROLIFERATIVE GLOMERULONEPHRITIS, severe:

immune complex deposits generated by antecedent infection with group A β−hemolytic streptococci (poststreptococcal glomerulonephritis)

...PROLONGED PT (prothrombin time):

Liver disease, especially Laennec's cirrhosis

...PROSTATITIS, bacterial:

Escherichia coli and *Proteus* spp. are commonly encountered pathogens. *Enterobacter* spp., enterococcus, *Klebsiella* spp., and *Staphylococcus aureus* are less commonly encountered pathogens

Acute:

both acute and chronic bacterial prostatitis usually are caused by the most common etiologic agents of UTI. The *Enterobacteriaceae* (*E. coli, Klebsiella,* and *Proteus*) and *Pseudomonas* are the most common causes. *S. faecalis* and *Staphylococcus epidermidis* are less frequent causes of prostatitis

Chronic:

both acute and chronic bacterial prostatitis usually are caused by the most common etiologic agents of UTI. The *Enterobacteriaceae* (*E. coli, Klebsiella,* and *Proteus*) and *Pseudo-*

The Most Common
CAUSES OF:

monas are the most common causes. *S. fae-calis* and *Staphylococcus epidermidis* are less frequent causes of prostatitis

...PROTEINURIA IN AN OTHERWISE HEALTHY CHILD OR ADOLESCENT:
orthostatic proteinuria

...PROM (Premature Rupture Of Membranes, placental):
idiopathic, amniocentesis, local defects or area of weakness, genital pathogens which can cause infection, previous PROM, polyhydramnios, abruptio placenta, smoking, coitus, bleeding, multiple induced abortions, incompetent cervix, preterm labor (recognized or unrecognized)

...PSEUDODEMENTIA:
a major depression

...PSEUDOMEMBRANOUS COLITIS:
complication of antibiotic use (most commonly ampicillin, clindamycin, and cephalosporins. Then penicillins other than ampicillin, erythromycin, and sulfur drugs. Rarely tetracycline, cloramphenicol, and enterally administered aminoglycosides), *Clostridium difficile*

...PSVT (Paroxysmal Supraventricular Tachycardia):
AV nodal reentry (responsible for approximately 60% of cases)

...PSYCHOSIS, postoperative:
due to Drugs: meperidine hydrochloride (Demerol), cimetidine, and corticosteroids are the most common precursors

...PUERPERAL MASTITIS:
Staphylococcus aureus from the infant's nose and throat

...PULMONARY HEMOSIDEROSIS:

unknown; in some cases, especially in young
children, the disease is related to ingestion of
cow's milk

...PULMONARY HYPERTENSION, hyperkinetic:
left-to-right shunt of circulation

...PULMONARY INSUFFICIENCY in the early postoperative
period following major abdominal surgery:
atelectasis

...PULMONARY NODULES, solitary:
most are sequelae to granulomatous disease
such as tuberculosis, histoplasmosis, coccidioidomycosis, or nocardia. Less common
causes include necrobiotic nodules as may be
be seen with rheumatoid diseases, arteriovenous malformations, even bland or septic emboli, which are more commonly multiple.
Pseudonodules due to superficial skin lesions
or nipple shadows not uncommonly cause un-
due concern

...PULPITIS (inflammation of the dental pulp):
pulpal inflammation and infection secondary
to caries

...PYELONEPHRITIS:
vesicoureteral reflux is the most common
cause of pyelonephritis. *Escherichia coli* is
the most commonly encountered organism.
Enterobacter spp., *Klebsiella* spp., and *Proteus* spp. are also commonly encountered
pathogens. Enterococcus, *Pseudomonas aeruginosa*, and *Staphylococcus epidermidis* are
less commonly encountered pathogens

Acute: *E coli*
Emphysematous Pyelonephritis:

113

The Most Common
CAUSES OF:

this is secondary to a gas-producing bacteria (most often *E. coli*)

Xanthogranulomatous pyelonephritis:

E. coli and *P. mirabilis* are the organisms most frequently cultured from this infection

...QUINSY (peritonsillar cellulitis and abscess):

a Group A β–hemolytic streptococcus. Anaerobic microorganisms such as bacteroides also cause peritonsillar infection

...RADIATION INJURY TO THE COLON:

radiation of the cervix, uterus, bladder, or ovaries

...RAPIDLY PROGRESSIVE GLOMERULONEPHRITIS:

immune complex (usually post-streptococcal; others idiopathic), angiitis, anti-glomerular basement membrane antibodies

...RAYNAUD'S PHENOMENON:

Secondary causes:

connective tissue diseases

...RECTOVAGINAL FISTULA:

in Patients with recurrent carcinoma of the cervix:

tumor necrosis

...RECURRENT HEMATURIA OF GLOMERULAR ORIGIN:

Berger's disease

...RELAPSING FEVER, tick-borne:

in Africa: *Borrelia duttonii*
in Asia: *Borrelia persica*
in North America:

Borrelia turicatae, B. hermsii, and *B. parkeri*

in Spain: *Borrelia hispanica*

...RENAL ARTERY OCCLUSION:

the common causes include emboli due to subacute infective endocarditis, atrial or ventricular thrombi, arteriosclerosis, polyarteritis

114

nodosa, trauma, and, in the neonate, umbilical artery catheterization

...**RENAL ARTERY STENOSIS:**

atherosclerosis, fibromuscular dysplasia

...**RENAL DISEASE:**

End stage:

in Children and Adolescents:

Medullary cystic disease (nephronophthisis)

...**RENAL FAILURE:**

Acute:　　acute tubular necrosis

Acquired, in infants and children:

hemolytic-uremic syndrome

in Hospitalized patients:

prerenal azotemia (50% of cases). Common causes of prerenal azotemia include intravascular volume depletion (hemorrhage, gastrointestinal losses [e.g., diarrhea, vomiting, nasogastric suction], renal losses [e.g., osmotic diuresis, diuretics, adrenal insufficiency], skin losses [e.g., burns, excessive sweating], sequestration in third spaces [e.g., pancreatitis, peritonitis, massive trauma with crush injury]); reduced cardiac output (cardiogenic shock, congestive heart failure, pericardial tamponade, massive pulmonary embolism); systemic vasodilatation (anaphylaxis, antihypertensive drugs, sepsis, drug overdose); systemic or renal vasoconstriction (anesthesia, surgery, alpha adrenergic agonists or high dose dopamine, hepatorenal syndrome); impaired renal autoregulation (nonsteroidal antiinflammatory drugs, angiotensin-converting enzyme inhibitors); hyperviscosity syndromes (multiple myeloma or macroglobulinemia, polycythemia)

115

The Most Common
CAUSES OF:
Chronic:

in Childhood:

congenital nephropathies

and Death

in Adults with renal cystic disease:

adult polycystic kidney disease

...RENAL INSUFFICIENCY, progressive:

in the First decade of life:

renal dysplasia

...RENAL TRAUMA:

in Children: a blunt blow to the abdomen or a deceleration injury (e.g., jumping from a height)

...RENAL TUBULAR ACIDOSIS:

Type I (Distal RTA):

primary (Mendelian dominant inheritance); secondary (autoimmune[Sjogren's, systemic lupus erythematosus], genetic disorders [sickle cell anemia]); disorders causing nephrocalcinosis (idiopathic hypercalciuria, primary hyperparathyroidism, hyperthyroidism, medullary sponge kidney); toxin-induced nephropathy (amphotericin B, lithium)

Type II (Proximal RTA):

isolated proximal tubular defect (drugs [acetazolamide], genetic); with Fanconi's syndrome (Mendelian recessive error of metabolism [cystinosis], as a metabolic consequence of chronic hypocalcemia and secondary hyperparathyroidism, malabsorption syndromes, or drugs or toxins [e.g., lead]); after renal injury from medullary cystic disease, multiple myeloma, postrenal transplant, or nephrotic syndrome

Type IV (Hyperkalemic RTA):

aldosterone deficiency (Addison's disease,

chronic heparin administration); drugs (spironolactone, amiloride, triamterene); generalized collecting duct dysfunction frequently associated with renal insufficiency (Lupus nephritis, obstructive uropathy, chronic pyelonephritis, renal transplantation, chronic glomerulonephritis)

...RESPIRATORY ACIDOSIS:

Acute: obstruction of the airway, neuromuscular disorders and diseases of the central nervous system are common causes of acute respiratory acidosis, according to Devlin

Chronic: seen in patients with chronic obstructive lung disease, such as emphysema

in Surgical Patients:

chronic pulmonary disease, respiratory depression, or the effects of anesthesia

...RESPIRATORY ALKALOSIS:

hyperventilation due to anxie ("hyperventilation syndrome") is probably the most common cause, according to Devlin. Other common causes include overventilation of patients on assisted ventilation, primary CNS disorders, salicylism, hepatic cirrhosis, hepatic coma, hypoxemia, fever, and gram-negative septicemia

...RESPIRATORY DISTRESS IN THE NEWBORN, unexplained:

Bacterial cause:

Group B β–hemolytic streptococcus

...RHEUMATOID ARTHRITIS:

etiology is unknown. The immunologic changes may be initiated by multiple factors

...RIGHT VENTRICULAR FAILURE:

left ventricular failure

The Most Common
CAUSES OF:

...RUPTURE OF THE SPLEEN, traumatic:

    Nonpenetrating:

        automobile accident

    Penetrating: knife wounds and gunshot wounds

...SCOLIOSIS IN ADOLESCENTS:

        idiopathic. Other causes include congenital
        failure of spinal development, musculoskele-
        tal disease (e.g., cerebral palsy), neurofibro-
        matosis, Marfan syndrome, juvenile rheuma-
        toid arthritis, trauma (e.g., fracture and
        destruction of vertebrae and severe burns),
        and structural defects (e.g., different leg
        lengths)

...SECONDARY HYPERSPLENISM:

        portal hypertension

...SECONDARY HYPERTENSION IN CHILDREN:

        renal disease. Virtually any renal disease, glo-
        merular or interstitial, may be the
        cause.Vascular causes are uncommon. Exam-
        ples include coarctation of the aorta, renal ar-
        tery stenosis, and renal artery occlusion. En-
        docrine causes of hypertension are very
        uncommon and are conditions associated with
        excess catecholamines or aldosterone. These
        include pheochromocytoma, primary or sec-
        ondary aldosteronism, and congenital adrenal
        hyperplasia with 11-hydroxylase or 17-
        hydroxylase deficiency. Neurologic disease
        as a cause of hypertension is often hard to
        document

...SECONDARY LYMPHEDEMA:

    in Developed countries:

        obstruction by malignancies, postsurgical
        lymphedema, lymphatic destruction from ther-
        apeutic radiation

118

The Most Common
CAUSES OF:

in Less well-developed countries:

Wuchereria bancrofti

...STD (sexually transmitted disease):

Chlamydia trachomatis

...SEIZURE: idiopathic, trauma, infection, stroke, CVA (cerebrovascular accident), tumor, vasculitis, parasite, poisons, drugs, (meningitis, uremia, encephalitis, hypoxia, electrolyte imbalance, hypoglycemia)

in Infants and young children:

an acute infection

in the Neonate:

due to a birth injury or a congenital defect

in Older children:

idiopathic epilepsy

...SEPSIS:

associated with Catheter use:

coagulase-positive and -negative staphylococci, candida (normal skin flora)

in Infants and children:

H. influenzae type b and *N. meningitidis*

in Neonates: Gram-positive cocci, especially group B β–hemolytic streptococcus (*Streptococcus agalactiae*), but also *S. aureus* and *S. epidermidis*, Gram-negative rods, especially *E. coli* and *K. pneumoniae*, Gram-positive rods (e.g., *L. monocytogenes*)

in Children: *Hemophilus influenza*

Postsplenectomy:

pneumococcus

...SEPTIC ARTHRITIS:

in Neonates: Group B streptococcus, *S. aureus*, and enteric gram-negative rods

119

The Most Common
CAUSES OF:

in Older children:

> *S. aureus. H. influenzae* type b is also common, especially in children younger than 5 years. Other causes include group A streptococcus, *S. pneumoniae*, and *N. meningitidis*. *N. gonorrhoeae* occurs in adolescents

...SEPTIC SHOCK, bacterial:

> this is most often due to gram-negative septicemia, although infection by gram-positive bacteria can also cause shock. Trauma, diabetes mellitus, hematologic diseases, corticosteroid therapy, immunosuppressive drugs, and radiation therapy increase susceptibility to infection and thus predispose to septic shock. Organisms include *Klebsiella-Aerobacter*, *Escherichia coli*, *Pseudomonas*, *Proteus*, *Bacteroides fragilis*, *Staphylococcus*, Paracolon, *Streptococcus*, mixed culture

...SEPTICEMIA:

> Enterobacter spp., *Escherichia coli*, *Klebsiella* spp., meningococcus, pneumococcus, *Proteus* spp., and *Staphylococcus aureus* are commonly encountered pathogens. *Pseudomonas aeruginosa*, *Staphylococcus epidermidis*, and β–hemolytic streptococcus are less commonly encountered pathogens. Approximately 30% of septicemias result from polymicrobial infections

due to *Bacteroides*:

> *Bacteroides fragilis*

Clostridial: *Clostridium perfringens*

Gram-negative:

> this is most often due to *E. coli* but can also be caused by *Klebsiella, Enterobacter, Serratia,*

120

The Most Common
CAUSES OF:

Pseudomonas aeruginosa, Bacteroides, and *Proteus*

Gram-positive: this is uncommon, but is occasionally caused by streptococci, staphylococci, pneumococci, clostridia, or other organisms

...SERIOUS BLOOD LOSS IN OBSTETRICS:

postpartum hemorrhage

...SERUM SICKNESS:

penicillin, although other antibiotics and drugs, such as propylthiouracil and barbiturates, can also cause this syndrome

...SEVERE PROLIFERATIVE GLOMERULONEPHRITIS:

immune complex deposits generated by antecedent infection with group A β–hemolytic streptococci (poststreptococcal glomerulonephritis)

...SEXUAL AMBIGUITY:

the adrenogenital syndrome due to 21-hydroxylase deficiency

...SEXUALLY TRANSMITTED DISEASE IN THE UNITED STATES:

infection with *Chlamydia trachomatis*

...SHIGELLOSIS in the US:

Shigella. sonnei, with *S. flexneri* and *S. sonnei* showing cyclic-type patterns

...SHOCK:

In the first 24 hours after Abdominal Surgery:

bleeding (hemoperitoneum). Postoperative hemoperitoneum is usually the result of a technical problem with hemostasis, but coagulation defects sometimes play a role

Septic, bacterial:

this is most often due to gram-negative septicemia, although infection by gram-positive

121

The Most Common
CAUSES OF:

bacteria can also cause shock. Trauma, diabetes mellitus, hematologic diseases, corticosteroid therapy, immunosuppressive drugs, and radiation therapy increase susceptibility to infection and thus predispose to septic shock. Organisms include *Klebsiella-Aerobacter*, *Escherichia coli*, *Pseudomonas*, *Proteus*, *Bacteroides fragilis*, *Staphylococcus*, Paracolon, *Streptococcus*, mixed culture

...SHORT STATURE in children:

constitutional delay of growth and development, familial (genetic) short stature, GH deficiency (fewer than 5%), primary hypothyroidism; rarely Cushing's disease, primordial growth failure, chronic systemic disease, and psychosocial deprivation.

...SHUNTS ASSOCIATED WITH PULMONARY HYPERTENSION:

ventricular septal defect, atrial septal defect, patent ductus arteriosus

...SINUSITIS:

S. pneumoniae, unencapsulated strains of *H. influenzae*, *B. catarrhalis* (now *Moraxella*), and *Staphylococcus aureus*. *Staphylococcus epidermidis* and β– hemolytic streptococcus are less commonly encountered pathogens

Acute:

Bacterial: *S. pneumoniae* and *H. influenzae*

...SOLITARY PULMONARY NODULES:

most are sequelae to granulomatous disease such as tuberculosis, histoplasmosis, coccidioidomycosis, or nocardia. Less common causes include necrobiotic nodules as may be be seen with rheumatoid diseases, arteriovenous malformations, even bland or septic em-

122

boli, which are more commonly multiple.
Pseudonodules due to superficial skin lesions
or nipple shadows not uncommonly cause un-
due concern

...SPINAL CORD COMPRESSION:

extramedullary malignant disease (most often
metastatic cancer originating in the lung,
breast, prostate, or kidney)

...SPLENIC VEIN THROMBOSIS:

pancreatitis

...SPONTANEOUS PNEUMOTHORAX:

subpleural emphysematous bleb rupture. Also
therapeutic needle punctures, trauma, perforation from pulmonary abscesses or septic in-
farctions; perforation of the esophagus

...STAPHYLOCOCCAL INFECTION in humans:

Staphylococcus aureus

...STATUS EPILEPTICUS:

stopping anticonvulsant medication

...STRANGULATED COLONIC OBSTRUCTION:

volvulus

...STENOSIS, vascular:

atherosclerotic lesions

...STRICTURE:

Urethral, postinflammatory:

in Males: gonorrhea (almost 60%)

...STRIDOR, in infancy:

laryngomalacia (infantile larynx)

...STROKE:

cerebrovascular infarction (most commonly
due to thrombosis of an atherosclerotic
plaque), hemorrhage (aneurysm rupture, associated with hypertension), lacunar vessel disease (infarction)

...SUBARACHNOID HEMORRHAGE:

trauma

123

The Most Common
CAUSES OF:

Non-traumatic:

        rupture of a berry aneurysm

...SUBDURAL HEMATOMA:

        a moving head striking a fixed object

Chronic: approximately 60% follow head trauma. Other causes include ruptured aneurysms and rapid deceleration injuries

...SUBMANDIBULAR SPACE INFECTION (Ludwig's Angina):

        usually develops from dental or peridontal infection, especially of the 2nd and 3rd mandibular molars. It may occur in association with problems caused by poor dental hygiene (e.g., gingivitis and dental sepsis), tooth extractions, or trauma (e.g., fractures of the mandible, lacerations of the floor of the mouth, peritonsillar abscess)

...SUDDEN DEATH:

        coronary artery disease

...SYNCOPE IN SICK SINUS SYNDROME:

        cardiac asystole and profound bradycardia. In a smaller percentage of cases, symptoms may be the result of tachycardia

...SYNERGISTIC NECROTIZING CELLULITIS:

        while *Streptococcus pyogenes* (Group A streptococcus) alone may occasionally cause these infections, usually they are caused by a mixture of aerobic and anaerobic bacteria, the most common isolates being aerobic streptococci other than Group A, aerobic gram-negative bacilli, anaerobic gram-positive cocci, and *Bacteroides* species

...TACHYCARDIA:

Paroxysmal Supraventricular Tachycardia (PSVT):

        AV nodal reentry (responsible for approxi-

The Most Common
CAUSES OF:

                              mately 60% of cases)

Wide QRS: ventricular tachycardia (VT)

...THALASSEMIA:

gene deletion, which is the most common cause of α-thalassemia; an abnormality in the transcription or processing of messenger RNA (mRNA), which occurs more frequently in β-thalassemia; thalassemic hemoglobinopathy, in which a structurally abnormal globin chain is produced in subnormal amounts (e.g., Hgb Lepore, Hgb E, Hgb Constant Spring)

   α-(Alpha) Thalassemia:

gene deletion

...THROMBOCYTOPATHY:

drugs are the most common cause of qualitative platelet disorder; includes chemotherapeutic agents, thiazides, alcohol, aspirin, nonsteroidal anti-inflammatory agents, high molecular weight dextran

...THROMBOCYTOPENIA:

  Immune-mediated:

    in Childhood:

idiopathic

  in the Newborn:

congenital infections, bacterial sepsis, immune-mediated causes, and disseminated intravascular coagulation

...THROMBOSIS OF THE SPLENIC VEIN:

pancreatitis

...THYROID STORM:

in the past, before adequate preparation with antithyroid drugs, surgical treatment was the most common precipitating factor. Presently thyroid storm is a rare complication of surgi-

The Most Common
CAUSES OF:

cal treatment and is more frequently precipitated by trauma, infection, diabetic acidosis, or toxemia of pregnancy

...THYROIDITIS, acute:

Staphylococcus aureus, *Streptococcus hemolyticus*, and pneumococcus

...TIA (Transient Ischemic Attack):

tumor, focal seizure, MS (multiple sclerosis), confusional states, migraine

...TICK-BORNE RELAPSING FEVER:

in Africa:	*Borrelia duttonii*
in Asia:	*Borrelia persica*
in North America:	

Borrelia turicatae, B. hermsii, and *B. parkeri*

in Spain: *Borrelia hispanica*

...TONSILLITIS: β - hemolytic streptococcus is a commonly encountered pathogen. *Klebsiella* spp. is less commonly encountered

...TRANSPLACENTAL INFECTIONS PRIOR TO BIRTH:

cytomegalovirus, *Treponema pallidum* (the agent of syphilis), human immunodeficiency virus [HIV; the agent of acquired immune deficiency syndrome (AIDS)], rubella virus, *Toxoplasma gondii*, echovirus, *Listeria monocytogenes*

...TRAUMA, renal:

in Children: a blunt blow to the abdomen or a deceleration injury (e.g., jumping from a height)

...TRAUMATIC VAGINITIS:

injury or chemical irritation

...TRAVELER'S DIARRHEA:

E. coli. Species of *Shigella*, *Salmonella*, and *Campylobacter* as well as *E. histolytica* and *Giardia lamblia* are other known causes of traveler's diarrhea

...TRICUSPID STENOSIS AND INSUFFICIENCY:

rheumatic fever, carcinoid syndrome, congenital anomalies

...TUBERCULOSIS:

several species of the genus *Mycobacterium* may cause lung disease, but 95% of cases of lung disease are due to *M. tuberculosis*. *Mycobacterium bovis* and *Mycobacterium avium* are seldom found in humans. Several "atypical" species of *Mycobacterium* that are chiefly soil dwellers have become clinically more important in recent years, because they are less responsive to preventive and therapeutic measures

...TUBULAR NECROSIS, acute:

renal hypoperfusion leading to ischemia with inadequate restoration of renal perfusion accounts for 50% of cases. Ischemic damage may occur also in the absence of systemic hypotension, as is the case in more than 50% of patients with postsurgical ATN. The other major cause of ATN is nephrotoxic injury from either exogenous (25%) or endogenous (20%) toxins. Approximately 70% of patients with ATN will have more than one possible cause for their renal failure

...TYPHOID FEVER:

Salmonella typhi

...ULCERS:

Decubitus:

Hospital acquired:

these are nearly always the result of inadequate nursing care

The Most Common
CAUSES OF:
Genital:

in the United States:

genital herpes, followed by syphilis. Other causes include lymphogranuloma venereum (LGV), chancroid, and granuloma inguinale (donavanosis) - all of which are uncommon in the United States. (Gonorrhea is one sexually transmitted disease that does not cause genital ulcer syndromes.)

...UNCONJUGATED HYPERBILIRUBINEMIA IN THE NEONATAL PERIOD:

a physiologic delay in the ability of the liver to clear, metabolize, and excrete the relatively large bilirubin burden at birth

...UNDERREPORTING OF HEALTH PROBLEMS, in elderly population:

ageist view, depression, intellectual decline, fear (of unknown), inaccessibility to health care system

...UPPER GASTROINTESTINAL HEMORRHAGE:

duodenal ulcer, gastric ulcer, diffuse erosive gastritis, esophageal varices, Mallory-Weiss tear of the gastroesophageal junction, gastric carcinoma

in Cirrhotic patients:

varices, erosive gastritis, peptic ulcer disease, and esophageal tears (Mallory-Weiss syndrome)

...URETHRAL STRICTURE:

in Males:

Acquired:due to prior instrumentation (most common) or external trauma

Postinflammatory:

gonorrhea (almost 60%)

...URETHRITIS:

The Most Common
CAUSES OF:

Acute: the major single specific etiology of acute urethritis is *Neisseria gonorrhoeae.* Urethral inflammation of all other etiologies is referred
to collectively as non-gonococcal urethritis
(NGU). NGU is twice as common as gonorrhea in the United States and in much of the
developed world as well. In some underdeveloped areas, however, gonorrhea accounts for
80 percent of the cases of acute urethritis.

Non-specific (NGU; Non-Gonococcal):

Chlamydia trachomatis (30-50% of cases),
serotypes D through K; *Ureaplasma urealyticum* (formerly the T strain of *Mycoplasma*)
also fairly common, has been recovered from
81% of men with *Chlamydia*-negative NGU
(Mandell), causing about 10% of cases
(Braunstein); Herpes simplex virus; Nonspecific, various causes include chemical, physical, etc.; Reiter's syndrome. Rare causes include *Trichomonas vaginalis*(isolated from 3-
15% of patients with NGU [Mandell]), tuberculosis, and syphilis

after Urologic surgery:

E. coli, other gram-negative rods, and enterococci

...URINARY INCONTINENCE, female:

inflammatory lesions (cystitis [usually a trigo-
nitis], urethritis), hormonal (estrogen loss),
congenital, acquired (fistulae, diverticula, urethral obstruction), detrussor dyssynergia, diseases of the nervous system (multiple sclerosis, trauma, diabetes mellitus), anatomic stress
incontinence

...URINARY TRACT INFECTION:

The Most Common
CAUSES OF:

the most common causes are gram-negative bacteria, particularly *Escherichia coli*. *E. coli* accounts for 80-90% of uncomplicated acute UTI in the ambulatory patient. Less common are *Enterobacter aerogenes, Proteus vulgaris, Proteus mirabilis, Pseudomonas aeruginosa,* and *Streptococcus faecalis*. Organisms such as Proteus, Klebsiella, Enterobacter, Pseudomonas, Enterococci, Serratia, and Staphylococcus assume more importance in hospitalized patients with recurrent infection, obstruction, calculi, immunosuppression, or following urinary tract instrumentation. *Staphylococcus saprophyticus* is responsible for 10-15% of acute UTI in young women. *Staphylococcus aureus* bacteriuria is uncommon and usually indicates the presence of an extrarenal source of infection (endocarditis, osteomyelitis, skin abscess) leading to hematogenous renal involvement. *Mycobacterium tuberculosis* and *Candida albicans* are other uncommon causes of hematogenous UTI

...URINARY TRACT OBSTRUCTION:

in Infants and children:

posterior urethral valves. Less frequent causes of obstruction include ureteral valves, a ureterocele, or congenital stenosis at the ureteropelvic junction

in Men after age 55:

prostatic hyperplasia

...VAGINAL BLEEDING COMPLICATING PREMATURE LABOR:

cervical dilation

...VAGINAL CYSTS IN INFANTS:

130

The Most Common
CAUSES OF:

ectopic ureter

...VAGINAL DISCHARGE (leukorrhea):

> *Gardnerella* infection (infections of the lower reproductive tract. Estrogen depletion (senile or atrophic vaginitis) and estrogen or psychic stimulation are other causes

...VAGINAL INJURY:

in Adult Women:

> a "lost" tampon

...VAGINITIS: *Candida albicans*. Other causes are *G. vaginalis*, *T. vaginalis*, and foreign bodies

Traumatic: injury or chemical irritation

...VARICES:

Duodenal: in a recent review, intrahepatic portal hypertension as a result of cirrhosis accounted for 30% of the cases, splenic vein obstruction secondary to pancreatitis, tumor, or thrombosis accounted for 25%, and an additional 25% were caused by portal vein obstruction as a result of thrombosis, infection, or tumor. Rarer causes included veno-occlusive disease, inferior vena cava obstruction, arteriovenous aneurysm involving the hepatic artery and portal vein, and postoperative shunt thrombosis

Esophageal: alcoholic cirrhosis, although any condition producing portal hypertension, even in the absence of hepatic disease (i.e., portal vein thrombosis or idiopathic portal hypertension), may result in variceal bleeding

...VASCULAR ANOMALIES OF THE BRAIN:

> arterio-venous malformations, cavernous angiomas, telangectasia, and venous angiomas

...VASCULAR DISEASE which causes pulmonary vascular obstruction:

131

The Most Common
CAUSES OF:

scleroderma or rheumatoid arthritis

...VASCULAR STENOSIS:

atherosclerotic lesions

...VENEREAL DISEASE:

Neisseria gonorrhea

in England: Non-gonococcal urethritis

...VESICAL OBSTRUCTION IN MALES:

enlarged prostate gland

...VIRAL INFECTION in the post-surgical immunosuppressed patient:

CMV (cytomegalovirus)

...VIRAL PNEUMONIA IN ADULTS:

influenza A virus

...VIRILIZATION OF THE FEMALE NEWBORN:

21-hydroxylase deficiency

...VULVOVAGINITIS:

candidiasis (*Candida albicans*) and *T. vaginalis*. Other microorganisms causing this syndrome include *G. vaginalis, U. urealyticum,* and *M. hominis*

...WATER-BORNE INFECTIOUS DIARRHEA:

G. lamblia, a flagellate protozoan

...WATERHOUSE-FRIDERICHSEN SYNDROME:

Neisseria meningitidis

...WATERY DIARRHEA in the elderly:

fecal impaction (as very liquid fecal matter passes around the obstruction)

...WHEEZING IN CHILDREN:

asthma

Young children:

viral respiratory infections

...WIDE QRS TACHYCARDIA:

ventricular tachycardia (VT)

...WOUND BREAKDOWN:

The Most Common
CAUSES OF:

local sepsis
...WOUND DEHISCENCE:
    Technical causes (in surgery):
        infection and excessively tight sutures
...WOUND INFECTION, anaerobic:
    Bacteroides fragilis
after Surgery on the colon:
    E. coli
...XANTHOGRANULOMATOUS PYELONEPHRITIS:
    E. coli and *P. mirabilis* are the organisms
    most frequently cultured from this infection

References

Amin, R. in Scully, RE, MD. *Case Records of the Massachusetts General Hospital.* 1989;320:43

Beck, WW: *Obstetrics and Gynecology.* (The National Medical Series for Independent Study). New York, John Wiley & Sons, Inc., 1989.

Benson, RC: *Handbook of Obstetrics and Gynecology.* Los Altos, Lange Medical Publications, 1983.

Braunstein, H: *Outlines and Review of Pathology.* St. Louis, C.V. Mosby Company, 1987.

Braunwald, E, ed: *Harrison's Principles of Internal Medicine,* 11th ed.. New York, McGraw-Hill Book Company, 1987.

Braunwald, E, ed: *Harrison's Principles of Internal Medicine* Companion Handbook, 11th ed.. New York, McGraw-Hill Book Company, 1988.

Bullock, J: *Physiology.* (The National Medical Series for Independent Study). Media, Harwal Publishing Company, 1984.

133

The Most Common
CAUSES OF:

Carithers, RL, Jr. Treatment of Alcoholic Liver Disease. *Practical Gastroenterology.* 1989;13:51

Casciato, DA, ed: *Manual of Clinical Oncology*, 2nd ed. Boston, Little, Brown and Company, 1988.

Casey, MJ. Abnormal Genital Bleeding. In: Peckham, BM and Shapiro, SS, eds.: *Signs and Symptoms in Gynecology* Philadelphia, JB Lippincott, 1983.

Chandrasoma, P: *Key Facts in Pathology*. New York, Churchill Livingstone, Inc., 1986.

Cooke, RA: *Colour Atlas of Anatomical Pathology*. New York, Churchill Livingstone, 1987.

Creighton University Lecture Series, Introduction to Clinical Medicine course, Microbiology course, Pathology course, 1988-89.

Creighton University Lecture Series, Department of OB/Gyn, 1989.

Day, AL, MD. Subarachnoid hemorrhage. *AFP.* 1989;40:95

Devlin, TM, ed.: *Textbook of Biochemistry With Clinical Correlations*, 2nd ed. New York, John Wiley & Sons, 1986.

Dworkin, PH: *Pediatrics* (The National Medical Series for Independent Study). New York, John Wiley & Sons, Inc., 1987.

Evans, MI: *Obstetrics and Gynecology* (Pre-Test Series). New York, McGraw Hill, Inc., 1989.

Gomella, LG: *Surgery On Call*. Norwalk, Appleton & Lange, 1990.

Graef, JW, ed.: *Manual of Pediatric Therapeutics* 4th ed. Boston, Little, Brown and Company, 1988.

Gregory, I: *Psychiatry*. Boston, Little, Brown and Company, Inc., 1983.

Heger, JW: *Case Studies In Cardiology For The House Officer*. Baltimore, Williams & Wilkins, 1988.

Hiyama, DT, ed.: *The Mont Reid Surgical Handbook* St. Louis, Mosby Year Book, 1990.

134

Hsu, B: *Physiology*. Boston, Little, Brown and Company, 1987.

Jacob, LS: *Pharmacology* (The National Medical Series for Independent Study). Media, Harwal Publishing Company, 1984.

Jarrell, BE: *Surgery* (The National Medical Series for Independent Study). Media, Harwal Publishing Company, 1986.

Kingsbury, DT, ed: *Microbiology* (The National Medical Series for Independent Study). Media, Harwal Publishing Company, 1985.

Kravath, RE, ed.: *Pediatrics* (Pre-Test Series). New York, McGraw Hill Book Company, 1987.

Krug, RS: *Behavioral Sciences* (Oklahoma Notes Series). New York, Springer-Verlag, 1987.

Lederle, FA, MD. Management of Small Abdominal Aortic Aneyrysms. *Annals of Internal Medicine*. 1990;113:731.

Levine, TB, MD. Congestive Heart Failure: Early signs and symptoms. *Medical Student*. November/December 1990, p. 17.

LiVolsi, VA, ed: *Pathology* (The National Medical Series for Independent Study). Media, Harwal Publishing Company, 1984.

Mandell, GL, ed.: *Principles and Practice of Infectious Diseases*. New York, Churchill Livingstone, Inc., 1990.

McCue, RW, MD. Carpal Tunnel Syndrome: Etiology and Therapy. *Medical Student*. 1989;16:4.

Medical Student. Epistaxis: Diagnosis and Treatment. *Medical Student*. November/December, 1990, p. 20.

The Merck Manual of Diagnosis and Therapy. Rahway, Merck Sharp & Dohme Research Laboratories, 1987.

Miscellanea Medica. *JAMA*. 1991;265:562.

Myers, AR, ed.: *Medicine* (The National Medical Series for Independent Study). Media, Harwal Publishing Company, 1986.

Nelson, WE, ed.: *Nelson Textbook of Pediatrics*, 13th ed. Philadelphia, W.B. Saunders Company, 1987.

O'Connor, PS. in Day, A, MD. Subarachnoid hemorrhage. *AFP*.

The Most Common
CAUSES OF:

July, 1989, p. 99.

Pichichero, ME, MD. Controversies in the Treatment of Streptococcal Pharyngitis. *AFP*. 1990;42:1567.

Radetsky, M. in Pichichero, ME, MD. Controversies in the Treatment of Streptococcal Pharyngitis. *AFP*. 1990;42:1567.

Reed, Barbara D. Postpartum Hemorrhage. *AFP*. 1988;37:111-
120.

Robbins, SL: *Pathologic Basis of Disease*. Philadelphia, W.B.
Saunders Company, 1984.

Rubin, E, ed.: *Pathology*. Philadelphia, J.B. Lippincott Company, 1988.

Rudolph, AM, ed.: *Pediatrics*, 18th ed. Norwalk, Appleton &
Lange, 1987.

Sabiston, DC: *Sabiston's Essentials of Surgery*. Philadelphia,
W.B. Saunders Company, 1987.

Schrock, TR, ed.: *Handbook of Surgery*, 9th ed. Greenbrae,
Jones Medical Publications, 1989.

Scialabba, FA, MD. Saccular Aneurysms of the Thoracic Aorta.
AFP. 1990;41:1475.

Schwartz, SI: *Principles of Surgery*. New York, McGraw-Hill
Book Company, 1989.

Sierles, FS: *Behavioral Science for the Boreds*. Miami, MedMaster, Inc., 1987.

Stillman, RM: *Surgery Diagnosis and Therapy*. East Norwalk,
Appleton and Lange, 1989.

Straub, WH, ed.: *Manual of Diagnostic Imaging*, 2nd ed. Boston,
Little, Brown and Company, 1989.

Szauter, KM. Management of Hepatic Encephalopathy. *Practical Gastroenterology*. 1989;13:40.

Tisher, CC, ed.: *Nephrology for the House Officer*. Baltimore,
Williams & Wilkins, 1989.

Tomb, DA: *Psychiatry for the House Officer*. Baltimore, Williams & Wilkins, 1988.

The Most Common
CAUSES OF:

Trask, AL, MD, FACS. Trauma Care: The race against time. *Medical Student*. 1990;17:4.

Way, LW: *Current Surgical Diagnosis and Treatment*. Norwalk, Appleton and Lange, 1988.

Woods, SM, ed.: *Psychiatry*, 5th ed. (Pre-Test Series). New York, McGraw Hill Inc., 1989.

The Most Common

Complications...

The Most Common
COMPLICATIONS:

...of ABSCESSES OF THE LUNG:

> failure to heal is the most common complication, and requires resection. Other complications are local spread, causing loss of additional parenchyma or even loss of an entire lobe; hemorrhage into the abscess, which can be massive; bronchopleural fistula; and emphysema, tension pneumothorax, pyopneumothorax, and pericarditis. Metastatic abscesses may occur, especially to the brain. Late complications are residual bronchiectasis, chronic abscess, chronic bronchopleural fistula, and recurrent pneumonitis

...of ACQUIRED IMMUNE DEFICIENCY SYNDROM (AIDS):

Pulmonary complication:

> *Pneumocystis carinii* pneumonia

...of ACUTE MYOCARDIAL INFARCTION:

Arrhythmias and conduction disturbances (by incidence):

> ventricular premature contractions (33-71%), atrial premature contractions (10-57%), sinus tachycardia (20-53%), sinus bradycardia (14-28%), atrial fibrillation or flutter (13-28%), ventricular tachycardia (4-28%), accelerated idioventricular rhythm (9-13%), second degree A-V block, Type I (4-10%), ventricular fibrillation (3-10%), right bundle branch block (5-8%), complete heart block (4-8%), left bundle branch block (2-7%), asystole (1-5%), supraventricular tachycardia (0-4%), second degree A-V block, Type II (0.5-2%)

...of AIDS (Acquired Immune Deficiency Syndrome):

Pulmonary complication:

> *Pneumocystis carinii* pneumonia

...of ALCOHOLISM:

141

The Most Common
COMPLICATIONS:

alcoholic liver disease

...of AMEBIASIS: the invasion of the vascular system of the
bowel with vascular transport to the liver

...of AMEBIC COLITIS (SERIOUS COMPLICATION):
amebic abscess of the liver

...of ANESTHESIA, Spinal:

hypotension; post dural-puncture headache

...of ANTIVENOM ADMINISTRATION FOLLOWING
SNAKE ENVENOMATION:
later development of serum sickness

...after BREAST BIOPSY:
Early complications:
hematoma formation, which may go on to become an abscess
Late complications:
cosmetically disfiguring scar retraction.
(Poorly placed subcutaneous sutures or drains
are the most common reasons)

...of BRUCELLOSIS:
involvement of the bones and joints, including
spondylitis of the intervertebral area of the
lumbar spine and localized suppuration in
large joints. In addition, peripheral neuritis,
meningitis, orchitis, suppurative endocarditis,
and pulmonary lesions may develop

...of CAROTID BODY TUMORS:
extension into local structures

...of CHOLELITHIASIS (acute complication):
acute cholecystitis

...of CLEFT PALATE:
speech disorders, dental caries, malocclusion,
and otitis media are among the frequently encountered complications

142

...of COCCIDIOIDOMYCOSIS, pulmonary:
> cavitation

...of CONGENITAL RUBELLA:
> deafness, cataracts, glaucoma, congenital heart disease, and mental retardation, but numerous other defects have been described. Some complications, such as a progressive encephalopathy, do not become apparent until the child is older

...of CROHN'S DISEASE:
> intestinal obstruction, abscesses and fistulas, perianal disease. Others include perforation, hemorrhage, and intractable symptoms

...related to COLONOSCOPY:
> bleeding and perforation

...of DIVERTICULAR DISEASE:
> diverticulitis

...of DUODENAL ULCER:
> hemorrhage, perforation, and duodenal obstruction. Less common complications are pancreatitis and biliary obstruction

...of ENDOSCOPY FOR UPPER GASTROINTESTINAL HEMORRHAGE:
> aspiration

...of GONORRHEA, genital:
> in Females: the most common complication, occurring in about 15 percent of women, is pelvic inflammatory disease (salpingitis)

...of HYPERTENSIVE HEART DISEASE (major complication):
> hemorrhage

...of INCARCERATED OR STRANGULATED HERNIA:
Postoperative complication:
> wound infection

...following INFLUENZA INFECTION:

143

The Most Common
COMPLICATIONS:

pneumonia, most often caused by secondary bacterial infection of an already weakened individual

...of LYME DISEASE:

Neurologic complication:

aseptic meningitis. Also encephalitis and cranial nerve disorders. A radiculoneuritis and myelitis have been observed

...of LUNG ABSCESS:

failure to heal is the most common complication, and requires resection. Other complications are local spread, causing loss of additional parenchyma or even loss of an entire lobe; hemorrhage into the abscess, which can be massive; bronchopleural fistula; and emphysema, tension pneumothorax, pyopneumothorax, and pericarditis. Metastatic abscesses may occur, especially to the brain. Late complications are residual bronchiectasis, chronic abscess, chronic bronchopleural fistula, and recurrent pneumonitis

...after MASTECTOMY:

wound and flap infections

...of MECKEL'S DIVERTICULUM:

in Children:

ulceration of the mucosa of the diverticulum or adjacent ileum, hemorrhage, inflammation, band obstruction, intussusception, hernial entrapment, and miscellaneous

...of MUMPS: a painful orchitis with parenchymal hemorrhage

in Childhood: meningoencephalitis.

...of PANCREATICODUODENECTOMY (the Whipple procedure):

hemorrhage, abscess, and pancreatic ductal

144

The Most Common
COMPLICATIONS:
leakage

...of PARENTERAL NUTRITION (medical complications):
water overload, hyperglycemia, hypoglycemia, and hepatic cholestasis

...PERIOPERATIVE:
the most common perioperative complications involve the pulmonary system

...of PHARYNGITIS (Streptococcal):
Suppurative complications:
acute otitis media and acute sinusitis. Other suppurative complications include peritonsillar cellulitis or abscess, retropharyngeal abscess, and suppurative cervical lymphadenitis

...POSTOPERATIVE:
of Incarcerated or strangulated hernia:
wound infection
after Major surgical procedures:
respiratory complications
Pulmonary: atelectasis
in Patients who die after surgery:
pneumonia

...of PREGNANCY:

acute pyelonephritis (one of most common)
in Pregnant diabetic women:
Severe: diabetic ketoacidosis, retinopathy nephropathy, cardiovascular problems, noncompliant patient and/or physician failure, preterm labor;
Other: emotional stress, infections, hypoglycemia, starvation ketosis, hypertension, fetal macrosomia, polyhydramnios

...of PREMATURE RUPTURE OF MEMBRANES (PROM, placental):
Fetal and Neonatal:

The Most Common
COMPLICATIONS:

congenital pneumonia, sepsis, meningitis, fetal deformation syndrome due to oligohydramnios, cord prolapse (especially if breech), pulmonary hypoplasia, fetal distress

Maternal: intrauterine infection (amnionitis), sepsis

...of PROM (premature rupture of membranes, placental):

Fetal and Neonatal:

congenital pneumonia, sepsis, meningitis, fetal deformation syndrome due to oligohydramnios, cord prolapse (especially if breech), pulmonary hypoplasia, fetal distress

Maternal: intrauterine infection (amnionitis), sepsis

...PULMONARY, following surgery:

atelectasis

...of PULMONARY COCCIDIOIDOMYCOSIS:

cavitation

...of RENAL BIOPSY, percutaneous:

bleeding that is usually self-limited. Significant bleeding requiring transfusion, percutaneous arterial embolization of a bleeding vessel, or nephrectomy is uncommon with an occurrence rate of 2.1%. The mortality rate of 0.07% is comparable to that of percutaneous liver biopsy or coronary angiography

...of RUBELLA, congenital:

deafness, cataracts, glaucoma, congenital heart disease, and mental retardation, but numerous other defects have been described. Some complications, such as a progressive encephalopathy, do not become apparent until the child is older

...of SHOCK (SEVERE COMPLICATION):

acute tubular necrosis of the kidney

...of SPINAL ANESTHESIA:

146

The Most Common
COMPLICATIONS:

hypotension; post dural-puncture headache

...of STRANGULATED OR INCARCERATED HERNIA:

    Postoperative complication:

        wound infection

...of TRANSFUSION:

        fever is the most common immediate transfusion reaction and is due chiefly to recipient reaction against white cells in the donor blood

    Lethal complication:

        viral hepatitis acquired from the donor is the commonest lethal complication of blood transfusion

    Massive transfusion:

        hypothermia. Others include citrate toxicity, hyperkalemia, acidosis, hyperammonemia, coagulopathy, infection

...of TYPHOID FEVER:

        intestinal perforation with peritonitis. Other problems are bleeding and thrombophlebitis, usually of the saphenous vein, cholecystitis, pneumonia, and focal abscesses in various organs and tissues

...of ULCERATIVE COLITIS:

    Anorectal complications:

        anal fissures are most common (about 12% of patients), and anorectal abscesses and fistulas are seen in 5% of patients

...of VARICELLA ZOSTER INFECTION:

    encephalopathy, cerebellitis, Guillain-Barre syndrome, aseptic meningitis, pneumonia, thrombocytopenic purpura, purpura fulminans, cellulitis, abscess formation, and arthritis

...following SURGICAL SPLENECTOMY:

    atelectasis of the left lower lung

The Most Common
COMPLICATIONS:
...following TRANSPLANTATION:

> infection (bacterial, fungal, and viral of all types)

...of the WHIPPLE PROCEDURE (pancreaticoduodenectomy):

> hemorrhage, abscess, and pancreatic ductal leakage

References

Beck, WW: *Obstetrics and Gynecology*. (The National Medical Series for Independent Study). New York, John Wiley & Sons, Inc., 1989.

Braunstein, H: *Outlines and Review of Pathology*. St. Louis, C.V. Mosby Company, 1987.

Creighton University Lecture Series, Introduction to Clinical Medicine course, Pathology course, 1988-89.

Dworkin, PH: *Pediatrics* (The National Medical Series for Independent Study). New York, John Wiley & Sons, Inc., 1987.

Hiyama, DT, ed.: *The Mont Reid Surgical Handbook* St. Louis, Mosby Year Book, 1990.

Jarrell, BE: *Surgery* (The National Medical Series for Independent Study). Media, Harwal Publishing Company, 1986.

Kingsbury, DT, ed: *Microbiology* (The National Medical Series for Independent Study). Media, Harwal Publishing Company, 1985.

Kravath, RE, ed.: *Pediatrics* (Pre-Test Series). New York, McGraw Hill Book Company, 1987.

The Most Common
COMPLICATIONS:

Rich, MW, ed.: *Coronary Care for the House Officer*. Baltimore, Williams & Wilkins, 1989.

Rubin, E, ed.: *Pathology*. Philadelphia, J.B. Lippincott Company, 1988.

Sabiston, DC: *Sabiston's Essentials of Surgery*. Philadelphia, W.B. Saunders Company, 1987.

Schrock, TR, ed.: *Handbook of Surgery*, 9th ed. Greenbrae, Jones Medical Publications, 1989.

Shanies, HM, PhD, MD. Pneumocystis Carinii Pneumonia. *Emergency Medicine*. 15 May, 1989, p. 71.

Stillman, RM: *Surgery Diagnosis and Therapy*. East Norwalk, Appleton and Lange, 1989.

Tisher, CC, ed.: *Nephrology for the House Officer*. Baltimore, Williams & Wilkins, 1989.

Way, LW: *Current Surgical Diagnosis and Treatment*. Norwalk, Appleton and Lange, 1988.

The Most Common

Conditions...

The Most Common
CONDITIONS:

...ASSOCIATED WITH:

Aortic Insufficiency:
> chronic rheumatic valvular disease or syphilitic heart disease. Less commonly SBE, valvular rupture, dissecting aneurysm, Marfan's disease, psoriatic and ankylosing spondylitis, interventricular septal defects

Catalepsy, waxy flexibility type:
> the catatonic stupor of schizophrenia

Cortical Renal Necrosis, bilateral:
> pregnancy, especially after placenta abruptio; after administration of certain drugs; in infection, burns, trauma, hemorrhage, hyperacute rejection

Diverticulosis: bleeding

Dysfunctional Uterine Bleeding (DUB):
> anovulation and continuous or unopposed estrogen secretion. Occasionally associated with poor quality ovulatory cycles

Hepatocellular injury:
> hepatitis

a Hooded Cervix:
> in utero drug exposure

Ileus: the postoperative period

Lymphangiosarcoma:
> following radical mastectomy, but may also result from other causes of lymphedema

Lymphatic obstruction with lymphedema:
> mastectomy for breast carcinoma, elephantiasis (filariasis), and radiation

Megacolon: seen most often with chronic partial colonic obstruction and constipation

severe Placental Abruption:
> maternal hypertension, chronic vascular disease, pregnancy-induced hypertension. Less

153

The Most Common
CONDITIONS:

frequent associations include trauma and sudden decompression of the uterus

Thiamine deficiency:

alcoholism

Right colon obstruction:

large bulky tumors that have less of a tendency to encircle the bowel

Ventral hernia which presents as a bulge in the area of a surgical incision:

a vertical incision

...WHICH CAUSE:

Lung abscess: tuberculosis, fungal infections, and carcinoma

...CONFUSED WITH:

Appendicitis: gastroenteritis in adults and mesenteric lymphadenitis in children and young adults. Also perforated peptic ulcer, colonic diverticulitis, intestinal obstruction, perforated carcinoma of the colon, Meckel's diverticulitis, and regional enteritis.

...WHICH LIMIT PEOPLE'S ACTIVITY:

diseases of the musculoskeletal system, circulatory system, nervous system and organs of special sense, respiratory system and mental disorders.

...WHICH MUST BE DIFFERENTIATED FROM:

Biliary stricture:

choledocholithiasis

...WHICH PRECEDE SINUSITIS:

viral upper respiratory infection, allergy (allergic rhinitis), and asthma. Other contributing factors include rapid changes in altitude, swimming, trauma, and immunologic defects

...WHICH PREDISPOSES A PATIENT TO SEPTIC SHOCK:

septicemia with gram-negative organisms

...IN WHICH:

154

The Most Common
CONDITIONS:

Coronary thrombosis is seen:
> atherosclerosis

Dysplasia arises:
> in hyperplastic squamous epithelium, and in areas of squamous metaplasia, sites other than squamous epithelium such as dysplastic changes in the mucosal cells

Hydropic swelling is seen:
> ischemia, high fever disease and patients with hypokalemia

Neonatal Exchange Transfusion is needed:
> Rh hemolytic disease of the newborn

Neutrophilia is seen:
> in association with bacterial infections and with infarction of tissues

Pseudomonas aeruginosa infection occurs:
> in the hospital environment

Rheumatoid Factor is seen:
> adult rheumatoid arthritis, also juvenile rheumatoid arthritis, Sjogren's syndrome, systemic lupus erythematosus, and occasionally other inflammatory diseases, including leprosy and infectious mononucleosis

The Most Common
CONDITIONS:

References

Beck, WW: *Obstetrics and Gynecology*. (The National Medical Series for Independent Study). New York, John Wiley & Sons, Inc., 1989.

Braunstein, H: *Outlines and Review of Pathology*. St. Louis, C.V. Mosby Company, 1987.

Creighton University Lecture Series, Pathology course, 1988-89.

Dworkin, PH: *Pediatrics* (The National Medical Series for Independent Study). New York, John Wiley & Sons, Inc., 1987.

Evans, MI: *Obstetrics and Gynecology* (Pre-Test Series). New York, McGraw Hill, Inc., 1989.

Gregory, I: *Psychiatry*. Boston, Little, Brown and Company, Inc., 1983.

Jarrell, BE: *Surgery* (The National Medical Series for Independent Study). Media, Harwal Publishing Company, 1986.

Rubin, E, ed.: *Pathology*. Philadelphia, J.B. Lippincott Company, 1988.

Sabiston, DC: *Sabiston's Essentials of Surgery*. Philadelphia, W.B. Saunders Company, 1987.

Sierles, FS: *Behavioral Science for the Boreds*. Miami, MedMaster, Inc., 1987.

Stillman, RM: *Surgery Diagnosis and Therapy.* East Norwalk, Appleton and Lange, 1989.

Way, LW: *Current Surgical Diagnosis and Treatment*. Norwalk, Appleton and Lange, 1988

The Most Common

Cytotoxic Agents
Which Cause...

...ALLERGIC REACTIONS:

L-asparaginase, bleomycin, melphalan, nitrogen mustard. Occasionally Adriamycin and daunorubicin, cyclophosphamide, methotrexate, cisplatin, procarbazine

...ALOPECIA:
actinomycin D, Adriamycin and daunorubicin, cyclophosphamide (high dose), VP-16-213 (etoposide). Occasionally bleomycin, methotrexate, nitrogen mustard, vincristine. Rarely alkylating agents (oral), decarbazine (imidazole carboxamide), fluorouracil, hydroxyurea, mitomycin C, nitrosoureas

...ANAPHYLAXIS:

L-asparaginase, bleomycin

...APNEA: alkylating agents with succinylcholine

...ARRHYTHMIAS:

Adriamycin and daunorubicin, cyclophosphamide (high dose)

...AZOOSPERMIA:

alkylating agents (especially cyclophosphamide, nitrogen mustard, thiotepa), methotrexate

...AZOTEMIA: See hyperuricemia, renal toxicity, retroperitoneal fibrosis (ureteral obstruction)

...BONE PAIN: procarbazine (arthralgia), hormonal therapy for breast cancer

...CATARACTS: busulfan

...COAGULOPATHY:

actinomycin D, Adriamycin and daunorubicin, L-asparaginase, mithramycin

...CONJUNCTIVITIS:

fluorouracil, methotrexate. Occasionally drugs associated with Stomatitis

...CONSTIPATION:

vincristine, vinblastine, vindesine

159

The Most Common
CYTOTOXIC AGENTS
WHICH CAUSE:

...CYSTITIS AND HEMATURIA:

cyclophosphamide. Rarely mercaptopurine

...DIARRHEA: actinomycin D, Adriamycin and daunorubicin, fluorouracil, methotrexate. Rarely dacarbazine (imidazole carboxamide), mercaptopurine, procarbazine

...DISULFIRAM (ANTABUSE) - LIKE REACTION:

procarbazine with alcohol

...DRUG INTERACTIONS:

Alkylating agents with succinylcholine:

prolonged curariform effect

Cyclophosphamide with allopurinol:

increased myelotoxicity (reasons?)

Mercaptopurine with allopurinol:

increased myelotoxicity

Methotrexate with phenylbutazone, probenecid, salicylates:

enhanced methotrexate effect

Nitrosoureas with cimetidine:

increased myelotoxicity

Procarbazine has monoamine oxidase inhibitor activity

...FEVER: bleomycin, dacarbazine (imidazole carboxamide), mithramycin, methotrexate. Rarely Adriamycin and daunorubicin, mercaptopurine, nitrogen mustard, thioguanine, thiotepa

...FLUID RETENTION:

corticosteroids, diethylstilbestrol, testosterone derivatives

...GYNECOMASTIA:

busulfan, diethylstilbestrol, tamoxifen, MOPP (Mustargen, Oncovin (vincristine), procarbazine, and prednisone) combination

...HEART FAILURE:

Adriamycin and daunorubicin, See Fluid retention. Rarely cyclophosphamide(high dose), chlorambucil

160

The Most Common
CYTOTOCXIC AGENTS
WHICH CAUSE:

...HEMATOTOXICITY (most cytotoxic drugs can cause pancy-
topenia):

Megaloblastosis:

antimetabolites (especially cytarabine, mercaptopurine, hydroxyurea)

Myelotoxicity (mild to absent):

L-asparaginase, bleomycin, hexamethylmela-
mine, hormones, mitotane (o,p'-DDD), streptozocin, vincristine

Thrombocytopenia (uncommon):

cyclophosphamide (low dose), vinblastine

...HYPERCALCEMIA:

hormonal therapy for breast cancer

...HYPERGLYCEMIA:

L-asparaginase, corticosteroids, cyclophosphamide, vinca alkaloids

...HYPERKALEMIA:

chemotherapy for Burkitt's lymphoma

...HYPERTENSIVE CRISIS:

procarbazine with sympathomimetic amines
or foods containing tyrosine

...HYPERURICEMIA:

mercaptopurine; radiotherapy or chemotherapy for lymphomas and leukemias

...HYPOCALCEMIA:

mithramycin. Rarely bone healing with hormonal therapy for breast cancer

...HYPOGYLCEMIA:

streptozocin

...HYPOMAGNESEMIA:

cisplatin

...HYPONATREMIA (inappropriate ADH):

cyclophosphamide, vincristine

...IMMUNOSUPPRESSION:

most drugs

The Most Common
CYTOTOXIC AGENTS
WHICH CAUSE:

...LACRIMATION (dacryocystitis, lacrimal duct stenosis):
    fluorouracil

...LIVER TOXICITY:

Moderate or marked:
    L-asparaginase, 5-azacytidine, mercaptopurine, methotrexate

Mild or rare: cytarabine, chlorambucil, dacarbazine (imidazole carboxamide), mithramycin, mitomycin C, nitrosoureas, streptozocin, testosterone derivatives, thioguanine

...MENSTRUAL IRREGULARITIES:
    same as Azoospermia

...MUSCLE CRAMPS:
    procarbazine, vinblastine, vincristine, VP-16-213 (etoposide)

...MUSCLE LYSIS:
    5-azacytidine

...NAUSEA OR VOMITING:
    actinomycin D, cyclophosphamide (high dose), dacarbazine (imidazole carboxamide), hexamethylmelamine, mithramycin, nitrogen mustard, nitrosoureas, mitotane (o,p'-DDD), procarbazine, cisplatin. Occasionally Adriamycin and daunorubicin, chlorambucil, cyclophosphamide, fluorouracil (loading dose), vinblastine

...NEOPLASIA (induction of second malignancy):

Carcinogenic in animals:
    Adriamycin and daunorubicin, nitrosoureas, procarbazine

Leukemia, acute nonlymphocytic:
    alkylating agents

Lymphomas: mercaptopurine (azathioprine)

Squamous cell carcinomas:
    mercaptopurine (azathioprine)

162

Urinary bladder carcinoma:

> cyclophosphamide

Vaginal carcinoma:

> diethylstilbestrol with in utero exposure

...NERVOUS SYSTEM TOXICITY:

> cytarabine (intrathecal), L-asparaginase, bleomycin (high dose), fluorouracil, hexamethyl-melamine, methotrexate (all routes), nitrogen mustard, nitrosoureas, mitotane (o,p'-DDD), procarbazine, cisplatin, vincristine, vindesine. Rarely 5-azacytidine, dacarbazine (imidazole carboxamide), hydroxyurea, nitrogen mustard, vinblastine

...OSTEOPOROSIS:

> corticosteroids, methotrexate (chronic therapy)

...PANCREATITIS:

> L-asparaginase

...PULMONARY TOXICITY:

> bleomycin, busulfan, nitrosoureas. Rarely chlorambucil, cyclophosphamide, melphalan, mitomycin C, methotrexate, procarbazine

...RENAL TOXICITY:

Prominent: methotrexate (high dose), cisplatin, streptozocin and other nitrosoureas

Mild: L-asparaginase, mithramycin, mitomycin C, mercaptopurine, methotrexate. Rarely Adriamycin and daunorubicin

...RETROPERITONEAL FIBROSIS:

> busulfan

...SKIN AND NAIL CHANGES:

> actinomycin, Adriamycin and daunorubicin, L-asparaginase, bleomycin, busulfan, fluorouracil, methotrexate, vinblastine

Uncommon changes:

163

The Most Common
CYTOTOXIC AGENTS
WHICH CAUSE:

actinomycin D, Adriamycin and daunorubicin, L-asparaginase, chlorambucil, cyclophosphamide, hydroxyurea, mithramycin, mitomycin C, mercaptopurine, nitrogen mustard, mitotane (o,p'-DDD), procarbazine, thioguanine

Inflammation following subcutaneous infiltration:

actinomycin D, Adriamycin and daunorubicin, dacarbazine, mithramycin, mitomycin C, nitrosoureas, nitrogen mustard, vinblastine, vincristine

Radiation recall phenomena (erythema or moist desquamation over a previous radiation port):

actinomycin D, Adriamycin and daunorubicin, bleomycin, methotrexate, procarbazine

...STOMATITIS (mucositis):

antitumor antibiotics, cyclophosphamide, fluorouracil. Rarely cytarabine, hydroxyurea, mercaptopurine

...TONGUE, BLACK HAIRY:

Adriamycin and daunorubicin, fluorouracil

...URINE, RED: Adriamycin and daunorubicin

References

Braunwald, E, ed: *Harrison's Principles of Internal Medicine*, 11th ed.. New York, McGraw-Hill Book Company, 1987.
Casciato, DA, ed: *Manual of Clinical Oncology*, 2nd ed. Boston, Little, Brown and Company, 1988.

The Most Common

Form Of...

The Most Common
FORM OF:

...ACQUIRED HYPOGONADOTROPIC AMENORRHEA:

psychogenic, occurring in association with either acute or chronic emotional stress

...ALCOHOL CONSUMED IN SUBSTANCE ABUSE:

beer

...AMEBIC COLITIS:

chronic amebic colitis > acute amebic colitis

...AMNESIA, psychogenic:

localized amnesia (a total loss of memory for a circumscribed period of time during which a traumatic incident or experience is often found to have occurred). Less commonly there may be *generalized* amnesia (for the entire previous life, including loss of knowledge of personal identity and, rarely, even loss of ability to use language or understand the functions of common objects). Unusual forms of this disorder include *systematized* amnesia, in which the memory loss involves only specific, closely related events (e.g., an episode of violence) but memory is retained for unrelated events occurring at the same time, and *continuous* amnesia, in which current experiences are forgotten as they occur

...ANTHRAX IN THE US:

cutaneous anthrax; malignant pustule form (95%) > septicemic or pneumonic, or gastrointestinal forms

...ARTERIAL DISORDER:

arterial occlusive disease

...ARTHRITIS: degenerative joint disease (osteoarthritis)

...ATROPHY: secondary to reduced functional demand

...BERGER'S DISEASE (IgA nephropathy):

a focal glomerulonephritis, which is indistin-

The Most Common
FORM OF:

guishable histologically from the nephritis of
Henoch-Schonlein purpura

...BRUCELLOSIS: undulant fever, and rarely, extreme pyrexia
and death

...CAMPHYLOBACTEROSIS:
gastroenteritis

...CANCER IN CHILDHOOD:
leukemia, brain tumor

Black children:
leukemia, central nervous system, lymphoma
including Hodgkin's, soft tissue sarcoma,
Wilms' tumor, neuroblastoma, eye and germ
cell

White children:
leukemia, central nervous system, lymphoma
including Hodgkin's, neuroblastoma, soft tissue sarcoma, Wilms' tumor, bone, eye, germ
cell, liver

...CANDIDIASIS:
Cutaneous: paronychia and onychomycosis, particularly
in people who frequently immerse their hands
or feet in water

Mucocutaneous:
Early in life:
oral thrush

...CARCINOMA OF THE ESOPHAGUS:
Squamous cell carcinoma:
a polypoid fungating lesion that protrudes into
the lumen (60%), a necrotic cancerous ulceration that excavates deeply into surrounding
structures and may erode into the respiratory
tree and the aorta, or permeate the mediastinum and pericardium (25%), and a diffuse infiltrative form that tends to spread within the
wall of the esophagus, causing thickening, ri-

gidity, and narrowing of the lumen with ulceration of the mucosa

...CHRONIC DRUG-INDUCED TUBULOINTERSTITIAL
NEPHRITIS:

analgesic nephropathy

...CLINICAL PRESENTATION OF LARGE BOWEL OB-
STRUCTION:

crampy abdominal pain, obstipation, and, later
on, nausea and vomiting

...COCCIDIOIDOMYCOSIS:

acute self-limited coccidioidomycosis: either
clinically silent or manifested as a nonspecific
flu syndrome

...CONGENITAL HEART DISEASE:

ventricular septal defect (20%), atrial septal
defect (10-15%), coarctation of the aorta (10-
15%), pulmonic valvular stenosis (10%), aortic valvular stenosis (10%), patent ductus arteriosus (10%), transposition of the great vessels (10%), atrioventricular septal defects (<
5%)

...CONJUNCTIVITIS, NEONATAL:

conjunctivitis in the newborn is secondary to
inflammation caused by silver nitrate and to
infection with *Neisseria gonorrhoeae* (gonococcal conjunctivitis), *Chlamydia trachomatis*
(inclusion conjunctivitis caused by *C. trachomatis* serotypes D through K), and *Staphylococcus aureus*. Less common causes include infection with group A or B
streptococcus, *Pseudomonas aeruginosa*, and
other bacteria, or herpesvirus hominis type 2.
N. gonorrhoeae, C. trachomatis, group B
streptococcus, and herpesvirus hominis are ac-

169

The Most Common
FORM OF:

quired on passage through a colonized or infected birth canal; other bacteria are usually acquired after birth

...CONTRACEPTION USED BY ADOLESCENTS:
the oral contraceptive pill

...CONTRACEPTIVE USED OUTSIDE THE UNITED STATES:
injectable progesterone

...CUTANEOUS CANDIDIASIS:
paronychia and onychomycosis, particularly in people who frequently immerse their hands or feet in water

...DEGENERATIVE CHANGE of uterine leiomyomas:
hyaline degeneration. Others include cystic degeneration, necrosis, carneous degeneration, mucoid degeneration, rarely sarcomatous degeneration

...DEGENERATIVE DEMENTIA:
Primary: Alzheimer's disease

...DEMYELINATING DISEASE:
sudanophilic leukodystrophy, sudanophilic leukodystrophy of Pelizaeus-Merzbacher type (aplasia axialis extracorticalis congenita), progressive subcortical encephalopathy (encephalitis periaxialis diffusa, Schilder's disease), spinocerebellar ataxia (Friedreich's ataxia), accompanied by variable mental retardation (or dementia when the onset is late)

...DISSOCIATIVE DISORDER:
psychogenic amnesia

...ECHINOCOCCIASIS:
pastoral echinococciasis

...EPILEPSY: tonic-clonic seizures (grand mal)

...FAMILIAL HYPERLIPIDEMIA:
in Children: familial hypercholesterolemia (classic type II

170

The Most Common
FORM OF:

hyperlipoproteinemia)

...FUNCTIONING ECTOPIC THYROID TISSUE that achieves
clinical significance:
lingual thyroid

...GAUCHER'S DISEASE:
type I, or adult Gaucher's disease > type II (infantile Gaucher's disease) and type III (juvenile Gaucher's disease)

...GALLBLADDER DISEASE, Symptomatic:
chronic cholecystitis (it is associated with
gallstones in nearly every case)

...GESTATIONAL TROPHOBLASTIC NEOPLASIA (GTN):
nonmetastatic GTN

...HEMOPHILIA: hemophilia A (1:5000) > hemophilia B
(1:30,000)

...HEPATITIS:
in Hemophiliacs:
non-A non-B hepatitis
Transfusion related:
non-A, non-B

...HERPES SIMPLEX VIRUS WHICH CAUSES GENITAL IN-
VOLVEMENT:
herpes simplex virus type 2

...HODGKIN'S DISEASE SEEN IN POORLY DEVELOPED
COUNTRIES:
the childhood form of Hodgkin's disease

...HYPERLIPIDEMIA, Familial:
in Children: familial hypercholesterolemia (classic type II
hyperlipoproteinemia)

...HYPERTENSION IN CHILDREN:
primary hypertension (also called idiopathic
or essential hypertension)

...HYPERTHERMIA, localized:
cutaneous burns

...HYPOGONADOTROPIC AMENORRHEA:

The Most Common
FORM OF:

Acquired: psychogenic, occurring in association with either acute or chronic emotional stress

Congenital: Kallman's syndrome

...IgA NEPHROPATHY (Berger's disease):
a focal glomerulonephritis, which is indistinguishable histologically from the nephritis of Henoch-Schonlein purpura

...INCEST: probably sibling, then father-daughter, and mother-son

...INJURY TO NERVES DURING CHILDBIRTH:
facial nerve injury and tearing of the brachial plexus

...INTRACRANIAL TUMORS:
gliomas, meningiomas, secondary metastatic tumors

...JOINT DISEASE IN ADULTS:
osteoarthritis

...LISTERIOSIS:
in Adults: meningitis

...LOCALIZED HYPERTHERMIA:
cutaneous burns

...METAPLASIA: replacement of a glandular epithelium by a squamous one. Other forms include replacement of one glandular epithelium by another, metaplasia of transitional epithelium to glandular epithelium, etc.

...MUCOCUTANEOUS CANDIDIASIS:
Early in life: oral thrush

...NATURAL BIRTH:
head-first

...NEONATAL CONJUNCTIVITIS:
conjunctivitis in the newborn is secondary to inflammation caused by silver nitrate and to infection with *Neisseria gonorrhoeae* (gonococcal conjunctivitis), *Chlamydia trachomatis*

172

(inclusion conjunctivitis caused by *C. trachomatis* serotypes D through K), and *Staphylococcus aureus*. Less common causes include infection with group A or B streptococcus, *Pseudomonas aeruginosa*, and other bacteria, or herpesvirus hominis type 2. *N. gonorrhoeae*, *C. trachomatis*, group B streptococcus, and herpesvirus hominis are acquired on passage through a colonized or infected birth canal; other bacteria are usually acquired after birth

...NEPHROGENIC DIABETES INSIPIDUS:

acquired > congenital. Acquired causes include chronic renal disease (medullary cystic disease, polycystic kidney disease, obstructive uropathy, pyelonephritis, severe chronic renal failure), pharmacologic agents (demeclocycline, lithium, glyburide, tolazamide, propoxyphene, methoxyflurane, amphotericin B, vinblastine, colchicine), electrolyte disorders (hypercalcemia, hypokalemia), dietary abnormalities (poor protein intake, excessive water intake, poor salt intake), and miscellaneous (amyloidosis, sarcoidosis, multiple myeloma, Sjogren's syndrome, sickle cell disease)

...NEPHROTIC SYNDROME:

in Adults: primary membranous glomerulonephritis (accounts for 30%-50%). Lipoid nephrosis accounts for about 20% of cases. Focal glomerulosclerosis is seen in about 5%-12% of renal biopsies in adult patients with nephrotic syndrome. Crescentic glomerulonephritis and amyloidosis are rarely encountered forms of nephrotic syndrome.

The Most Common
FORM OF:

in Children: minimal change disease (lipoid nephrosis or nil lesion), (80%). The remaining 20% of cases occur with primary glomerulopathies, with systemic diseases, or secondary to toxic injuries. Primary membranous glomerulonephritis accounts for less than 1% of cases in children.

...NYSTAGMUS: horizontal jerk nystagmus

...PERFORATION OF THE GALLBLADDER:
localized perforation. Also free intraperitoneal perforation (less common) and into a surrounding viscus

in Acute Cholecystitis:
pericholecystic abscess

...PNEUMONIA: Bronchopneumonia

Bacterial: pneumococcal pneumonia (caused by *Streptococcus pneumoniae*) accounts for about 80 percent of the cases

...POLYCYSTIC KIDNEYS:
the adult form is autosomal dominant. It is much more common than the infantile form

...PRIMARY DEGENERATIVE DEMENTIA:
Alzheimer's disease

...PSYCHOGENIC AMNESIA:
localized amnesia (a total loss of memory for a circumscribed period of time during which a traumatic incident or experience is often found to have occurred). Less commonly there may be *generalized* amnesia (for the entire previous life, including loss of knowledge of personal identity and, rarely, even loss of ability to use language or understand the functions of common objects). Unusual forms of this disorder include *systematized* amnesia, in

which the memory loss involves only specific, closely related events (e.g., and episode of violence) but memory is retained for unrelated events occurring at the same time, and *continuous* amnesia, in which current experiences are forgotten as they occur

...PSYCHOTHERAPY:

individual therapy

...PUERPERAL INFECTION:

endometritis (childbed fever)

...RENAL DISEASE:

hypertensive renal disease (benign essential)

...RENAL TRAUMA:

renal contusions or ecchymoses constitute approximately 85% of renal trauma. Minor injuries also include subcapsular hematomas and superficial cortical lacerations

...RESPIRATORY DISTRESS IN THE NEWBORN:

the idiopathic syndrome, presumed to be due to functional and anatomical immaturity of fetal lungs

...RETARDATION:

Secondary: Down's syndrome. Less frequently poor prenatal care, certain maternal health problems, birth complications, malnutrition, and exposure to toxic substances

...SALMONELLOSIS:

gastroenteritis

...SECONDARY RETARDATION:

Down's syndrome. Less frequently poor prenatal care, certain maternal health problems, birth complications, malnutrition, and exposure to toxic substances

...SEIZURES IN THE NEONATAL PERIOD:

Subtle seizures -which manifest as rhythmic

The Most Common
FORM OF:

eye deviation or blinking, lip smacking, "bicycling," or apnea. This is followed by generalized tonic, multifocal clonic, focal clonic, and myoclonic seizures

...SEPARATION ANXIETY DISORDER:

school refusal or school phobia

...SKELETAL DYSPLASIA:

achondroplasia

...SKIN REACTIONS IN DRUG ALLERGY:

exanthematous eruptions, urticaria, angioedema, and photosensitivity. Less commonly bullous eruptions (epidermal necrolysis, Stevens-Johnson syndrome) can be fatal

...SQUAMOUS CELL CARCINOMA OF THE ESOPHAGUS:

a polypoid fungating lesion that protrudes into the lumen (60%), a necrotic cancerous ulceration that excavates deeply into surrounding structures and may erode into the respiratory tree and the aorta, or permeate the mediastinum and pericardium (25%), and a diffuse infiltrative form that tends to spread within the wall of the esophagus, causing thickening, rigidity, and narrowing of the lumen with ulceration of the mucosa

...SUICIDE ATTEMPT:

drug ingestion

...TARDIVE DYSKINESIAS:

orofacial dyskinesia, consisting of incessant facial tics, grimaces, lip smacking, etc., and *buccal-lingual-masticatory dyskinesia*, which resembles chewing motions with intermittent tongue protrusion. Less commonly there may be *choreiform* (rapid and jerky) movements of the limbs, *athetoid* (slow, sinuous, writhing) movements of the fingers or toes, or swaying movements of the trunk

...THYROIDITIS: Hashimoto's thyroiditis (chronic) > subacute thyroiditis, acute suppurative thyroiditis (most uncommon)

Chronic: Hashimoto's disease, or chronic lymphocytic thyroiditis

...TRANSMISSION OF TOXOPLASMOSIS:
ingestion of oocysts, ingestion of tissue cysts, and congenital acquisition

...TULAREMIA: ulceroglandular

...TUMORS, intracranial:
gliomas, meningiomas, secondary metastatic tumors

...WOUND INFECTION following mastectomy:
wound and flap infections due to necrosis of the wound edges, either from tension or from burns with electrocautery

References

Beck, WW: *Obstetrics and Gynecology*. (The National Medical Series for Independent Study). New York, John Wiley & Sons, Inc., 1989.

Braunstein, H: *Outlines and Review of Pathology*. St. Louis, C.V. Mosby Company, 1987.

Braunwald, E, ed: *Harrison's Principles of Internal Medicine*, 11th ed.. New York, McGraw-Hill Book Company, 1987.

Dworkin, PH: *Pediatrics* (The National Medical Series for Independent Study). New York, John Wiley & Sons, Inc., 1987.

Gregory, I: *Psychiatry*. Boston, Little, Brown and Company,

The Most Common
FORM OF:

Inc., 1983.

Jarrell, BE: *Surgery* (The National Medical Series for Independent Study). Media, Harwal Publishing Company, 1986.

Kingsbury, DT, ed: *Microbiology* (The National Medical Series for Independent Study). Media, Harwal Publishing Company, 1985.

Kravath, RE, ed.: *Pediatrics* (Pre-Test Series). New York, McGraw Hill Book Company, 1987.

Krug, RS: *Behavioral Sciences* (Oklahoma Notes Series). New York, Springer-Verlag, 1987.

Myers, AR, ed.: *Medicine* (The National Medical Series for Independent Study). Media, Harwal Publishing Company, 1986.

Nelson, WE, ed.: *Nelson Textbook of Pediatrics*, 13th ed. Philadelphia, W.B. Saunders Company, 1987.

Robbins, SL: *Pathologic Basis of Disease*. Philadelphia, W.B. Saunders Company, 1984.

Rubin, E, ed.: *Pathology*. Philadelphia, J.B. Lippincott Company, 1988.

Sabiston, DC: *Sabiston's Essentials of Surgery*. Philadelphia, W.B. Saunders Company, 1987.

Schwartz, SI: *Principles of Surgery*. New York, McGraw-Hill Book Company, 1989.

Stillman, RM: *Surgery Diagnosis and Therapy*. East Norwalk, Appleton and Lange, 1989.

Tisher, CC, ed.: *Nephrology for the House Officer*. Baltimore, Williams & Wilkins, 1989.

Tomb, DA: *Psychiatry for the House Officer*. Baltimore, Williams & Wilkins, 1988.

Way, LW: *Current Surgical Diagnosis and Treatment*. Norwalk, Appleton and Lange, 1988.

The Most Common

Manifestations Of...

The Most Common
MANIFESTATIONS OF:

...AMNESIA, psychogenic:

localized amnesia (a total loss of memory for a circumscribed period of time during which a traumatic incident or experience is often found to have occurred). Less commonly there may be *generalized* amnesia (for the entire previous life, including loss of knowledge of personal identity and, rarely, even loss of ability to use language or understand the functions of common objects). Unusual forms of this disorder include *systematized* amnesia, in which the memory loss involves only specific, closely related events (e.g., and episode of violence) but memory is retained for unrelated events occurring at the same time, and *continuous* amnesia, in which current experiences are forgotten as they occur

...BACTEREMIA, gonococcal:

polyarthritis, dermatitis, and fever. Shock seldom occurs

...BACTERIAL MENINGITIS IN ADULTS:

the most common physical finding is a stiff neck, which is characterized by pain and resistance on flexion. Lethargy and drowsiness are common signs; confusion, agitated delirium, and stupor occur less frequently

...BREAST CANCER:

breast lump, then spontaneous nipple discharge. Other presenting manifestations include skin changes, axillary lymphadenopathy, or signs of locally advanced or disseminated disease.

...CENTRAL NERVOUS SYSTEM (CNS) INFECTION WITH VARICELLA:

181

The Most Common
MANIFESTATIONS OF:

acute cerebellar ataxia

...CONGENITAL RUBELLA:

deafness, cataracts, glaucoma, congenital heart disease, and mental retardation, but numerous other defects have been described. Some complications, such as a progressive encephalopathy, do not become apparent until the child is older

...CUSHING'S DISEASE:

Psychiatric manifestations:

an organic affective syndrome of agitated depression, with depressed but labile mood, loss of libido, insomnia, fatigue, irritability, anxiety, episodes of disturbed behavior, difficulty concentrating, and risk of suicide

...CUSHING'S SYNDROME:

hypertension, diabetes, hypokalemic alkalosis, osteoporosis, buffalo hump, truncal obesity, muscle weakness, peripheral muscle wasting, striae, easy bruisability, hirsutism, acne, menstrual irregularities, emotional lability

...CYSTIC FIBROSIS:

respiratory insufficiency due to abnormal mucous gland secretion in the airways, producing secondary infection, cough, dyspnea, bronchiectasis, and fibrosis; malabsorption due to pancreatic insufficiency and abnormal mucous gland secretions in the gastrointestinal tract, producing fatty stools, vitamin deficiencies, failure to gain weight, and retarded growth. Other manifestations and complications include electrolytes in sweat; respiratory complications (hemoptysis, pneumothorax, cor pulmonale); intestinal problems (meconium ileus, rectal prolapse, intussusception); repro-

182

ductive effects (sterility in men, thick spermicidal cervical mucus in women); focal biliary cirrhosis; pancreatic effects (abnormal glucose tolerance, type II diabetes); nasal effects (sinusitis, nasal polyposis); musculoskeletal effects

...DEFIBRINATION SYNDROME (Disseminated Intravascular Coagulation, DIC):

in the Surgical patient:

diffuse bleeding from many sites at surgery and from needle punctures

...DESQUAMATIVE INTERSTITIAL PNEUMONITIS (DIP):

dyspnea. Other symptoms include fatigue, anorexia, weight loss, cyanosis, and digital clubbing. Copious crackles are audible on auscultation, especially at lung bases

... DIC (Defibrination Syndrome, Disseminated Intravascular Coagulation):

in the Surgical patient:

diffuse bleeding from many sites at surgery and from needle punctures

...DISSEMINATED INTRAVASCULAR COAGULATION (Defibrination Syndrome, DIC):

in the Surgical patient:

diffuse bleeding from many sites at surgery and from needle punctures

...ENCEPHALITIS:

early signs and symptoms are nonspecific and typical of acute systemic illness, with fever, headache, vomiting, and upper respiratory symptoms. Neurologic signs and symptoms develop abruptly. Most commonly there is a decreased level of consciousness, which may range from confusion to deep coma. Seizures, paralysis, and abnormal reflexes are also com-

The Most Common
MANIFESTATIONS OF:

mon. Increased intracranial pressure can result in papilledema

Neurologic signs:

decreased level of consciousness, which may range from confusion to deep coma. Seizures, paralysis, and abnormal reflexes are also common. Increased intracranial pressure can result in papilledema

...ENDOGENOUS HYPERCORTISOLISM (CUSHING'S DISEASE):

Psychiatric manifestations:

an organic affective syndrome of agitated depression, with depressed but labile mood, loss of libido, insomnia, fatigue, irritability, anxiety, episodes of disturbed behavior, difficulty concentrating, and risk of suicide

...EWING'S SARCOMA:

pain that is followed by localized swelling

...FOOD POISONING:

Gastrointestinal:

diarrhea, nausea, vomiting, and abdominal pain

...GASTROINTESTINAL FOOD POISONING:

diarrhea, nausea, vomiting, and abdominal pain

...GLYCOSIDE TOXICITY:

Cardiac manifestations:

atrioventricular junctional rhythm, premature ventricular depolarizations, bigeminal rhythm, and second-degree atrioventricular blockade. However, it is claimed that digitalis can cause virtually every variety of arrhythmia

...HYPERCORTISOLISM, endogenous (CUSHING'S DISEASE):

Psychiatric manifestations:

184

The Most Common
MANIFESTATIONS OF:
an organic affective syndrome of agitated depression, with depressed but labile mood, loss of libido, insomnia, fatigue, irritability, anxiety, episodes of disturbed behavior, difficulty concentrating, and risk of suicide

...INFECTION by:

Chlamydia trachomatis:

in Infants:

inclusion conjunctivitis, pneumonia

Listeria monocytogenes:

in Neonates:

meningitis

...GIANT SACCULAR ANEURYSM ON THE INTERNAL CAROTID COMPLEX:

palsies of cranial nerves III, IV, and VI; seizures (due to compression of the medial aspect of the temporal lobe)

...INFECTIOUS PROCESS, ongoing:

fever

...LEAD NEUROTOXICITY in the adult:

a peripheral neuropathy, typically affecting the radial and peroneal nerves and resulting in wrist and foot drop, respectively

...MALIGNANT MASTOCYTOSIS:

Early manifestation of systemic disease:

urticaria pigmentosa

...MENINGITIS, bacterial:

in Adults: the most common physical finding is a stiff neck, which is characterized by pain and resistance on flexion. Lethargy and drowsiness are common signs; confusion, agitated delirium, and stupor occur less frequently

...PSYCHOGENIC AMNESIA:

localized amnesia (a total loss of memory for a circumscribed period of time during which a

The Most Common
MANIFESTATIONS OF:

traumatic incident or experience is often found to have occurred). Less commonly there may be *generalized* amnesia (for the entire previous life, including loss of knowledge of personal identity and, rarely, even loss of ability to use language or understand the functions of common objects). Unusual forms of this disorder include *systematized* amnesia, in which the memory loss involves only specific, closely related events (e.g., and episode of violence) but memory is retained for unrelated events occurring at the same time, and *continuous* amnesia, in which current experiences are forgotten as they occur

...RENAL TRAUMA:

in Children: hematuria. Other common symptoms are abdominal pain and tenderness, which may mimic an acute abdomen or renal colic. A flank mass may be present

...RUBELLA, congenital:

deafness, cataracts, glaucoma, congenital heart disease, and mental retardation, but numerous other defects have been described. Some complications, such as a progressive encephalopathy, do not become apparent until the child is older

...SHOCK: anuria

...SICKLE CELL NEPHROPATHY:

in Children: a renal concentrating and acidification defect. Microscopic or gross hematuria, the latter sometimes severe, may occur in children with sickle cell trait as well as in those with homozygous sickle cell disease

...SYSTEMIC LUPUS ERYTHEMATOSUS:

186

joint involvement (polyarthralgias)

Cardiac involvement:

pericarditis, although all layers of the heart may be involved

Renal manifestation:

glomerulonephritis. Occasionally an interstitial nephritis or (rarely) a vasculitis is associated with the disease

...TARDIVE DYSKINESIA:

repetitive sucking or smacking movements of the mouth or repetitive movements of the tongue. Loss commonly, affected persons exhibit choreiform movements of the limbs and athetoid twisting of the trunk

...TERTIARY SYPHILIS:

syphilitic cardiovascular disease

...TOXOCARIASIS:

in older Children and Adults:

granulomatous endophthalmitis causing unilateral squinting and loss of visual acuity

...TOXOPLASMOSIS:

in normal, otherwise Healthy individuals:

lymphadenopathy involving the cervical lymph nodes, although most cases of toxoplasmosis are asymptomatic. Others include pharyngitis, fever, rash, hepatomegaly, splenomegaly, and atypical lymphocytosis. Severe cases may develop meningoencephalitis, visceral involvement, pneumonitis, myocarditis, hepatitis and chorioretinitis

...TRAUMA, renal:

in Children: hematuria. Other common symptoms are abdominal pain and tenderness, which may mimic an acute abdomen or renal colic. A flank mass may be present

187

The Most Common
MANIFESTATIONS OF:
...TULAREMIA: Regional lymphadenitis
...ULCER DISEASE:
 duodenal ulcers, then gastric ulcers

References

Braunstein, H: *Outlines and Review of Pathology*. St. Louis, C.V. Mosby Company, 1987.

Casciato, DA, ed: *Manual of Clinical Oncology*, 2nd ed. Boston, Little, Brown and Company, 1988.

Creighton University Lecture Series, Pathology course, 1988-89.

Dworkin, PH: *Pediatrics* (The National Medical Series for Independent Study). New York, John Wiley & Sons, Inc., 1987.

Gregory, I: *Psychiatry*. Boston, Little, Brown and Company, Inc., 1983.

Jarrell, BE: *Surgery* (The National Medical Series for Independent Study). Media, Harwal Publishing Company, 1986.

Katzung, BG, ed.: *Basic and Clinical Pharmacology*, 3rd ed. Norwalk, Appleton & Lange, 1987.

Kingsbury, DT, ed.: *Microbiology* (The National Medical Series for Independent Study). Media, Harwal Publishing Company, 1985.

Myers, AR, ed.: *Medicine* (The National Medical Series for Independent Study). Media, Harwal Publishing Company, 1986.

Rubin, E, ed.: *Pathology*. Philadelphia, J.B. Lippincott Company, 1988.

Way, LW: *Current Surgical Diagnosis and Treatment*. Norwalk, Appleton and Lange, 1988.

Woods, SM, ed.: *Psychiatry*, 5th ed. (Pre-Test Series). New York, McGraw Hill Inc., 1989.

The Most Common

Neoplasms Of...

The Most Common
NEOPLASMS OF:

...ABDOMEN:

Abdominal wall:

Malignant:

sarcomas. They tend to arise in the deeper layers

in Children: common tumors include Wilms' tumor, neuroblastoma. Rare tumors include rhabdomyosarcoma, Hodgkin's disease and non-Hodgkin's lymphoma, hepatoblastoma and hepatocellular carcinoma, germ cell tumors, leukemic infiltration and metastases

Viscera:

Metastatic to:

regional lymph nodes, then the liver

...associated with ectopic ACTH PRODUCTION:

Malignant neoplasms: cancers of the lung, particularly small cell (oat cell) carcinoma. It also complicates carcinoid tumors, thymomas and neuroendocrine tumors, such as pheochromocytomas, neuroblastomas, and medullary carcinomas of the thyroid. Others: pancreatic and liver tumors

...AIDS PATIENTS:

Kaposi's sarcoma

...ANUS:

Malignant: squamous cell carcinoma (over 90%). The other tumor types each represent less than 2 percent

...APPENDIX: carcinoid

Malignant: carcinoid tumor, adenocarcinoma

...BILIARY TRACT:

Malignant: carcinoma of the gallbladder

...BLACK PERSONS:

The Most Common
NEOPLASMS OF:

Malignant:

    Lymphohematopoietic:

        plasma cell myeloma

    Sarcoma: fibrosarcoma

...BLADDER: urothelial tumors (transitional cell carcinomas) (>90%). Then squamous cell carcinomas (8%). Adenocarcinoma, sarcoma, lymphoma, and carcinoid tumors are rare

Malignant:

    Sarcoma: sarcoma botryoides

...BONE:

    Benign: exostoses (osteochondromas), followed by benign giant cell tumors

    Malignant: metastatic > primary

        Primary: osteosarcoma, followed by Ewing's sarcoma, chondrosarcoma, and malignant giant cell tumors. These four neoplasms together constitute the vast bulk of bone cancers (Rubin reports that chondrosarcoma is #2)

          in Pediatric patients:

            osteogenic sarcoma

    Metastatic from:

        tumors of the breast, prostate, lung, thyroid, and kidney

    Metastatic to:

    Ewing's sarcoma:

        the lung. Metastases to other bones or lymph nodes rarely develop. Central nervous system metastases, particularly meningeal, have been reported but are very rare

...BOTH SEXES:

    Malignant: lung cancer, skin cancer

...in which BRACHYTHERAPY IS USED:

    Malignant neoplasms:

        cancers of the oral cavity, oropharynx, uterine

192

The Most Common
NEOPLASMS OF:

cervix, and prostate

...BRAIN: primary (70-75%) > metastatic (25-30%)

Primary:

in Adults: Grade IV astrocytoma (most commonly Glioblastoma Multiforme) that arise in the hemispheres, meningioma

in Children:

Low grade (i.e., grades I and II) midline astrocytomas

by Category of tumor:

glioma (40-50%) [glioblastoma 25-30%], astrocytoma (8-12%), ependymoma (2-3%), oligodendroglioma (2-3%)]; meningioma (12-15%); acoustic nerve tumor (5-10%); medulloblastoma (2-3%)

by Individual tumor:

glioblastoma multiforme (an astrocytic glioma), meningioma, astrocytoma (a glioma), ependymoma (a glioma), Pituitary adenoma, Schwannoma, lymphoma, medulloblastoma (a glioma), oligodendroglioma (a glioma), papilloma of choroid (a glioma)

Metastatic from:

lung (bronchogenic carcinoma), breast carcinoma, kidney carcinoma, gastrointestinal carcinoma, melanocarcinoma, testicular carcinoma, choriocarcinoma

...BREAST:

Benign: fibroadenoma

Malignant: infiltrating ductal carcinoma

Men: ductal adenocarcinoma

Women: ductal adenocarcinoma (78%), lobular carcinoma (9%), comedocarcinoma (5%), medul-

The Most Common
NEOPLASMS OF:

lary carcinoma (4%), colloid carcinoma (3%), papillary carcinoma (rare), inflammatory carcinoma (1%), Paget's disease of the breast (always associated with ductal carcinoma in women)

Metastatic to (incidence):
bone (30-50%), liver (30-50%), lung (35%), skin, regional lymph nodes (supraclavicular and internal mammary lymphatics), brain (30% according to Casciato; least common site according to Stillman)

in Adolescents:
fibroadenoma

Tumors, Palpable (not necessarily neoplastic):
in Patients under 30 years of age:
fibroadenoma, papillomatosis, breast abscess, cystosarcoma phyllodes, and mesothelial neoplasms
in Patients over 30 years of age:
breast cysts, fibrocystic disease, breast cancer, breast abscess, fat necrosis, or cystosarcoma phyllodes

...CENTRAL NERVOUS SYSTEM (CNS):
Rubin reports that metastatic tumors are more common than primary; Casciato reports 60% of brain tumors are primary and that 40% are metastatic

Primary:
Adults: astrocytoma (62%) [astrocytoma:G3-4 - glioblastoma multiforme = 50%, astrocytoma: G1-2 = 12%]; meningioma (15%); acoustic schwannoma (10%); oligodendroglioma (4%); medulloblastoma (2%); and rarely histiocytic lymphoma, pinealoma, and jugular body paraganglioma

194

Children: astrocytoma (spongioblastoma) (30%), brain-stem glioma (20%), medulloblastoma (20%), ependymoma (9%), craniopharyngioma (3%)

...CERVIX: 95% of cervical cancers are squamous cell carcinomas; most of the remainder are adeno-carcinomas

Malignant: squamous cell carcinoma (~80%), adenocar-cinoma (18%), sarcoma (2%)

Metastatic to: once invasive cancer is established, the tumor spreads primarily by local extension into other pelvic structures and sequentially along lymph node chains. Uncommonly, patients with lo-cally advanced tumors may have evidence of blood-borne metastases, most often to the lung, liver, or bone

Invasive: squamous carcinoma, adenocarcinoma. Rare-ly small cell carcinoma, verrucous carcinoma, sarcoma, and lymphoma

...CHEST WALL:

Benign: chondroma. It occurs at the costochondral junction

...CHILDHOOD: hematologic malignancies - acute lymphocytic leukemia (ALL); CNS tumors. Carcinomas are exceedingly rare in children

Malignant: leukemia > CNS tumors > Hodgkin's disease and lymphoma > soft tissue sarcomas > neuro-blastoma > Wilms' tumor > bone tumors > re-tinoblastoma

Acute leukemia: lymphoblastic (acute lymphoblastic leukemia [ALL]) (70%), myelocytic or monocytic (15%), and the remainder are undifferentiated

Ages 5 to 9 years: acute leukemia

Ages > 9 years:

The Most Common
NEOPLASMS OF:
soft tissue and bone tumors

Brain tumor:
    Malignant:
          medulloblastoma

Epithelial origin:
    Malignant:
          liver tumors

Liver: hepatoblastoma
Solid tumors: brain tumors, neuroblastoma

...COLON:
    Benign: epithelial polyps (many [perhaps up to 90%] are non-neoplastic and are referred to as hyperplastic polyps. However, some are true neoplasms and are called "adenomatous polyps.")

    Malignant: adenocarcinomas
    Adult: adenomatous polyps

...COLON AND RECTUM:
    Primary:
        Malignant:
          adenocarcinoma (98%). Lymphomas and soft tissue sarcomas are rare

    Metastatic to: Regional lymph nodes, liver (70%), lung (25-40%), and bone (5-10%), followed by many other sites including the serosal membrane of the peritoneal cavity, brain (1%), and others

...CNS (Central Nervous System):
          metastatic
    Adults: astrocytoma (62%) [astrocytoma:G3-4 - glioblastoma multiforme = 50%, astrocytoma: G1-2 = 12%]; meningioma (15%); acoustic schwannoma (10%); oligodendroglioma (4%); medulloblastoma (2%); and rarely histiocytic

lymphoma, pinealoma, and jugular body paraganglioma

Children: astrocytoma (spongioblastoma) (30%), brain-
stem glioma (20%), medulloblastoma(20%),

ependymoma (9%), craniopharyngioma(3%)

...DUODENUM:
  Malignant (rare):

adenocarcinomas

...ENDOMETRIUM:
  Malignant:

adenocarcinoma

...EPIDIDYMIS: adenomatoid tumor

...ESOPHAGUS:
  Benign: leiomyoma, but fibromas, lipomas, hemangiomas, neurofibromas, lymphangiomas, and
squamous papillomas may also arise in this location

  Malignant: with rare exceptions, malignant lesions of the
esophagus are squamous cell carcinomas
(could be up to 98%). The remainder are
adenocarcinomas (could be up to 5-10%), undifferentiated carcinomas (could be up to 5-
10%). Sarcomas (leiomyosarcoma and fibrosarcoma) and melanocarcinoma are so rare as
to be medical curiosities. Small cell cancers
and lymphomas are also rare

  Carcinoma:

squamous cell carcinoma, adenocarcinoma,
mucoepidermoid carcinoma, and adenocystic
carcinoma

  Metastatic to: the liver and lungs (visceral metastases); direct spread is to the larynx, trachea, thyroid
glands, recurrent laryngeal nerves, and pericardium

The Most Common
NEOPLASMS OF:

...FATAL, IN MEN AND WOMEN:
> cancer of the lung

...FEMALES: lung, breast, colon and rectum, uterus, leukemia and lymphoma, ovary, urinary, pancreas, skin, oral

Malignant: lung, breast, colon and rectum (Rubin reports the incidence of lung cancer overtaking that of breast cancer in women). (Stillman reports that skin cancer is #1 and breast cancer is #2)

which causes Death:
(years of Age):
Less than 15:
> leukemia, CNS, connective tissue, bone, kidney

15-34: breast, leukemia, uterus, CNS, Hodgkin's
35-54: breast, lung, bowel, ovary, uterus
55-74: lung, breast, bowel, ovary, pancreas
More than 75:
> bowel, breast, lung, pancreas, uterus

All ages: lung, breast, bowel (colon), ovary, pancreas
(1988 data: lung ↑ to #1 in women)

...in which FEVER OCCURS:
Malignant: Hodgkin's disease, renal cell carcinoma, and osteogenic sarcoma, although many other tumors occasionally are complicated by fever

...associated with FEVER OF UNKNOWN ORIGIN:
Malignant: lymphoproliferative neoplasms and obscure adenocarcinomas (biliary tree, pancreas, kidney) are the most common types of malignant disease associated with fever of unknown cause

...THE FIRST YEAR OF LIFE:
> mesoblastic nephroma; others rare.

...THE GASTROINTESTINAL TRACT:

198

which causes Death:

    colon carcinoma, adenocarcinoma of the pancreas

...GENITAL TRACT, females:

Malignant: endometrial carcinoma OR cervical carcinoma, cancer of the uterine corpus

...GENITOURINARY TRACT:

Malignant: #1 not available. Vesical neoplasms are the second most common cancer of the genitourinary tract

in Infancy:

    Malignant:

        sarcoma botryoides

...GERM CELLS:

in Children: sacrococcygeal germ cell tumors

Females:

    Benign: teratoma

    Malignant:

        dysgerminoma

which secrete GONADOTROPINS:

    germ cell tumors, gestational trophoblastic tumors (choriocarcinoma, hydatidiform mole) and pituitary tumors. Less commonly, gonadotropin secretion is observed with hepatoblastomas in children and cancers of the lung, colon, breast, and pancreas in adults.

...HEAD AND NECK:

    squamous cell carcinoma

Malignant: the great majority of malignant neoplasms of the mucosa of the head and neck are squamous cell carcinomas of various degrees of differentiation

Metastatic to: regional lymph nodes

Hypopharynx:

    Nodal metastases:

The Most Common
NEOPLASMS OF:

the upper, mid, and lower jugular chain nodes; the retropharyngeal nodes of Rouviere; and, less frequently, the nodes along the spinal accessory nerve in the posterior triangle

...HEART: benign (75-80%) > malignant (20-25%); benign myxoma is the most common lesion

Primary: myxoma

Benign: myxoma (75-80%). Others include rhabdomyomas (Purkinje hamartoma; most common in childhood), papillary tumor of heart valve (Lambl excrescence), fibromas, lipomas, and teratomas

Malignant:
predominantly cardiac sarcomas: rhabdomyosarcoma and angiosarcoma are most common. Others are fibrosarcoma, liposarcoma, neurosarcoma, leiomyosarcoma, teratoma, mesothelioma, lymphoma, and other even greater rarities

Metastatic from:
carcinoma (67%; lung, breast), sarcoma (20%), and melanoma (12%), according to Way. Jarrell lists melanoma, lymphoma, and leukemia as the tumors which most often metastasize to the heart

...associated with HYPERCALCEMIA FROM BONY INVOLVEMENT:

Malignant neoplasms:
breast and multiple myeloma

...associated with HYPERCALCEMIA WITHOUT METASTASES TO BONE:

Malignant neoplasms:
lung cancer

...HYPOPHARYNX:

Malignant: squamous carcinoma (>95%)

200

The Most Common
NEOPLASMS OF:

Metastatic to:
>Nodal metastases:
>>the upper, mid, and lower jugular chain nodes; the retropharyngeal nodes of Rouviere; and, less frequently, the nodes along the spinal accessory nerve in the posterior triangle

...HYPOTHALAMIC-PITUITARY AREA:
>in Children: craniopharyngiomas

...associated with INAPPROPRIATE PRODUCTION OF ADH (ANTI-DIURETIC HORMONE):
>Malignant neoplasms:
>>small cell carcinomas of the lung. Also reported with carcinomas of the prostate, gastrointestinal tract, and pancreas, thymomas, lymphomas, and Hodgkin's disease

...INFANCY AND EARLY CHILDHOOD:
>lymphoblastic leukemia, neuroblastoma, nephroblastoma (Wilms' tumor), hepatoblastoma, retinoblastoma, rhabdomyosarcoma, teratoma, and ependymoma

...INFANTS AND CHILDREN UNDER 5 YEARS OF AGE:
>embryomas or blastomas. These include the eight most common tumors of infancy and early childhood: lymphoblastic leukemia, neuroblastoma, nephroblastoma (Wilms' tumor), hepatoblastoma, retinoblastoma, rhabdomyosarcoma, teratoma, and ependymoma

...causing INTESTINAL OBSTRUCTION:
>adenocarcinoma of the colon or rectum. Other malignant tumors include carcinoid or lymphoma

...INTRACRANIAL, NEUROBLASTIC:
>medulloblastoma

The Most Common
NEOPLASMS OF:
...KIDNEY:

Benign: renal adenoma

    Parenchyma, solid tumor:
        renal adenoma

Malignant: renal adenocarcinoma (aka: renal cell carcinoma, clear cell carcinoma, Grawitz's tumor, or hypernephroma)

    Sarcomas:
        leiomyosarcoma is the most common. Others include rhabdomyosarcoma, liposarcoma, and fibrosarcoma, although all are very infrequent neoplasms

Metastatic from:
        lung, stomach and breast

Metastatic to:
    (Renal Adenocarcinoma, Renal Cell Carcinoma):
        lungs (30%), adjacent renal hilar lymph nodes (25%), ipsilateral adrenal (12%), opposite kidney (2%), and bones (mainly long bones)

    (by incidence):
        lung (50-75%), bone (30-50%), liver (35-40%), brain (5-10%)

in Childhood: Wilms' tumor

    Malignant:
        Wilm's tumor (nephroblastoma)

    Age < 1 month:
        congenital mesoblastic nephroma

Collecting system of the kidney:
        over 90% of these tumors are urothelial transitional cell carcinomas. Less than 5% of tumors in this location are squamous carcinomas (often associated with chronic inflammation and stone formation) or adenocarcinomas

Renal pelvis:

The Most Common
NEOPLASMS OF:

transitional cell carcinoma (90%)

...KIDNEY TRANSPLANT PATIENTS:

transplant patients have an increased risk of malignancy from immunosuppressive drugs. The most common are squamous and basal cell skin cancers. Cancers of the gastrointestinal (GI) tract are also common, particularly colon and stomach, and there is an increased risk of genitourinary malignancy

...LARGE INTESTINE:

Benign:	epithelial polyps (many [perhaps up to 90%] are non-neoplastic and are referred to as hyperplastic polyps. However, some are true neoplasms and are called "adenomatous polyps.")
Malignant:	adenocarcinomas
Adult:	adenomatous polyps

...LARYNX:

Malignant:	squamous cell carcinoma

...LIVER: metastatic > primary

Benign:	hemangioma, hepatocellular adenoma, focal nodular hyperplasia

Malignant, primary:

hepatocellular carcinoma (parenchymal cells) (70-90%), cholangiocarcinoma (hepatic bile ducts) (10-30%), hemangiosarcoma (Kupffer cells or sinus lining cells) (rare), mixed forms (rare)

Metastatic to (incidence):

(Hepatocellular Carcinoma):

lung (20%), bone (10%)

in Children:	hepatoblastoma
in Men:	malignant
in Women:	benign

203

The Most Common
NEOPLASMS OF:

...LUNG: metastatic
   Benign: hamartomas (mixed tumors) (8% coin le-
              sions). Other types are rare and include fi-
              brous mesotheliomas, xanthomatous and in-
              flammatory pseudotumors, benign granular
              cell myoblastomas, and miscellaneous rare le-
              sions of epithelial origin (papilloma, polyps,
              etc.), of mesodermal origin (hemangioma, ar-
              teriovenous fistulas, lipomas), and unknown
              origin (granuloma, plasma cell tumor)
   Malignant: Sources vary somewhat. The following are
              histologic types and ranges (with authors cit-
              ed): Braunwald (Harrison's) indicates that the
              most common histologic type found in males
              is epidermoid cancer (squamous cell), while
              adenocarcinoma is the most common type
              found in females. The histologic incidence is
              reported as epidermoid (squamous cell carci-
              noma) (33%), adenocarcinoma (25%), small
              cell carcinoma (25%), large cell carcinoma
              (16%), bronchoalveolar carcinoma (a variant
              of adenocarcinoma; 3%). Braunstein reports
              similar incidence ranges, but reports squa-
              mous cell as one half of lung cancers. Cascia-
              to lists essentially similar ranges. Jarrell dif-
              fers by reporting adenocarcinoma as the most
              common lung carcinoma (30-50%) and squa-
              mous cell carcinoma second (25-40%), with
              similar ranges for remaining tumors. Schrock
              may clarify everything by citing that epider-
              moid (squamous cell) carcinomas comprise
              25-35%, and adenocarcinomas *once account-
              ed for* 15% of all lung cancers but recent epi-
              demiologic data suggest this is changing dra-

matically, with recent reports showing that up to 46% of lung cancers are adenocarcinomas. Others tumors include mixed histology (20%) (adenosquamous is the most frequent), and uncommonly bronchial carcinoids, cystic adenoid carcinomas, carcinosarcomas, and mesotheliomas. Also giant cell (anaplastic) carcinoma and bronchoalveolar carcinoma (both rare)

in Men: epidermoid cancer (squamous cell carcinoma)
in Women:
    adenocarcinoma

Metastatic from:
    colon, kidneys, uterus and ovaries, testes, malignant melanoma, pharynx, and bone

Metastatic to (% are incidences):
    lung cancer commonly metastasizes to the cervical and abdominal lymph nodes, bone (30-50%), liver (30-50%), lung (35%), adrenal glands, kidneys, brain (15-30%). The exact sequence of metastases differs somewhat with different pathologic types, but the patterns are the same

Adenocarcinoma: (by frequency)
    liver (45%), mediastinal lymph nodes(40%), bone(40%), brain (30%)

Large Cell: (by frequency)
    bone (40%), mediastinal lymph nodes (40%), liver (30%), brain (30%)

Small cell: (by frequency)
    mediastinal lymph nodes (95%), liver (50%), brain (40%), bone (35%), bone marrow (30%)

Squamous: (by frequency)
    mediastinal lymph nodes (30%), liver (30%), bone (25%), brain (20%), bone marrow (5%)

The Most Common
NEOPLASMS OF:
Calcified lesions:

> lesions that are completely or heavily calcified are most likely benign. Malignant lesions with calcifications are most often squamous cell carcinomas. Adenocarcinomas are next most common. Calcification in malignant lesions generally consists of small flecks located eccentrically or at the periphery of the nodule

...LYMPHATIC SYSTEM:

> metastatic tumor

Benign: cystic hygroma

...MALES: lung, prostate, colon and rectum, urinary (renal and bladder cancer ~9%), leukemia and lymphoma, oral, skin, pancreas

Malignant: lung cancer, colorectal cancer

    in 1930:   stomach cancer

    Ages 20 to 40 years:

> testicular cancer

which cause Death:

(years of Age):

Less than 15:

> leukemia, CNS, lymphoma, connective tissue, bone

15-34:   leukemia, CNS, lymphoma, skin, Hodgkin's

33-54:   lung, bowel, CNS, pancreatic adenocarcinoma, leukemia

55-74:   lung, bowel, prostate, pancreas, stomach

More than 75:

> lung, prostate, bowel, pancreas, bladder

All ages: lung, colorectal, prostate, pancreas, leukemia

Over 50 years of age:

Malignant:

> lung, prostatic carcinoma

...MEDIASTINUM:

The Most Common
NEOPLASMS OF:

benign (75%) > malignant

Anterior mediastinum:
> thymoma

Germ cell neoplasm (very rare - less than 1% of all mediastinal tumors):

   Malignant:
> seminoma

Middle mediastinum:
> middle mediastinal lesions are usually cystic in nature. The two most common are pericardial cysts and bronchogenic cysts

Posterior mediastinum:
> posterior mediastinal lesions are neurogenic tumors located in the paravertebral gutter. About 10-20% are malignant. Seventy-five percent of these neurogenic tumors occur in children under 4 years of age. Malignancy is most likely to occur if the tumor arises in childhood

Teratoma: benign (80%) > malignant

...MEN: lung, prostate, colon and rectum, urinary (renal and bladder cancer ~9%), leukemia and lymphoma, oral, skin, pancreas

Malignant: lung cancer, colorectal cancer

  in 1930: stomach cancer

  Ages 20 to 40 years:
> testicular cancer

which cause Death:

  (years of Age):

  Less than 15:
> leukemia, CNS, lymphoma, connective tissue, bone

  15-34: leukemia, CNS, lymphoma, skin, Hodgkin's

  33-54: lung, bowel, CNS, pancreatic adenocarcino-

The Most Common
NEOPLASMS OF:

ma, leukemia

    55-74:   lung, bowel, prostate, pancreas, stomach

    More than 75:

        lung, prostate, bowel, pancreas, bladder

    All ages: lung, colorectal, prostate, pancreas, leukemia

Over 50 years of age:

    Malignant:

        lung, prostatic carcinoma

...MINOR SALIVARY GLANDS:

    Malignant: adenoid cystic carcinoma, followed by adeno-carcinoma and mucoepidermoid carcinoma

...NASAL CAVITY AND PARANASAL SINUSES:

        squamous cell carcinoma. Adenocarcinoma, sarcoma, melanoma, lymphoma and minor salivary gland tumors also occur. Esthesio-neuroblastoma is an uncommon malignant neoplasm that arises from olfactory mucosa at the superior aspect of the nasal cavity

    Malignant: squamous cell carcinoma. Others are adenoid cystic and mucoepidermoid carcinomas, malignant mixed tumors, adenocarcinomas, lymphomas, fibrosarcomas, osteosarcomas, chondrosarcomas, and melanomas. Esthesioneuroblastoma is an uncommon malignant neoplasm that arises from olfactory mucosa at the superior aspect of the nasal cavity

    Metastatic from:

        hypernephroma

...NEUROBLASTOMA:

    Metastatic to: bone, bone marrow, liver, skin, and lymph nodes

...NEWBORNS:

    Solid tumor: sacrococcygeal germ cell tumors

...ORAL MUCOSA:

208

The Most Common
NEOPLASMS OF:

Malignant:

squamous cell carcinoma (>95%). Others include adenocarcinoma, melanoma, and sarcomas

...OROPHARYNX:

squamous carcinoma

...OVARY:

benign (80%) > malignant. Benign dermoid cyst (benign cystic teratoma) is the most common <u>type</u> of ovarian neoplasm (this is of germ cell origin). Epithelial tumors are by far the most common tumors of the ovaries, comprising approximately 60-75% of ovarian neoplasms (serous epithelial tumors - 20-50%, mucinous epithelial tumors - 15-20%, Brenner tumors are uncommon - ≤ 2% of ovarian neoplasms). Others include germ cell tumors (15-20%), sex cord (gonadal) - stromal (5-10%) (granulosa-theca cell tumors - 5% of all ovarian tumors, fibromas arising in the ovarian stroma - 5% of all types), and metastatic (5-10%)

Benign:

benign dermoid cyst (benign cystic teratoma) is the most common <u>type</u> of ovarian neoplasm (this is of germ cell origin)

Malignant

serous cystadenocarcinoma (≥ 65% of all ovarian cancers), endometrioid carcinoma (10-25%), mucinous cystadenocarcinoma (~15%); all of these are <u>epithelial</u> tumors). Epithelial tumors account for 95% of malignant ovarian tumors: Serous cystadenocarcinoma is the most common of these (40-65% or more of all ovarian cancers); endometrioid tumors - 20% of all ovarian cancers; mucinous cystadenocarcinomas - 5-10% of all ovarian

The Most Common
NEOPLASMS OF:

cancers; clear cell adenocarcinoma is uncommon. Sex cord (Gonadal) - Stromal tumors account for 2% of malignant ovarian tumors. Germ cell tumors account for 1%: Dysgerminoma accounts for ~2% of all ovarian cancers; endodermal sinus (yolk sac) tumor is the second most frequent cancer of germ cell origin

Metastatic from:

stomach (Krunkenberg's tumor), gastrointestinal tract (colon, biliary tract, and pancreas), breast, and genital tract

Metastatic to: (incidence)

liver (10-15%), lung (10%), bone (2-5%), brain (1%)

Epithelial:

serous (20-50% of ovarian tumors), mucinous (15-20% of all ovarian tumors), endometrioid (10-25% of all primary ovarian adenocarcinomas), clear cell carcinomas (5-11% of primary ovarian tumors), Brenner tumors (1.7% of all ovarian neoplasms), mixed mesodermal tumors (rare)

Mucinous:

mucinous cystadenocarcinomas represent about 10% of mucinous tumors

Serous:

serous cystadenocarcinomas ≥ 65%, benign serous cystadenomas - 20%, borderline serous tumors (carcinomas of low malignant potential) - 9-15%

Germ Cell origin:

benign cystic teratoma (95%)

Benign: benign cystic teratoma (95%)

Malignant:

dysgerminoma accounts for 50% of these (and 2% of all ovarian neoplasms), endodermal sinus (yolk sac) tumor - 20%. Choriocarcinoma may arise in the ovary from the teratogenous development of germ cells, but is rare. Others (rare) include embryonal carcinoma; polyembryoma; and mixed germ cell tumors containing various combinations of dysgerminoma, teratoma, endodermal sinus tumor, and choriocarcinoma

seen during Pregnancy:

Cystic: benign cystic teratomas (about 40% are of this variety), serous and mucinous cystadenomas, and endometrial cysts

Solid tumor:

dysgerminoma

...PANCREAS:

Malignant: duct cell adenocarcinoma (75%), giant cell carcinoma (5%), cystadenocarcinoma (5%), colloid carcinoma or mucinous adenocarcinoma (2%). Other tumor types include acinar cell carcinoma, adenosquamous cancer (adenoacanthoma), pancreaticoblastoma, papillary cystic carcinoma, anaplastic carcinoma, carcinoids, microadenocarcinoma (resembles carcinoid tumors: widespread metastases occur early), lymphomas, and sarcomas, nonfunctional islet cell tumors, and peptide-producing tumors such as insulinomas and Zollinger-Ellison tumors

Metastatic to: liver (50-70%), lung (25-40%), bone (5-10%), brain (1-5%)

...PARAPHARYNGEAL SPACE:

retromandibular parotid tumors, neurogenic tumors (e.g., neurilemmoma, neurofibroma), or carotid body tumors

The Most Common
NEOPLASMS OF:

...PAROTID GLAND:

    Malignant: mucoepidermoid carcinoma.

...PENIS:

    Malignant: squamous cell carcinoma, usually well differentiated, constitutes nearly all penile cancers (over 95%). Rare penile cancers include melanoma, sarcomas, and metastatic tumor

    Metastatic to: tumor disseminates through the lymphatic system and the blood to distant organs, most often to the lungs, and less frequently to bone and other sites

...PEOPLE WITH GONADOTROPIC SYNDROMES:

    germ cell tumors, gestational trophoblastic tumors (choriocarcinoma, hydatidiform mole) and pituitary tumors. Less commonly, gonadotropin secretion is observed with hepatoblastomas in children and cancers of the lung, colon, breast, and pancreas in adults.

...PEOPLE WITH INAPPROPRIATE ADH SECRETION:

    small cell carcinomas of the lung. Also reported with carcinomas of the prostate, gastrointestinal tract, and pancreas, thymomas, lymphomas, and Hodgkin's disease

...PEOPLE WITH PARANEOPLASTIC ENDOCARDITIS:

    solid tumors. This condition may occasionally be seen with leukemias and lymphomas

...PEOPLE WITH PLEURAL EFFUSION CAUSED BY MALIGNANT DISEASE:

    Primary neoplasms:

        in Men: lung

        in Women:

            breast

...PERICARDIUM:

    Metastatic from:

212

pulmonary and breast carcinoma

...PERIPHERAL NERVOUS SYSTEM:

Primary:

Nerve sheath origin:

schwannoma, neurofibroma

Neuronal origin:

adrenal medulla, sympathetic ganglion

...PERITONEUM: metastatic lesions

Metastatic from:

adenocarcinoma of the gastrointestinal tract, pancreas, or ovary. However, sarcomas, lymphomas, leukemias, and carcinoid tumors all may involve the peritoneum

...PHEOCHROMOCYTOMA:

benign (90%) > malignant (10%) when the pheochromocytoma is of adrenal origin. Malignant lesions with metastases occur more frequently (46%) when the primary lesion is extraadrenal

...PINEAL GLAND:

dysgerminoma, although gliomas, choriocarcinoma, and melanomas also occur

...PITUITARY:

according to Straub, although nonsecreting pituitary adenomas are probably the most commonly occurring pituitary tumors, they usually remain undetected during life, and prolactin-hormone (PH)-secreting adenomas are the most common clinically detected pituitary tumors

Adenoma:

Hypersecretory:

prolactin-secreting adenoma and growth hor-

The Most Common
NEOPLASMS OF:

mone-secreting adenoma

...PLACENTA

Benign: chorioangioma

...PROSTATE: adenocarcinomas (95%)

Malignant: adenocarcinoma (almost all). Sarcomas and transitional, small, and squamous cell carcinomas are rare

Metastatic to (incidence):
bone (50-75%), lung (15-50%), liver (15%). Metastases to the brain (2%), and other soft tissues are rare

...RETROPERITONEUM:
malignant (85%) (if renal tumors are excluded). Approximately one sixth of cases are Hodgkin's disease and one sixth are non-Hodgkin's lymphoma. Sarcomas often appear in the retroperitoneum, particularly rhabdomyosarcoma (in children), leiomyosarcoma, and liposarcoma. Germ cell tumors, adenocarcinomas, and rare neuroblastomas account for most of the remainder of cases. Carcinomas of the breast, lung, and gastrointestinal tract can metastasize to retroperitoneal structures by way of the bloodstream or the spinal venous plexus

...SALIVARY GLANDS:

Benign: the mixed salivary gland tumor, or pleomorphic adenoma (70% of parotid tumors and 50% of all salivary gland tumors). Warthin's tumor (papillary cystadenoma lymphomatosum) (5% of parotid neoplasms), oncocytomas, monomorphic adenomas (rare)

Malignant: mucoepidermoid carcinoma, acinic cell carcinoma, adenoid cystic carcinoma. Less com-

The Most Common
NEOPLASMS OF:

mon tumors include carcinoma arising in a pleomorphic adenoma and primary squamous cell carcinoma (1% of salivary cancers)

Minor glands:
  adenoid cystic carcinoma, followed by adenocarcinoma and mucoepidermoid carcinoma

...SCROTUM: skin squamous cell carcinoma, occasionally basal cell carcinoma

...SKIN: basal cell carcinoma
  Malignant: basal cell carcinoma, squamous cell carcinoma

  Anal: squamous cell cancer

...SMALL INTESTINE:
  benign > malignant

  Benign: polyps. Others include lipomas, leiomyomas, hemangiomas, fibromas, and neurofibromas

  Malignant: adenocarcinoma (rare in the small bowel), carcinoid, lymphoma, sarcoma, and metastases from distant malignancies

  Sarcoma: Leiomyosarcoma
  Symptomatic tumors:
    benign > malignant

...SOFT TISSUE:

  Sarcoma: liposarcoma, fibrosarcoma
    in the Pediatric age group:
      rhabdomyosarcoma

...SPINAL CORD, intramedullary:
  astrocytoma (cervico-thoracic), ependymoma (lumbosacral)

...STOMACH: malignant (benign are uncommon)
  Benign: leiomyomas and polyps are the two most common. Others include fibromas, neurofibromas, aberrant pancreas, and angiomas
  Malignant: adenocarcinoma (~95%). 5% are lymphomas

215

The Most Common
NEOPLASMS OF:

(3%) or leiomyosarcomas (2%). Carcinoids, squamous cancers, and other types rarely occur

Lymphoma:
diffuse histiocytic lymphoma (aka: follicular center, large, noncleaved type)

Sarcoma: leiomyosarcoma, fibrosarcoma, and endothelial sarcoma

Metastatic from:
generalized lymphomatosis and leukemia

Metastatic to (incidence):
liver (35-50%), lung (20-30%), bone (5-10%), brain (1-5%)

...TESTICLE: malignant tumors of germ cell origin: seminomatous (35%) or nonseminomatous (teratocarcinoma - 38%, embryonal carcinoma - 20%, teratoma - 5%, rarely choriocarcinoma - 2%). Non-germ cell tumors such as Sertoli cell tumors and Leydig cell tumors are rare and usually benign

Malignant:
Age over 60 years:
lymphomas

in Young males:
germ cell cancers (seminoma, embryonal cell, teratoma, and others). Other types, which account for less than 5 percent of cases, include rhabdomyosarcoma, lymphoma, and melanoma. Rarely, Sertoli cell tumor, interstitial cell tumor, or other mesodermal tumors develop

Metastatic from:
prostatic carcinoma, lung cancer, melanoma, or leukemia

in Infancy: yolk sac tumor (entodermal sinus tumor)

...associated with THROMBOPHLEBITIS:

216

Malignant neoplasms:

    carcinoma of the lung, pancreas, and gastrointestinal tract. Tumors of the breast, ovary, prostate, and other organs may also lead to this complication

...THYMUS: two-thirds of thymic tumors are considered to be benign, and of these, 10% are simple cysts

...THYROID:

Malignant: papillary carcinoma (60-85%), follicular cancer (10-20%), anaplastic giant and spindle cell cancers (10-15%), medullary thyroid cancers (3-7%). Hurthle cell cancer is an uncommon tumor. Other tumors found in the thyroid include Hodgkin's disease, lymphomas, a variety of soft tissue sarcomas, and metastatic cancers of lung, colon, and other primary sites. Undifferentiated carcinomas (3%) include small cell (rare), giant cell, spindle cell, and squamous cell types

Metastatic from:

    hypernephroma (in one series); bronchogenic carcinomas account for 20 percent of secondary thyroid metastases (both entries from Schwartz)

Metastatic to: lung (65%), liver (60%), bone (40%), brain (1%)

Carcinoma: papillary carcinoma is most common (75%). Follicular carcinoma represents 15 to 30 percent of cases. Anaplastic and medullary carcinomas comprise the remaining small percentage

Follicular carcinoma:

Metastatic to:

    lung and bone

Radiation-induced:

The Most Common
NEOPLASMS OF:

papillary carcinoma

...TRACHEA:
Primary: Primary neoplasms of the trachea are rare. The most common is squamous cell carcinoma. Adenocystic carcinoma also affects the trachea. Other primary tracheal neoplasms include carcinosarcomas, pseudosarcomas, mucoepidermoid carcinomas, squamous papillomas, chondromas, and chondrosarcomas

Secondary: these are usually from the lung, the esophagus, or the thyroid gland

...URETER: more than 90% of ureteral tumors are urothelial transitional cell carcinomas

...URETHRA:
Malignant: squamous cell carcinoma, usually arising from the stratified squamous epithelium of the proximal (bulbous) urethra or distal (penile) urethra (80%); transitional cell carcinoma arising in the prostatic urethra (15%). Adenocarcinomas possible arise from Cowper's glands

...UROLOGIC SYSTEM:
Malignant: not available. Renal adenocarcinoma (aka: renal cell carcinoma, clear cell carcinoma, Grawitz's tumor, or hypernephroma) is the third most common

...UTERUS: leiomyoma
Benign: leiomyoma
Malignant: endometrial adenocarcinoma (~70%), adenocanthoma (20%), adenosquamous carcinoma (10%). A small percentage are clear cell, small cell, or squamous carcinomas and sarcomas

Metastatic to: Endometrial cancer spreads by direct extension. Hematogenous spread is an uncommon late finding in adenocarcinoma but occurs early in sarcoma. The lungs are the most frequent site of distant metastatic involvement

...VAGINA:

malignant (squamous cell carcinoma)

Malignant: squamous carcinoma (~85%), and the remainder are adenocarcinomas, melanomas and sarcomas

Secondary: extension of cervical cancer

...VISCERA:

Malignant: ovary #4, pancreas #9

in early Childhood:

neuroblastoma, then Wilms' tumor (nephroblastoma)

...VULVA:

Malignant: squamous cell carcinoma (>85%), melanoma (5-10%). Adenocarcinoma, sarcoma, basal cell carcinoma, and other tumors constitute the remainder

...WOMEN: lung, breast, colon and rectum, uterus, leukemia and lymphoma, ovary, urinary, pancreas, skin, oral

Malignant: lung, breast, colon and rectum (Rubin reports the incidence of lung cancer overtaking that of breast cancer in women). (Stillman reports that skin cancer is #1 and breast cancer is #2)

which causes Death:

(years of Age):

Less than 15:

leukemia, CNS, connective tissue, bone, kidney

15-34: breast, leukemia, uterus, CNS, Hodgkin's

35-54: breast, lung, bowel, ovary, uterus

55-74: lung, breast, bowel, ovary, pancreas

More than 75:

The Most Common
NEOPLASMS OF:
bowel, breast, lung, pancreas, uterus
All ages: lung, breast, bowel (colon), ovary, pancreas
(1988 data: lung ↑ to #1 in women)

References

Beck, WW: *Obstetrics and Gynecology*. (The National Medical Series for Independent Study). New York, John Wiley & Sons, Inc., 1989.

Benson, RC: *Handbook of Obstetrics and Gynecology*. Los Altos, Lange Medical Publications, 1983.

Braunstein, H: *Outlines and Review of Pathology*. St. Louis, C.V. Mosby Company, 1987.

Braunwald, E, ed: *Harrison's Principles of Internal Medicine*, 11th ed.. New York, McGraw-Hill Book Company, 1987.

Casciato, DA, ed: *Manual of Clinical Oncology*, 2nd ed. Boston, Little, Brown and Company, 1988.

Chandrasoma, P: *Key Facts in Pathology*. New York, Churchill Livingstone, Inc., 1986.

Creighton University Lecture Series, Introduction to Clinical Medicine course, Pathology course, 1988-89.

Dworkin, PH: *Pediatrics* (The National Medical Series for Independent Study). New York, John Wiley & Sons, Inc., 1987.

Jarrell, BE: *Surgery* (The National Medical Series for Independent Study). Media, Harwal Publishing Company, 1986.

LiVolsi, VA, ed: *Pathology* (The National Medical Series for Independent Study). Media, Harwal Publishing Company, 1984.

The Merck Manual of Diagnosis and Therapy. Rahway, Merck Sharp & Dohme Research Laboratories, 1987.

Myers, AR, ed.: *Medicine* (The National Medical Series for Inde-

220

pendent Study). Media, Harwal Publishing Company, 1986.

Robbins, SL: *Pathologic Basis of Disease.* Philadelphia, W.B. Saunders Company, 1984.

Rubin, E, ed.: *Pathology.* Philadelphia, J.B. Lippincott Company, 1988.

Sabiston, DC: *Sabiston's Essentials of Surgery.* Philadelphia, W.B. Saunders Company, 1987.

Schrock, TR: *Handbook of Surgery.* Chicago, Jones Medical Publications, 1989.

Schwartz, SI: *Principles of Surgery.* New York, McGraw-Hill Book Company, 1989.

Stillman, RM: *Surgery Diagnosis and Therapy.* East Norwalk, Appleton and Lange, 1989.

Straub, WH, ed.: *Manual of Diagnostic Imaging,* 2nd ed. Boston, Little, Brown and Company, 1989.

Tisher, CC, ed.: *Nephrology for the House Officer.* Baltimore, Williams & Wilkins, 1989.

Way, LW: *Current Surgical Diagnosis and Treatment.* Norwalk, Appleton and Lange, 1988.

The Most Common

Others...

The Most Common
OTHERS:

CARDIOVASCULAR

...ABNORMALITY:
>of Human heart valves:
>>mitral valve prolapse
>in patients with Peripheral Arterial Occlusive Disease:
>>hypertriglyceridemia

...ARRHYTHMIAS AND CONDUCTION DISTURBANCES COMPLICATING ACUTE MYOCARDIAL INFARCTION (by incidence):
>ventricular premature contractions (33-71%), atrial premature contractions (10-57%), sinus tachycardia (20-53%), sinus bradycardia (14-28%), atrial fibrillation or flutter (13-28%), ventricular tachycardia (4-28%), accelerated idioventricular rhythm (9-13%), second degree A-V block, Type I (4-10%), ventricular fibrillation (3-10%), right bundle branch block (5-8%), complete heart block (4-8%), left bundle branch block (2-7%), asystole (1-5%), supraventricular tachycardia (0-4%), second degree A-V block, Type II (0.5-2%)

...ARTERIES ASSOCIATED WITH INTIMAL THICKENING:
>coronary arteries, abdominal aorta

...ARTERY OF THE LEG WHICH IS OCCLUDED:
>the superficial femoral artery

...ATRIUM AFFECTED BY CARDIAC MYXOMA:
>left > right

...BACTERIA:
>Causing:
>>Lymphangitis and Lymphadenitis:
>>>staphylococci or β—hemolytic streptococci

225

The Most Common
OTHERS:
...CARDIAC DISEASE (form of):

    in young Children:

        congenital heart disease

    Preexisting, in pregnancy:

        rheumatic heart disease

...CARDIAC LESION in females:

        mitral valve prolapse

...CARDIAC TUMOR:

        direct extension of bronchogenic carcinoma

...CLINICAL FEATURE seen in kidneys in congestive heart failure:

        mild to moderate proteinuria

...COAGULOPATHY, congenital:

        Factor VIII deficiency (Hemophilia A - classical)

...CONDUCTION DISTURBANCES AND ARRHYTHMIAS COMPLICATING ACUTE MYOCARDIAL INFARCTION (by incidence):

    ventricular premature contractions (33-71%), atrial premature contractions (10-57%), sinus tachycardia (20-53%), sinus bradycardia (14-28%), atrial fibrillation or flutter (13-28%), ventricular tachycardia (4-28%), accelerated idioventricular rhythm (9-13%), second degree A-V block, Type I (4-10%), ventricular fibrillation (3-10%), right bundle branch block (5-8%), complete heart block (4-8%), left bundle branch block (2-7%), asystole (1-5%), supraventricular tachycardia (0-4%), second degree A-V block, Type II (0.5-2%)

...CONGENITAL ANOMALY:

    of the Heart: ventricular septal defect

        Cyanotic: Tetralogy of Fallot

The Most Common
OTHERS:

...CONGENITAL COAGULOPATHY:

        Factor VIII deficiency (Hemophilia A - classical)

...CONGENITAL HEART DISORDER:

        ventricular septal defect (VSD)

Cyanotic: Tetralogy of Fallot

...CONGENITAL VASCULAR ABNORMALITY:

        arteriovenous fistula

...CORONARY ARTERY which is predominant:

        right, then balanced between right and left, then left

...CYANOTIC CONGENITAL CARDIAC ABNORMALITY:

        Tetralogy of Fallot

...DISEASE:

    of the Heart and blood vessels which leads to death in the United States:

        atherosclerosis of the coronary arteries

...DISORDER:

    resulting in Arterial Obstruction:

        atherosclerosis

...DRUGS:

    associated with Raynaud's Phenomenon:

        nicotine, propranolol, and the ergot derivatives

...FATAL CONGENITAL HEART LESION IN NEWBORNS:

        hypoplastic left heart syndrome

...FINDING:

    in Cardiac involvement in Systemic Lupus Erythematosus:

        pericarditis, although all layers of the heart may be involved

...HEART VALVE AFFECTED BY:

    Acquired valvular deformities:

The Most Common
OTHERS:

the mitral and aortic valves. Right sided
valves are uncommonly affected

...INDICATIONS FOR:

Cardiac transplantation:

ischemic heart disease and cardiomyopathy

Intra-Aortic Balloon Pump (IABP) in the CCU:

cardiogenic shock complicating acute myocardial infarction. Patients with a surgically cor-
rectable mechanical defect (acute ventricular
septal defect, papillary muscle rupture, or ventricular aneurysm) are most likely to benefit.
An IABP may also be helpful in stabilizing
patients with severe, reversible myocardial
stunning following reperfusion with a thrombolytic agent or coronary angioplasty

...INSTRUMENTS used for noninvasive vascular testing:

Doppler ultrasound and plethysmography

...LESION:

Cardiac, in children with congenital rubella, and the TORCH
complex:

patent ductus arteriosus and various septal defects. Stenosis of the pulmonary artery and
complex cardiac anomalies are also found

causing Myocardial death:

atherosclerosis of the LAD (left anterior descending) coronary artery

in Rheumatic Heart Disease:

Valvular lesion:

the mitral valve alone is affected in 40-50% of
cases (stenosis and/or insufficiency); the aortic and mitral valves together in 35-40%; the
aortic valve alone in 15-20%; trivalvular disease (mitral, aortic, and tricuspid together) in

The Most Common

OTHERS:

2-3%; mitral and tricuspid together (uncommon); mitral, aortic, tricuspid, and pulmonary
together (rare). Tricuspid disease alone is rare
and the pulmonary valve is virtually never affected. With all valves the involvement may
induce either stenosis, insufficiency, or both.
Way indicates that the most common lesion is
<u>stenotic</u> scarring of the mitral valve. Howev-
er, Dworkin indicates that mitral <u>insufficiency</u>
is the most common lesion, followed by aortic
insufficiency, mitral stenosis (less common
and usually is the end result of multiple attacks of acute rheumatic fever), and least commonly, aortic stenosis. It would appear that
the incidence of stenosis or insufficiency may
be difficult to ascertain, since these lesions
commonly occur together as a result of the
rheumatic scarring. The incidence of valves
involved, on the other hand, is well established

complicating Tertiary Syphilis:
syphilitic aortitis

...METHOD OF:
Bypassing severe occlusive disease in the aorta and iliac arteries:
aortoiliac or aortofemoral grafting using artificial graft material

...NONSELECTIVE PORTAL-SYSTEMIC SHUNT PER-
FORMED:
end-to-side portacaval shunt, followed by the
mesocaval (mesenteric-caval) shunt and the
side-to-side portacaval shunt

229

The Most Common
OTHERS:

...ORGAN AFFECTED BY:

    Infarction: brain, retina, heart (left ventricle), spleen, kidney, small intestine, lower leg

...ORGANISM:

    which Causes:

        Endocarditis, right sided:

            Staphylococcus aureus, Diplococcus pneumoniae

        Pericarditis, purulent or fibrinopurulent:

            staphylococci, streptococci, or pneumococci

    which Infects:

        Cavernous sinus thrombosis:

            Staphylococcus aureus

...PATHOGENIC LESION ASSOCIATED WITH ANEURYSM:

        atherosclerosis

...PORTAL-SYSTEMIC SHUNT PERFORMED:

    Nonselective: end-to-side portacaval shunt, followed by the mesocaval (mesenteric-caval) shunt and the side-to-side portacaval shunt

    Selective: the distal splenorenal (Warren) shunt

...PREDISPOSING CONDITIONS FOR:

    Deep-vein thrombosis and pulmonary embolism:

        surgery, childbirth

...PRIMARY NEOPLASMS WHICH METASTASIZE TO THE:

    Heart: lung, breast, lymphoma, leukemia, melanoma

...PROCEDURE PERFORMED FOR:

    emergency Portacaval shunting:

        an end-to-side portacaval shunt or a mesocaval shunt

...PULMONARY DISEASE CAUSING PULMONARY HYPERTENSION:

        obstructive emphysema

...RADIOGRAPHIC FINDINGS ON CHEST X-RAY OF NON-DISSECTING ANEURYSM OF THE THORACIC AORTA:

> mediastinal widening or a focal bulge of the aortic contour. Displacement of the trachea or esophagus frequently occurs. Curvilinear calcifications are frequently seen in the wall of the aneurysm. The presence of a pleural effusion raises the possibility of leakage from the aneurysm

...RESULT OF HYPERTENSION SECONDARY TO TYRAMINE INGESTION WHEN ON MAO INHIBITORS:

> an intense, throbbing headache accompanied by other unpleasant sensations; cerebrovascular accidents, hyperpyrexia, and death have infrequently occurred

...SELECTIVE PORTAL-SYSTEMIC SHUNT PERFORMED:

> the distal splenorenal (Warren) shunt

...SHUNT PERFORMED:

Portal-systemic:

Nonselective:

> end-to-side portacaval shunt, followed by the mesocaval (mesenteric-caval) shunt and the side-to-side portacaval shunt

Selective: the distal splenorenal (Warren) shunt

Tetralogy of Fallot:

> Blalock-Taussig operation (i.e., anastomosis of the subclavian artery to a pulmonary artery branch) and the modified Blalock-Taussig operation (i.e., interposition of a tubular graft between the subclavian and pulmonary arteries)

...SOURCE OF:

The Most Common

OTHERS:
Emboli to the lower extremity:

the heart: atherosclerotic heart disease with arterial plaques and thrombi and mural thrombi, rheumatic valvular heart disease; abdominal aortic ulcerated plaques

...THERAPEUTIC AGENTS USED TO TREAT CHILDHOOD HYPERTENSION:

Thiazide diuretics (Chlorothiazide, hydrochlorothiazide); Vasodilators (hydralazine); β–adrenergic antagonists [β - blockers] (propranolol, metoprolol); central sympatholytics (methyldopa). Other agents, including newer β- blockers, prazosin, minoxidil, clonidine, guanabenz, and captopril are proving to be effective and well tolerated but are not officially approved for use in children

...TIME:
that Air Embolism occurs:

Arterial: occurs as a consequence of tears in pulmonary parenchyma, opening venous channels

Venous: during the course of brain or head and neck surgery performed with patient in a sitting position

of Death in pulmonary embolism:

ninety percent of deaths occur within 2 hours after the onset of initial symptoms

of Diagnosis of aortic aneurysm:

routine physical examination

that Myocardial infarction, perioperative, occurs:

during the first 3 postoperative days. The remainder occur during the next 3 days.

that Perioperative myocardial infarction occurs:

during the first 3 postoperative days. The re-

232

mainder occur during the next 3 days.

of Rupture of the heart after an MI:

within the first few days

...UNDERLYING DISEASE ASSOCIATED WITH MYCOTIC ANEURYSM:

bacterial infection

...VALVE AFFECTED BY BACTERIAL ENDOCARDITIS:

the mitral valve

...VALVE INVOLVED IN RHEUMATIC ENDOCARDITIS:

the mitral valve

...VALVULAR DISEASE in the United States:

myxomatous transformation of valve and mitral valve prolapse (synonyms: mucinous degeneration, vlue valve, floppy valve)

...VALVULAR LESIONS IN RHEUMATIC DISEASE:

the mitral valve alone is affected in 40-50% of cases (stenosis and/or insufficiency); the aortic and mitral valves together in 35-40%; the aortic valve alone in 15-20%; trivalvular disease (mitral, aortic, and tricuspid together) in 2-3%; mitral and tricuspid together (uncommon); mitral, aortic, tricuspid, and pulmonary together (rare). Tricuspid disease alone is rare and the pulmonary valve is virtually never affected. With all valves the involvement may induce either stenosis, insufficiency, or both. Way indicates that the most common lesion is <u>stenotic</u> scarring of the mitral valve. However, Dworkin indicates that mitral <u>insufficiency</u> is the most common lesion, followed by aortic insufficiency, mitral stenosis (less common and usually is the end result of multiple at-

The Most Common
OTHERS:

tacks of acute rheumatic fever), and least commonly, aortic stenosis. It would appear that the incidence of stenosis or insufficiency may be difficult to ascertain, since these lesions commonly occur together as a result of the rheumatic scarring. The incidence of valves involved, on the other hand, is well established

...VEINS AFFECTED BY PHLEBOTHROMBOSIS:

deep leg veins

...VENOUS VASCULAR AUTOGRAFTS used:

greater and lesser saphenous veins and occasionally the internal jugular vein or a forearm vein

DENTAL AND ORAL

...INFECTIONS OF THE ORAL CAVITY:

odontogenic infections

...MICROBES IN THE ORAL CAVITY:

viridans streptococci

DERMATOLOGY

...CARCINOMA OF THE GASTROINTESTINAL TRACT ASSOCIATED WITH ACANTHOSIS NIGRICANS:

tumors of the stomach

...EFFECTS OF EXPOSURE TO NICKEL:

dermatitis ("nickel itch")

...GASTROINTESTINAL CARCINOMA ASSOCIATED WITH

234

OTHERS:

...ACANTHOSIS NIGRICANS:

tumors of the stomach

...ORGANISM WHICH CAUSES:

Fungal infections of the skin in adolescents:

Microsporum, *Trichophyton*, *Epidermophyton*, and *Pityrosporum*

...SCENARIO FOR SCALD BURNS:

hot liquid in a cup or pot turned over in the kitchen

...SKIN PROBLEM IN ADOLESCENTS:

acne, fungal infections

...TIME THAT JAUNDICE SECONDARY TO ANTIPSYCHOTICS AND NON-MAO INHIBITOR ANTI-DEPRESSANTS OCCURS:

between the second and fourth weeks of therapy

EMERGENCIES/ACCIDENTS

...AGENT RESPONSIBLE FOR INJURY IN MOTOR VEHICLE ACCIDENTS:

kinetic energy

...BACTERIA WHICH CAUSES SEPTIC SHOCK:

Klebsiella-Aerobacter, *Escherichia coli*, *Pseudomonas*, *Proteus*, *Bacteroides fragilis*, *Staphylococcus*, Paracolon, *Streptococcus*, Mixed culture

...CONSEQUENCE OF BLUNT TRAUMA TO THE THORAX:

rib fractures

...DIAGNOSIS ASSOCIATED WITH SUICIDE:

depression

The Most Common
OTHERS:

...EMERGENCY IN NEONATES, acquired:
  Gastrointestinal:

  necrotizing enterocolitis

...EVENT WHICH PRECIPITATES SUICIDE:

  a conflict with parents. Others include a
  breakup with a girlfriend or boyfriend, a conflict with peers, pregnancy, etc.

...FATAL EVENT following the more usual surgical procedures
  such as herniorrhaphy and cholecystectomy:

  pulmonary embolism

...FINDING IN A PERSON WHO SURVIVES SHOCK:

  depleted lipid store in adrenal glands

...GASTROINTESTINAL EMERGENCY IN NEONATES, acquired:

  necrotizing enterocolitis

...INJURY:

  Resulting in an emergency ward visit by children:
    that due to a fall

  Treated in emergency departments for all children under 16
  years of age:

  poisoning #3

...ROUTE OF ANTIGEN ADMINISTRATION IN ANAPHY-
  LAXIS:

  parenteral route. Ingestion and inhalation are

  less common routes

...SCENARIO FOR SCALD BURNS:

  hot liquid in a cup or pot turned over in the

  kitchen

...TIME THAT HOUSE FIRES OCCUR:

  at night; in December through March

236

The Most Common
OTHERS:

<u>ENDOCRINE</u>

...ADRENAL CORTICAL ABNORMALITY PRESENT IN
THE PERIOPERATIVE SETTING:
> a relative hypoadrenalism referred to as secon-
> dary adrenal insufficiency, due to glandular
> suppression in patients taking daily exogenous
> glucocorticoids.

...ANOMALY:
of Thyroid development of clinical importance:
> persistence of the thyroglossal duct as a cyst.
> Others include the development of a lingual
> thyroid, suprahyoid, infrahyoid, and prethyr-
> oid tissue

...ANTIBODIES FOUND IN HASHIMOTO'S THYROIDITIS
(CHRONIC LYMPHOCYTIC THYROIDI-
TIS):
> antithyroglobulin and antimicrosomal antibod-
> ies

...COMPLAINT:
of Abdominal symptoms in hypothyroidism:
> constipation and changes in bowel habits
in Hashimoto's disease (lymphadenoid goiter):
> enlargement of the neck with pain and tender-
> ness in the region of the thyroid
in Lymphadenoid goiter (Hashimoto's disease):
> enlargement of the neck with pain and tender-
> ness in the region of the thyroid

...DEFECT OF THE ADRENOGENITAL SYNDROME (congenital adrenal hyperplasia):
> 21-hydroxylase deficiency

...DISEASE:

237

The Most Common
OTHERS:

Endocrine-metabolic, in childhood:

> insulin-dependent diabetes mellitus (IDDM),
> type I

...ENDOCRINE AUTOGRAFT used:

> parathyroid autotransplantation

...ENDOCRINE-METABOLIC DISEASE OF CHILDHOOD:

> insulin-dependent diabetes mellitus (IDDM),
> type I

...FEATURES OF CUSHING'S SYNDROME:

> hypokalemia, hyperglycemia, hypertension,
> and muscle weakness. The other prominent
> features of this syndrome, such as obesity,
> buffalo hump, and a moon facies are less common

...INDICATION FOR HOSPITALIZING PREGNANT DIABETIC PATIENTS:

> uncontrolled hyperglycemia, ketoacidosis,
> persistent ketonuria, proteinuria, hypertension,
> deterioration in renal function, pyelonephritis,
> excessive weight gain, preterm labor

...LESIONS WHICH PRODUCE GASTRIN IN ZOLLINGER-ELLISON SYNDROME:

> pancreatic non-B islet cell carcinomas (60%),
> solitary adenomas (25%), and hyperplasia or
> microadenomas (10%); the remaining cases
> (5%) are due to solitary submucosal gastrinomas in the first or second portion of the duodenum

...PEOPLE IN WHICH GRAVE'S DISEASE BECOMES CLINICALLY APPARENT:

> young patients

...SIDE EFFECT:

Endocrine and Endocrine-like:

OTHERS:

of antipsychotic and non-MAO inhibitor anti-depressant therapy:

weight gain. Others include amenorrhea or other menstrual changes, inappropriate lactation in females and galactorrhea in males, breast enlargement in either sex, alterations of glucose metabolism, peripheral edema due to fluid retention, alterations in various laboratory tests

...SYMPTOM:

of Grave's disease:

emotional lability, increased appetite, heat intolerance, weight loss, frequent loose stools, deterioration of behavior and school performance, and poor sleeping. Weakness and inability to participate in sports are sometimes noted

related to the Thyroid gland in people with a goiter:

an awareness of increasing size of the neck or the presence of a mass

...TESTS USED FOR ASSESSMENT OF THYROID FUNCTION:

Radioimmunoassay (RIA), thyroid gland imaging [technetium 99m (^{99m}Tc) scanning, ultrasound], T_3 resin uptake, Free thyroxine index (T_7), TRH stimulation test, thyroid receptor antibody tests, radioactive iodine uptake

...THYROID CONDITION IN CHILDHOOD AND ADOLESCENCE:

chronic lymphocytic thyroiditis (CLT) (commonly referred to as Hashimoto's thyroiditis)

The Most Common

OTHERS:

...TIME OF PRESENTATION OF INSULIN-DEPENDENT DIABETES MELLITUS (IDDM) IN CHILDREN:

in early adolescence

...TREATMENT FOR HYPOTHYROIDISM:

L-Thyroxine

GASTROINTESTINAL

...ACQUIRED GASTROINTESTINAL EMERGENCY IN NEONATES:

necrotizing enterocolitis

...ACUTE CONDITION REQUIRING ACUTE ABDOMINAL SURGERY:

acute appendicitis

...AEROBIC BACTERIA IN THE STOOL:

E. coli

...ANTIBIOTICS IMPLICATED IN PSEUDOMEMBRANOUS COLITIS:

ampicillin, clindamycin, and cephalosporins. Then penicillins other than ampicillin, erythromycin, and sulfur drugs. Rarely tetracycline, cloramphenicol, and enterally administered aminoglycosides

...BACTERIA:

in the normal human Colon:

Bacteroides fragilis

in wound infections after surgery on the colon:

E. coli

...CARCINOMA OF THE GASTROINTESTINAL TRACT ASSOCIATED WITH ACANTHOSIS NIGRI-

The Most Common
OTHERS:

CANS:

tumors of the stomach

...COMPLAINT OF ABDOMINAL SYMPTOMS IN HYPO-
THYROIDISM:

constipation and changes in bowel habits

...CONGENITAL HERNIA:

Bochdalek hernia

...DEVELOPMENTAL ANOMALY OF THE SMALL INTES-
TINE:

Meckel's diverticulum

...DISORDER:

of primary Esophageal motility in children:
gastroesophageal reflux. Others are rare, most
commonly achalasia

simulating Peptic ulcer:
chronic cholecystitis, in which cholecysto-
grams show either nonfunctioning of the gallbladder or stones in a functioning gallbladder;
pancreatitis, in which the serum amylase is elevated (not elevated in peptic ulcer disease
unless the ulcer penetrates the pancreas); functional indigestion, in which x-rays are normal;
and reflux esophagitis

...DRUGS USED TO TREAT UPPER GASTROINTESTINAL
TRACT INFECTIONS AFTER GASTROIN-
TESTINAL SURGERY:
a cephalosporin or a penicillin-
aminoglycoside combination

...EMERGENCY IN NEONATES, acquired:
Gastrointestinal:

necrotizing enterocolitis

...GASTROINTESTINAL CARCINOMA ASSOCIATED WITH

The Most Common
OTHERS:

ACANTHOSIS NIGRICANS:

tumors of the stomach

...GASTROINTESTINAL EMERGENCY IN NEONATES, acquired:

necrotizing enterocolitis

...INDICATIONS:

for Acute Abdominal surgery in childhood:
appendicitis

for Elective Surgery in Crohn's disease:
failure of symptoms to respond to medical

management

...METHOD OF MANAGING ANAL FISSURES:

surgical excision

...MICROBES in:

GI tract, normal adult:

Stomach: *Candida albicans, Lactobacillus* sp., although usually sterile

Duodenum and jejunum:
Candida albicans, Enterococcus sp., *Lactobacillus* sp., Diphtheroids

Distal ileum:
Enterobacteriaceae, Bacteroides sp.

Terminal ileum and colon:
Bacteroides fragilis, B. melaninogenicus, B. oralis, Fusobacterium necrophorum, F. nucleatum, Streptococcus faecalis, Escherichia coli, Klebsiella sp., *Enterobacter* sp., *Eubacterium limosum, Bifidobacterium bifidum, Lactobacillus* sp., *Proteus* sp., *Staphylococcus aureus, Clostridium perfringens, C. tetani, Candida albicans, Clostridium septicum, Clostridium innocuum, Clostridium ramosum,*

The Most Common
OTHERS:

Streptococcus sp. (Groups A,B,C, F, and G), *Pseudomonas aeruginosa, Salmonella enteritidis, Shigella* sp., *Salmonella typhi, Peptostreptococcus* sp., *Peptococcus* sp.

Colon, facultative anaerobes:

E. coli

Oral cavity: viridans streptococci

Stools:

of Bottle fed infants:

Lactobacillus acidophilus, gram-negative enteric rods, enterococci, and anaerobic rods such as *Clostridium* sp.

of Breast fed infants:

Lactobacillus bifidus, enteric rods, enterococci, and staphylococci

...MODE OF:

development of Anorectal abscess:

extension of a local traumatic abscess within the anorectal canal

spread of Colon cancer:

lymphatic spread

Discovery of tubular adenomas of the colon:

as incidental lesions at autopsy, or during endoscopic or barium enema studies performed for investigation of some other intestinal problem. Occasionally, however, they come to clinical attention because of bleeding. Rarely, large pedunculated lesions may be the leading point of an intussusception

...ORGANISM:

Cultured from anal rectal abscess fistulas:

E. Coli

Found in the Intestines (i.e. found in the most people, not #

243

The Most Common
OTHERS:

of bx):

Escherichia, Bacteroides, Aerobacter, Enterococci, Clostridia, Streptococci, Staphylococci, Paracolon, Aerobic Gram-positive rods, Pseudomonas, Proteus, Lactobacilli, Yeast, Alcaligenes

...ORGANS TO PROTRUDE INTO AN OMPHALOCELE:
the liver and small bowel

...PATHOGEN OF CHILDHOOD DIARRHEA in developed countries:

rotavirus

...PATHOLOGIC PROBLEMS OF MECKEL'S DIVERTICULUM:
ulceration, obstruction, and acute inflammation

...PATHOLOGIC STATE ASSOCIATED WITH DIVERTICULOSIS:
diverticulitis

...POLYPS OF THE COLON:
adenomatous polyp (aka: polypoid adenoma, tubular adenoma)

...PRESENTING SYMPTOMS:
in Symptomatic Small Bowel Tumors:
bleeding, perforation, or obstruction

...PROBLEMS:
Esophageal, in Infants:

gastroesophageal reflux

...RADIOGRAPHIC MANIFESTATION OF ACUTE DIVERTICULITIS:
barium outside the diverticulum

...RAPID NONINVASIVE TEST USED FOR DIAGNOSING CHOLELITHIASIS, DILATATION OF BILE DUCTS, OR ENLARGEMENT OF

THE PANCREAS:

ultrasonography

...ROUTE FOR NONRENAL LOSS OF POTASSIUM:

the gastrointestinal tract (i.e. vomiting, diarrhea (especially the watery-diarrhea syndrome), laxative abuse, and villous adenoma of the colon)

...SIZE OF ADENOMATOUS POLYPS OF THE COLON:

smaller than 1 cm in diameter

...SIZE OF CARCINOMAS OF THE STOMACH AT THE TIME OF DISCOVERY:

between 2 and 10 cm in diameter (80%) > less than 2 cm (~10%)

...SURGICAL PROCEDURE PERFORMED FOR:

Gastroesophageal reflux in children:

Nissen fundoplication

...SYMPTOM:

of Abdominal irradiation:

decreased appetite

of Acute diverticulitis:

left lower quadrant pain and a change in normal bowel habits, either constipation or diarrhea. Nausea and vomiting may also be present

of Anal Fissures:

excruciating pain during and after defecation

of Celiac disease in children:

diarrhea. Failure to thrive is frequently seen. Vomiting is more common in younger patients. There may be abdominal distention and irritability. Short-stature, iron-resistant anemia, and rickets may be seen in older children

245

The Most Common
OTHERS:

of Cow's milk and soy protein intolerance in children:
vomiting and diarrhea. Rectal bleeding may be seen if colitis is present. Edema secondary to excessive enteric protein loss may be dramatic and is often associated with anemia. Rhinorrhea, wheezing, and eczema may occasionally be seen and are frequently accompanied by eosinophilia and an elevated serum immunoglobulin E (IgE) level. Anaphylaxis rarely is observed but may be life threatening

of Diverticulitis, acute:
left lower quadrant pain and a change in normal bowel habits, either constipation or diarrhea. Nausea and vomiting may also be
present

of Gastroesophageal reflux in children:
vomiting

of Hemorrhoids:
protrusion, bleeding, dull pain, and pruritus

of Ulcerative colitis:
rectal bleeding, diarrhea, abdominal pain,
weight loss, and fever

...TIME:

that Meckel's diverticula is detected:
incidental finding at laparotomy, then as a result of a significant complication

of Presentation of:
severe, Abdominal Pain in acute occlusion of the superior mesenteric artery:
early in the course of the disease
Necrotizing enterocolitis in preterm infants:
within the first week of feeding

that Umbilical hernias close by:

> closure by the age of 2 years

...TRACHEOESOPHAGEAL MALFORMATION pattern:

> esophageal atresia (the proximal segment of the esophagus ends as a blind pouch in the midthorax [proximal pouch]) with a distal tracheo-esophageal fistula (distal segment of esophagus [connected to stomach] forms a connection to the bronchus near the carina) (86% of cases); the next two occur almost equally (in 6% of cases) and are pure esophageal atresia (proximal and distal blind pouches) without fistula, and tracheoesophageal fistula without atresia (H fistula); the most uncommon type (in 2% of cases) combines both a proximal and a distal tracheo-esophageal fistula with a proximal atresia

...TREATMENT FOR ANAL FISSURE:

> conservative, involving the use of stool softeners, agents to relax the anal sphincter such as warm sitz baths, and local application of anti-inflammatory agents.

...USE OF:

Cecostomy tube:

> colonic ileus

a Rectal tube: to relieve colonic distention from a colonic ileus or obstruction

GENETICS/CONGENITAL

...ABNORMALITY:

of Internal organ systems in Down syndrome:

The Most Common
OTHERS:

        cardiac defects, especially endocardial cushion defects and septal defects; gastrointestinal abnormalities (especially duodenal atresia and Hirschsprung's disease)

...ANOMALY:
  secondary to in utero exposure to Anticonvulsants:
      oral clefts and congenital heart defects
  Autosomal, among living persons:
      Down's syndrome (mongolism)
  of the Bladder, severe:
      exstrophy of the bladder
  Congenital, of the uterus:
      Rokitansky-Kuster-Hauser syndrome
  of the Penis: hypospadias
  of Thyroid development of clinical importance:
      persistence of the thyroglossal duct as a cyst. Others include the development of a lingual thyroid, suprahyoid, infrahyoid, and prethyroid tissue
  Urethral, in Males:
      hypospadias

...AUTOSOMAL ANOMALY AMONG LIVING PERSONS:
      Down's syndrome (mongolism)

...AUTOSOMAL TRISOMY:
      Down syndrome

...BLADDER ANOMALY, severe:
      exstrophy of the bladder

...CHROMOSOMAL ABNORMALITY:
  Clinically recognized:
      trisomy 21 (Down's syndrome)
  in Down's syndrome:
      trisomy of chromosome number 21 of group G, resulting in a total of 47 instead of the usu-

OTHERS:

al 46 chromosomes; translocation of an extra
chromosome 21 to another acrocentric chromosome - most frequently chromosome 14 or
21, in which case the total number remains
46; or mosaicism, in which some cells have
46 and some have 47 chromosomes

in Klinefelter's syndrome:

47,XXY karyotype (80%). The remainder are
mosaics or have more than two X chromosomes

in Maternal age over 35 years of age:

Trisomy 21. Others include other autosomal
trisomies (i.e., 13 and 18) and sex chromosomal abnormalities

in Newborn infants:

balanced translocations > trisomy 21 > trisomy 47,XXY = trisomy 47,XXX = trisomy
47,XYY > unbalanced translocations > mono-
somy X (45,X) and X deletion variants > trisomy 18 > trisomy 13 > other trisomies

...CHROMOSOMES AFFECTED BY TRISOMIES:

sex chromosomes > autosomes

...COAGULOPATHY, congenital:

Factor VIII deficiency (Hemophilia A - classical)

...CONGENITAL ANOMALY:

Fatal: hypoplastic left heart syndrome

of the Heart: ventricular septal defect

Cyanotic: Tetralogy of Fallot
of the Nervous system:

myelomeningocele

The Most Common
OTHERS:

of the Uterus: Rokitansky-Kuster-Hauser syndrome

...CONGENITAL COAGULOPATHY:

Factor VIII deficiency (Hemophilia A - classical)

...CONGENITAL DEFECT OF THE COMPLEMENT COMPONENTS:

C2 deficiency

...CONGENITAL ENZYME DEFICIENCY:

combined deficiency of sucrase and isomaltase. Congenital lactase deficiency is much less common, but a transient lactase deficiency frequently follows an episode of infectious gastroenteritis

...CONGENITAL HEART DISORDER:

ventricular septal defect (VSD)

Cyanotic: Tetralogy of Fallot

...CONGENITAL HERNIA OF THE DIAPHRAGM:

Bochdalek hernia. This is due to a Foramen of Bochdalek, a posterolateral diaphragmatic defect. The anterior diaphragmatic defect, the Foramen of Morgagni, is much less common

...CONGENITAL MALFORMATION:

In diabetes (maternal) during pregnancy:

caudal regression, situs inversus, renal anomalies (ureter duplex, agenesis, cystic kidney), heart anomalies (transposition of the great vessels, ventricular septal defect, atrial septal defect), CNS defects (anencephaly, spina bifida, hydrocephalus), anal/rectal atresia

...CONGENITAL VASCULAR ABNORMALITY:

arteriovenous fistula

...CYANOTIC CONGENITAL CARDIAC ABNORMALITY:

Tetralogy of Fallot

...CYTOGENIC ABNORMALITY:

Down's syndrome (trisomy 21)

...DEFECT OF THE COMPLEMENT COMPONENTS:

Congenital: C2 deficiency

...DEVELOPMENTAL ANOMALY OF THE SMALL INTESTINE:

Meckel's diverticulum

...DISEASE:

of Connective tissue, heritable:

Marfan syndrome, Ehler-Danlos syndrome,

and osteogenesis imperfecta

Lethal, inherited, of Caucasians:

cystic fibrosis

...DISORDER:

Clinically important, in Caucasian children:

Autosomal recessive:

cystic fibrosis

...FATAL CONGENITAL HEART LESION IN NEWBORNS:

hypoplastic left heart syndrome

...FINDING:

Chromosomal, in Down's Syndrome:

trisomy of chromosome number 21 of group

G, resulting in a total of 47 instead of the usual 46 chromosomes; translocation of material, in which case the total number remains 46; or mosaicism, in which some cells have 46 and some have 47 chromosomes

...GENETIC HYPERLIPIDEMIA IN CHILDHOOD:

familial hypercholesterolemia

...GENOTYPE OF TRUE HERMAPHRODITES:

The Most Common
OTHERS:

46,XX

...HEREDITARY COAGULATION DISORDER:
> hemophilia A and von Willebrand's disease (both are disorders involving coagulation factor VIII)

...HYPERLIPIDEMIA IN CHILDHOOD:

Genetic: familial hypercholesterolemia

...INDICATION:
> of a Genetic problem that is recognized in the school-aged child:
>> mental retardation

...INDUCERS OF DNA MUTATIONS:
> chemical mutagens

...KARYOTYPE OF PATIENTS WHO HAVE TURNER SYNDROME:
> monosomy of the X chromosome (45,X)

...LETHAL INHERITED DISEASE OF CAUCASIANS:
> cystic fibrosis

...MATERNAL INFECTION WHICH CAUSES CONGENITAL ANOMALIES AND MENTAL RETARDATION:
> not available. Rubella #2 according to Gregory.

...MYOPATHY:

Hereditary: muscular dystrophies, myotonic muscle disorders, metabolic myopathies, congenital myopathies

...ORGAN AFFECTED BY:

Congenital anomalies:
> the kidneys and genitourinary tract

Cystic Fibrosis:
> the gastrointestinal and respiratory systems

252

Thalidomide exposure:

>ears (microtia and anotia) and the heart

...ORGANS TO PROTRUDE INTO AN OMPHALOCELE:

>the liver and small bowel

...TIME:

that Bone marrow chromosome studies are used:

>in the evaluation of leukemias

...TISSUES USED FOR CHROMOSOME ANALYSIS:

>peripheral blood (the T cells)

...TRACHEOESOPHAGEAL FISTULA pattern:

>distal segment of esophagus (connected to stomach) forms a connection to the bronchus near the carina. The proximal segment ends as a blind pouch in the midthorax.

...TRANSMISSION (genetic) OF VON WILLEBRAND'S DISEASE (VWD):

>autosomal dominant trait with variable penetrance is the most common form, although genetically its transmission is variable

...TRISOMY, autosomal:

>Down syndrome

GENITOURINARY

...AGE OF MALES PRESENTING WITH SERTOLI-LEYDIG TUMORS OF THE TESTICLE:

>30 to 45 years of age

...ANOMALY:

of the Bladder, severe:

>exstrophy of the bladder

of the Penis: hypospadias

Urethral:

The Most Common
OTHERS:
in Males: hypospadias

...ANTIPSYCHOTIC ASSOCIATED WITH EJACULATORY
   DYSFUNCTIONS:

   thioridazine

...BACTERIA:
   Causing:
   Pyelonephritis:

   Escherichia coli. Other frequent causes include *Proteus,* enterococcus, and *Klebsiella.*

   Urethritis: *E. coli*, other gram-negative rods, and enterococci

...BLADDER ANOMALY, severe:
   exstrophy of the bladder

...CONTRACEPTION form used in U.S.:

   Irreversible: surgical sterilization

...COUNTERPART (in the female) OF EPISPADIAS IN
   MALES:

   bifid clitoris

...ORGANISM:
   Cultured from:
   Urine in Acute Pyelonephritis:

   Escherichia coli

...PATHOLOGY of the lower genital tract:
   infection

...RENAL PROBLEM SEEN BY OBSTETRICIANS:
   symptomatic bacteriuria

...SEQUELA OF RECURRENT PYELONEPHRITIS:
   Long-term sequela:
   hypertension

...SEXUALLY TRANSMITTED DISEASE:

   Chlamydial infection - Chlamydial cervicitis
   and urethritis (since *Chlamydia trachomatis* is
   hard to isolate and since the infection is not a

254

The Most Common

OTHERS:

reportable disease at this time, exact figures about its prevalence are not available)

Non-gonococcal:

Chlamydia trachomatis

Reported in the United States:

Neisseria gonorrhoeae (since *Chlamydia trachomatis* is hard to isolate and since the infection is not a *reportable* disease at this time, exact figures about its prevalence are not available)

...SEXUALLY TRANSMITTED PROTOZOAL INFECTION:

Trichomonas vaginalis

...STAGE OF PROSTATE ADENOCARCINOMA AT DETECTION:

Stage C

...SYMPTOM:

of Testicular cancer:

a painless enlargement usually noticed during bathing or after a minor trauma. Painful enlargement of the testis occurs in 30 to 50% of patients and may be the result of bleeding or infarction in the tumor.

...URETHRAL ANOMALY:

in Males: hypospadias

...VENEREAL DISEASE in the US and western Europe, diagnosed:

Chlamydia trachomatis, N. Gonorrhoeae

GERIATRICS

...ILLNESSES OF THE ELDERLY:

depression and organic mental disorders

The Most Common

OTHERS:
...PSYCHIATRIC PROBLEM in elderly:
>> depression, dementia

HEMATOLOGY AND ONCOLOGY

...ANTIBODIES:
>> which inactivate Coagulation factors:
>>> IgG usually. Most commonly against factors VIII and X.

...ANTIGENS:
>> involved in Hemolytic disease of the newborn (erythroblastosis fetalis):
>>> $Rh_0(D)$ - from the Rh blood group system

...COAGULATION ABNORMALITY in women with PIH (pregnancy-induced hypertension):
>> thrombocytopenia

...COAGULATION FACTORS INACTIVATED BY ANTIBODIES:
>> Factors VIII and X

...COMPLEMENT DEFICIENCY:
>> C2, C3, C6,7,8

...DISORDER:
>> Metabolic, of red blood cells:
>>> G6PD deficiency

...ENZYMES WHICH CAUSE ENZYMOPATHIC HEMOLYTIC ANEMIAS:
>> Glycolytic enzymes:
>>> pyruvate kinase (PK)
>> Hexose monophosphate shunt enzymes:
>>> glucose-6-phosphate dehydrogenase (G6PD)

...HEREDITARY COAGULATION DISORDER:

hemophilia A and von Willebrand's disease
(both are disorders involving coagulation factor VIII)

...METABOLIC DISORDER OF RED BLOOD CELLS:
G6PD deficiency
...RED BLOOD CELL METABOLIC DISORDER:
G6PD deficiency
...THERAPY EMPLOYED FOR CHILDHOOD AUTOIM-
MUNE HEMOLYTIC ANEMIA:
supportive care and judicious use of transfu-
sions and corticosteroids

HEPATIC AND BILIARY

...AGE OF INCIDENCE OF:
Hepatitis A: childhood, young adulthood

Hepatitis B: adulthood
...ANATOMICAL RELATIONSHIP:
between the Common bile duct and the pancreatic duct:
the ducts most commonly unite outside the
duodenum and traverse the duodenal wall and
papilla as a single duct, the ducts join the duodenal wall and have a short common channel, least commonly they enter the duodenum
independently
of the Cystic artery:
nearly always a branch of the right hepatic artery that passes behind the cystic duct
between the Cystic duct and the hepatic duct:

an acute angle
...BACTERIA:
Causing:

The Most Common
OTHERS:

Cholangitis:

> *E. coli*

Present in infections in the biliary tree:

> *E. coli, Streptococcus faecalis* (the aerobic gram-positive enterococcus), *Salmonella*, anaerobic organisms, especially *C. perfringens*

...COMPLAINT:

associated with Carcinoma of the Gallbladder:

> right upper quadrant pain

...ETIOLOGY OF HEPATIC CIRRHOSIS:

> alcohol abuse, followed by postnecrotic cirrhosis and biliary cirrhosis

...HEPATIC ABSCESSES:

in Third World Countries:

> amebic abscesses, then bacterial abscesses

in the Western World:

> bacterial abscesses, then amebic abscess

...INDICATIONS:

for Cholecystectomy:

> chronic cholecystitis

...METHOD OF:

Diagnosing:

Primary sclerosing cholangitis:

> exploratory laparotomy

...NON-BILIARY SURGERIES ASSOCIATED WITH POST-OPERATIVE ACUTE ACALCULOUS CHOLECYSTITIS:

Major cardiac and aortic surgery or renal transplantation

...ORGANISM:

which Causes:

Emphysematous Cholecystitis:

258

OTHERS:

virulent, gas-forming organism, usually a clostridial, coliform, or anaerobic streptococcal species

...PRESENTING SYMPTOMS:

in Choledochal Cyst:

intermittent jaundice

in Gallbladder Trauma:

right upper quadrant pain, right chest pain, biliary leakage through a penetrating wound, and shock

...RAPID NONINVASIVE TEST USED FOR DIAGNOSING CHOLELITHIASIS, DILATATION OF BILE DUCTS, OR ENLARGEMENT OF THE PANCREAS:

ultrasonography

...RESULT OF INOPERABLE HEPATOBLASTOMA:

most patients die within 1 year

...SIGNS OF:

Hepatic abscess due to *Entamoeba histolytica*:

hepatomegaly and point tenderness due to a single abscess in the upper outer quadrant of the right lobe

...SYMPTOMATIC DISORDER OF THE GALL BLADDER:

Chronic cholecystitis

...TIME:

that Biliary colic occurs:

1 to 2 hours postprandially, usually in the evening and almost never in the morning

of diagnosis of Gallbladder Trauma:

at laparotomy

The Most Common

OTHERS:
IMMUNOLOGY/ALLERGIC DISORDERS

...ANTIBODIES:
   which inactivate Coagulation factors:
   > IgG usually. Most commonly against factors VIII and X.

   found in Hashimoto's thyroiditis (chronic lymphocytic thyroiditis):
   > antithyroglobulin and antimicrosomal antibodies

...ANTIGENS:
   involved in Hemolytic disease of the newborn (erythroblastosis fetalis):
   > $Rh_0(D)$ - from the Rh blood group system

   causing Isoimmunization:
   > D, C, Kelly, E, Duffy, and Kidd

...COAGULATION FACTORS INACTIVATED BY ANTIBODIES:
   > Factors VIII and X

...COMPLAINT:
   in Hashimoto's disease (lymphadenoid goiter):
   > enlargement of the neck with pain and tenderness in the region of the thyroid

   in Lymphadenoid goiter (Hashimoto's disease):
   > enlargement of the neck with pain and tenderness in the region of the thyroid

...COMPLEMENT DEFICIENCY:
   > C2, C3, C6,7,8

...CONGENITAL DEFECT OF THE COMPLEMENT COMPONENTS:
   > C2 deficiency

...DEFECT OF THE COMPLEMENT COMPONENTS:

Congenital: C2 deficiency

...DISEASE:

of Peripheral nerves:

Presumed autoimmune, postinfectious:

Guillain-Barre syndrome. Others include some cases of Bell's palsy and sixth nerve palsy. Gradenigo syndrome (sixth nerve palsy associated with pain in the distribution of the fifth cranial nerve) is secondary to osteomyelitis of the petrous ridge of the sphenoid bone. Brachial plexus neuropathies have been associated with influenza vaccination

...EYE MUSCLE involved in Grave's Disease:

Inferior Rectus

...FINDING:

in Cardiac involvement in Systemic Lupus Erythematosus: pericarditis, although all layers of the heart may be involved

...FOODS:

which cause Allergic reactions:

milk, eggs, shellfish, peanuts and other nuts, cereal grains (gluten), citrus fruits, and the preservatives (metabisulfite) and dyes (yellow food dye no. 5) added to foods

...HEART VALVE INVOLVED IN RHEUMATIC ENDOCARDITIS:

the mitral valve

...IMMUNODEFICIENCY SYNDROME:

selective IgA deficiency

...IMMUNOPHENOTYPE OF CELLS IN CHILDREN WITH ACUTE LYMPHOCYTIC LEUKEMIA (ALL):

The Most Common
OTHERS:

CALLA-positive non-T, non-B cell ALL > CALLA-negative non-T, non-B cell ALL (3 to 4 times)

...JOINT AFFECTED BY JUVENILE RHEUMATOID AR-THRITIS, in pauciarticular JRA:

the knee

...LESION:

in Rheumatic Heart Disease:

mitral insufficiency, followed by aortic insufficiency. Mitral stenosis is less common and usually is the end result of multiple attacks of acute rheumatic fever. Least common is aortic stenosis. The tricuspid and pulmonary valves virtually never are affected

...PEOPLE IN WHICH GRAVE'S DISEASE BECOMES CLINI-CALLY APPARENT:

young patients

...POLLENS WHICH CAUSE ALLERGIC RHINITIS:

ragweed, other weeds, grasses, and trees

...ROUTE OF ANTIGEN ADMINISTRATION IN ANAPHY-LAXIS:

parenteral route. Ingestion and inhalation are less common routes

...SYMPTOM:

of Grave's disease:

emotional lability, increased appetite, heat intolerance, weight loss, frequent loose stools, deterioration of behavior and school performance, and poor sleeping. Weakness and inability to participate in sports are sometimes noted

...SYNDROME:

Immunodeficiency:

262

selective IgA deficiency

...THERAPY EMPLOYED FOR CHILDHOOD AUTOIM-
MUNE HEMOLYTIC ANEMIA:

supportive care and judicious use of transfusions and corticosteroids

...VALVE INVOLVED IN RHEUMATIC ENDOCARDITIS:

the mitral valve

...VALVULAR LESIONS IN RHEUMATIC DISEASE:

the mitral valve alone is affected in 40-50% of
cases (stenosis and/or insufficiency); the aortic and mitral valves together in 35-40%; the
aortic valve alone in 15-20%; trivalvular disease (mitral, aortic, and tricuspid together) in
2-3%; mitral and tricuspid together (uncommon); mitral, aortic, tricuspid, and pulmonary
together (rare). Tricuspid disease alone is rare
and the pulmonary valve is virtually never affected. With all valves the involvement may
induce either stenosis, insufficiency, or both.
Way indicates that the most common lesion is
<u>stenotic</u> scarring of the mitral valve. Howev-
er, Dworkin indicates that mitral <u>insufficiency</u>
is the most common lesion, followed by aortic
insufficiency, mitral stenosis (less common
and usually is the end result of multiple attacks of acute rheumatic fever), and least commonly, aortic stenosis. It would appear that
the incidence of stenosis or insufficiency may
be difficult to ascertain, since these lesions
commonly occur together as a result of the
rheumatic scarring. The incidence of valves
involved, on the other hand, is well estab-

The Most Common
OTHERS:

INFECTIOUS AND PARASITIC DISEASES/MICROBIOLOGY

...ABNORMALITY:

    in Trichinosis: eosinophilic leukocytosis

...ABSCESSES, hepatic, in the Western World:

    bacterial abscesses

...ADENOVIRUS SEROTYPES associated with acute respiratory disease in military recruits:

    serotypes 4, 7, and 21

...AEROBIC BACTERIA IN THE STOOL:

    E. coli

...AGE OF INCIDENCE OF:

    Hepatitis A: childhood, young adulthood

    Hepatitis B: adulthood

...ANTIBIOTICS:

    Implicated in pseudomembranous colitis:

        ampicillin, clindamycin, and cephalosporins. Then penicillins other than ampicillin, erythromycin, and sulfur drugs. Rarely tetracycline, chloramphenicol, and enterally administered aminoglycosides

    Used to treat diverticulitis:

        ampicillin

...APPEARANCE OF RICKETTSIEAE:

    pairs of rod shaped cells with tapered ends

...AREAS AFFECTED BY *ENTAMOEBA HISTOLYTICA* INFECTION:

    in areas with poor sanitation

...BACTERIA:

264

in the normal human Colon:

> *Bacteroides fragilis*

which are Glucose nonfermenting gram negative rods:

> *Pseudomonas, Acinetobacter anitratus*

...COMMUNICABLE DISEASE:

> tuberculosis (*Mycobacterium tuberculosis*)

...COMPLAINT:

in Clostridial myositis and cellulitis (gas gangrene):

> severe pain at the site of injury

in Gas Gangrene:

> severe pain at the site of injury

...CONSEQUENCES:

of Prenatal rubella infection:

> cataracts, deafness, congenital heart disease, brain damage (sometimes including microcephaly), and secondary retardation. Some cases of early infantile autism have also been
> associated with prenatal rubella

of *Trypanosoma cruzi* infection:

> chronic Chaga's disease

...DIAGNOSIS:

in self-referred Female Clinic Patients with sexually transmitted disease:

> vaginitis

...DIAGNOSTIC TECHNIQUE used to demonstrate "school of fish" or "chaining" of *Hemophilus ducreyi* gram-negative rods:

Gram stain of exudate from the chancre, Gram stain of the aspirate of the bubo

...DIFFERENTIAL AND SELECTIVE MEDIA used for separation of Enterobacteriaceae lactose fermentors and non-fermentors:

The Most Common
OTHERS:

eosin-methylene blue (EMB) and MacConkey agar

...DISEASE:
  of Peripheral nerves:
    Presumed autoimmune, postinfectious:

> Guillain-Barre syndrome. Others include some cases of Bell's palsy and sixth nerve palsy. Gradenigo syndrome (sixth nerve palsy associated with pain in the distribution of the fifth cranial nerve) is secondary to osteomyelitis of the petrous ridge of the sphenoid bone. Brachial plexus neuropathies have been associated with influenza vaccination

  Sexually transmitted:

> Chlamydial infection

  associated with Slow (unconventional) viruses:

> scrapie

...DOMESTIC ANIMALS INFECTED WITH RABIES:
  cattle, dogs, and cats

...DRUGS:
  Used to treat:
    Leprosy: dapsone
    Necrotizing fasciitis:

> penicillin and an aminoglycoside

    Upper gastrointestinal tract infections after gastrointestinal surgery:

> a cephalosporin or a penicillin-aminoglycoside combination

...EVENT ASSOCIATED WITH THE ONSET OF ACUTE PELVIC INFLAMMATORY DISEASE:

> a recent menstrual flow

...FLAVIVIRUS in the US:

St. Louis encephalitis (SLE)

...FOODS:

Contaminated with *Clostridium botulinum* toxin:

most commonly present in vegetables or other foods that have been improperly home-canned and stored without refrigeration, conditions that provide suitable anaerobic conditions for growth of the vegetative cells that elaborate

the neurotoxins (A-G)

...FUNGI WHICH CAUSE MYCETOMA:

Madurella mycetomatis, M. grisea, Leptosphaeria senegalenis, Petriellidium boydii, Aspergillus nidulans, and *Acremonium,* and *Curvularia* species

...HEART VALVE AFFECTED BY:

bacterial Endocarditis:

the mitral valve

...HEART VALVE INVOLVED IN RHEUMATIC ENDOCARDITIS:

the mitral valve

...HEMOLYSIN in *S. aureus* isolated from clinical specimens:

alpha hemolysin

...HEPATIC ABSCESSES:

in Third World Countries:

amebic abscesses, then bacterial abscesses

in the Western World:

bacterial abscesses, then amebic abscess

...HOSTS for rabies:

dogs, cats, cattle, skunks, bats, foxes, and squirrels

The Most Common

OTHERS:

...INFECTION:

Adenovirus: acute respiratory disease, usually seen in military training camps; pharyngoconjunctivitis, usually seen in the summer months

Adenovirus:

    in Children:

        pharyngoconjunctivitis

    in AIDS patients:

        Pneumocystosis carinii pneumonia. Mycobacterial infections also are found frequently - especially those caused by *Mycobacterium avium-intracellulare*. Cytomegalovirus disease is very common among AIDS patients and may be much more severe in these patients than it is in otherwise healthy people. Cryptococcal meningitis and cryptosporidial diarrhea tend to run a more aggressive course in AIDS patients

    Opportunistic:

        Pneumocystis carinii

CMV: congenital and neonatal subclinical diseases

Echovirus: aseptic meningitis, rash, fever, and enteritis, acute respiratory infection, myocarditis, pleurodyna, paralysis, and encephalitis

associated with Fever of Unknown Origin:

        tuberculosis and hepatobiliary infection are the most common types of infectious disease associated with fever of unknown cause

    in Children:

        tuberculosis, brucellosis, tularemia, salmonellosis, diseases due to rickettsiae or spirochetes, infectious mononucleosis, cytomegalic inclusion disease, and hepatitis

268

Human: toxoplasmosis may be the most common infection of mankind, according to Rubin

associated with a Papovavirus:

        skin warts (verrucae)

due to Intravenous drug abuse:

        cutaneous abscesses, cellulitis, and ulcers

Maternal, which causes congenital anomalies and mental retardation:

        cytomegalic inclusion body disease, rubella

Natal and Prenatal, resulting in mental retardation:

        cytomegalic inclusion disease, rubella, herpes simplex, toxoplasmosis, and syphilis

Opportunistic:

    in AIDS patients:

        Pneumocystis carinii

of the Oral cavity:

        odontogenic infections

associated with a Papovavirus:

        skin warts (verrucae)

Surgical: furuncles

Trichomonas vaginalis:

        vaginal infections

in Women ages 16-25 years of age (most common serious infection):

        acute PID (pelvic inflammatory disease)

...INTESTINAL PARASITE, identified, in the U.S.:

        Giardia lamblia

...ISOLATE FROM HUMAN MENINGOCOCCAL DISEASE, caused by *N. meningitidis* serogroup B or C:

        serotype 2

...LABORATORY TEST USED FOR THE IDENTIFICATION OF *S. aureus*:

        coagulase test

The Most Common
OTHERS:

...LESION:

    Cardiac, in children with congenital rubella, and the TORCH complex:

        patent ductus arteriosus and various septal defects. Stenosis of the pulmonary artery and complex cardiac anomalies are also found

    Ocular, in children afflicted with herpes simplex:

        keratoconjunctivitis

    complicating Tertiary Syphilis:

        syphilitic aortitis

...LOCATION for:

    Lymphatic filariasis:

        Asia

    Onchocerciasis:

        African tropics. Also Yemen and Latin America

    Trichuriasis: southeastern portion of the United States

...LONG-TERM SEQUELA OF RECURRENT PYELONEPHRITIS:

    hypertension

...MATERNAL INFECTION WHICH CAUSES RETARDATION:

    cytomegalic inclusion body disease

...MATERNAL INFECTION WHICH CAUSES CONGENITAL ANOMALIES AND MENTAL RETARDATION:

    not available. Rubella #2 according to Gregory.

...METHOD OF:

    Diagnosing:

        primary sclerosing Cholangitis:

           exploratory laparotomy

        Giardiasis:

270

identification of the parasite (trophozoite or cyst) in formed or unformed stool. The parasite also can be recovered from the duodenum if a string is passed, by mouth, into the duodenum (string test)

Pneumocystis carinii pneumonia, histopathologic diagnosis:

fiberoptic bronchoscopy, usually combined with bronchoalveolar lavage and/or transbronchial biopsy

acute Sinusitis:

radiography

Sporotrichosis:

culture, but serologic tests are also of value.

Direct examination of pus is seldom helpful

Introducing pathogens into the respiratory tract:

inhalation of aerosolized microorganisms

...MICROBES in:

GI tract, normal adult:

Stomach: *Candida albicans*, *Lactobacillus* sp., although usually sterile

Duodenum and jejunum:

Candida albicans, Enterococcus sp., *Lactobacillus* sp., Diphtheroids

Distal ileum:

Enterobacteriaceae, *Bacteroides* sp.

Terminal ileum and colon:

Bacteroides fragilis, *B. melaninogenicus*, *B. oralis*, *Fusobacterium necrophorum*, *F. nucleatum*, *Streptococcus faecalis*, *Escherichia coli*, *Klebsiella* sp., *Enterobacter* sp., *Eubacterium limosum*, *Bifidobacterium bifidum*, *Lactobacillus* sp., *Proteus* sp., *Staphylococcus au-*

The Most Common
OTHERS:

reus, *Clostridium perfringens*, *C. tetani*, *Candida albicans*, *Clostridium septicum*, *Clostridium innocuum*, *Clostridium ramosum*, *Streptococcus* sp. (Groups A,B,C,F, and G), *Pseudomonas aeruginosa*, *Salmonella enteritidis*, *Shigella* sp., *Salmonella typhi*, *Peptostreptococcus* sp., *Peptococcus* sp.

Colon, facultative anaerobes:

E. coli

Oral cavity: viridans streptococci

Stools:

of Bottle fed infants:

Lactobacillus acidophilus, gram-negative enteric rods, enterococci, and anaerobic rods such as *Clostridium* sp.

of Breast fed infants:

Lactobacillus bifidus, enteric rods, enterococci, and staphylococci

...MODE OF:

development of Anorectal abscess:

extension of a local traumatic abscess within the anorectal canal

acquiring Brucellosis:

in much of the World:

unpasteurized dairy products (in the United States brucellosis is an occupational disease of farmers, employees of abattoirs, and veterinarians; in the arctic and subarctic regions humans acquire brucellosis by eating raw bone marrow of infected reindeer)

Transmission of measles (rubeola) infection:

inhalation. It may also be passed through the placenta

272

The Most Common

OTHERS:

...NATAL AND PRENATAL INFECTIONS RESULTING IN
MENTAL RETARDATION:

> cytomegalic inclusion disease, rubella, herpes
> simplex, toxoplasmosis, and syphilis

...NEUROECTODERMAL DEFECT involved in bacterial meningitis:

> congenital sinus tract

...ORGAN AFFECTED BY:

Mumps infection:

> the parotid salivary glands. Less often the vi-
> rus attacks the pancreas, ovaries, testes, and
> other organs

...ORGANISM:

which Causes:

Peritonitis, primary:

in Adults:

> an enteric pathogen - usually *E. coli.* Entero-
> cocci and pneumococci are also seen

Postsplenectomy Sepsis:

> pneumococcus

Primary peritonitis:

in Adults:

> an enteric pathogen - usually *E. coli.* Entero-
> cocci and pneumococci are also seen

Puerperal Mastitis:

> *Staphylococcus aureus* from the infant's nose
> and throat

Relapsing fever, tick-borne:

in Africa:

> *Borrelia duttonii*

in Asia:

> *Borrelia persica*

in North America:

> *Borrelia turicatae,* B. *hermsii,* and *B. parkeri*

273

The Most Common
OTHERS:

in Spain:

Borrelia hispanica

Sinusitis: *S. pneumoniae*, unencapsulated strains of *H. influenzae*, and *B. catarrhalis*

Thyroiditis, acute:

Staphylococcus aureus, Streptococcus hemolyticus, and pneumococcus

Tick-borne relapsing fever:

in Africa:

Borrelia duttonii

in Asia:

Borrelia persica

in North America:

Borrelia turicatae, B. hermsii, and *B. parkeri*

in Spain:

Borrelia hispanica

Cultured from:

Anal Rectal Abscess Fistulas:

E. Coli

Urine in Acute Pyelonephritis:

Escherichia coli

Found in the Intestines (i.e. found in the most people, not # of bx):

Escherichia, Bacteroides, Aerobacter, Enterococci, Clostridia, Streptococci, Staphylococci, Paracolon, Aerobic Gram-positive rods, Pseudomonas, Proteus, Lactobacilli, Yeast, Alcaligenes

which Infects:

Cavernous sinus thrombosis:

Staphylococcus aureus

Parasitic:

associated with Pruritus:

> pinworm, scabies mites, lice, and roundworm larvae

which Produces:

> Myotoxin in Clostridial Myonecrosis (Gas Gangrene):
>
> > *C. perfringens* Type A (80-90% of cases), but myotoxin may also come from *C. novyi*, *C. septicum*, and rarely from three other species
>
> Toxin (myotoxin) in Clostridial Myonecrosis (Gas Gangrene):
>
> > *C. perfringens* Type A (80-90% of cases), but myotoxin may also come from *C. novyi*, *C. septicum*, and rarely from three other species

...ORIGIN OF BACTERIAL INFECTION AND NEONATAL SEPSIS:

> acquired via the birth canal or nosocomially. The infection almost always is bacteremic (often with seeding of the meninges via the blood) and associated with systemic symptoms

...PAPOVAVIRUS INFECTION in humans:

> the human wart virus

...PARASITIC ORGANISMS ASSOCIATED WITH PRURITUS:

> pinworm, scabies mites, lice, and roundworm larvae

...PARTICLES SEEN IN HEPATITIS B INFECTED SERUM:

> spherical particles

...PATHOGEN OF CHILDHOOD DIARRHEA in developed countries:

> rotavirus

...PEOPLE SEEN WITH GIANT CELL PNEUMONITIS SECONDARY TO MEASLES:

275

The Most Common
OTHERS:

Hosts unable to form antibody
...PREDISPOSING CONDITIONS for:

Septicemia due to *Bacteroides*:

peritoneal abscess, septic abortion, gynecologic surgery or manipulation, lower back or hip trauma, and infected decubitus ulcer

...RICKETTSIAL INFECTION in the United States:

Rocky Mountain spotted fever

...SEASON OF INFECTION BY:

adenovirus Pharyngoconjunctivitis:

summer months

...SEQUELA OF RECURRENT PYELONEPHRITIS:

Long-term sequela:

hypertension

...SEROLOGIC TEST for the diagnosis of:

antecedent *S. pyogenes* infection:

antistreptolysin O titers

Toxoplasma gondii:

detection of IgG antibody against *T. gondii* by indirect immunofluorescence

...SEXUALLY TRANSMITTED DISEASE:

Chlamydial infection - Chlamydial cervicitis and urethritis (since *Chlamydia trachomatis* is hard to isolate and since the infection is not a reportable disease at this time, exact figures about its prevalence are not available)

Non-gonococcal:

Chlamydia trachomatis

Reported in the United States:

Neisseria gonorrhoeae (since *Chlamydia trachomatis* is hard to isolate and since the infection is not a *reportable* disease at this time, exact figures about its prevalence are not available)

...SEXUALLY TRANSMITTED PROTOZOAL INFECTION:

Trichomonas vaginalis

...SIGNS OF:

Hepatic abscess due to *Entamoeba histolytica*:

hepatomegaly and point tenderness due to a
single abscess in the upper outer quadrant of
the right lobe

Infection with *Entamoeba histolytica*:

intermittent diarrhea with blood and mucus,

flatulence, and abdominal cramps

...SITUATION IN WHICH:

Non-A, Non-B hepatitis infection occurs:

following blood transfusion and parenteral

drug use

...SOURCE OF:

Clostridium botulinum toxin:

most commonly present in vegetables or other
foods that have been improperly home-canned
and stored without refrigeration, conditions
that provide suitable anaerobic conditions for
growth of the vegetative cells that elaborate
the neurotoxins (A-G)

Myotoxin in Clostridial Myonecrosis (Gas Gangrene):

C. perfringens Type A (80-90% of cases), but
myotoxin may also come from *C. novyi*, *C.
septicum*, and rarely from three other species

Salmonellosis in the US:

Poultry products (i.e, flesh and eggs), improperly cooked roast beef

Toxin (myotoxin) in Clostridial Myonecrosis (Gas Gangrene):

C. perfringens Type A (80-90% of cases), but

The Most Common
OTHERS:

myotoxin may also come from *C. novyi*, *C. septicum*, and rarely from three other species

...SYMPTOM:

Brain Abscess:headache, caused by increased intracranial pressure

of Enterobiasis:

pruritus ani

of Herpes simplex virus (HSV):

recurrent vesiculoulcerative genital lesions

of Osteomyelitis in older children:

fever and localized bone tenderness. Local swelling, redness, warmth, and suppuration may occur subsequently

of Sinusitis in younger children:

fever, purulent nasal discharge, and daytime cough that persists longer than 10 days. Suggestive signs of acute sinusitis include periorbital swelling, localized tenderness to pressure, and malodorous breath

of Trichinosis: fever, weakness, and muscle pain. Also eyelid edema, a maculopapular rash, and petechial hemorrhages in the conjunctiva and beneath the nails. Serious complications include congestive heart failure, delirium, psychosis, paresis, and coma. Hemoptysis and pulmonary consolidation are common.

...TIME:

of infestation with Head lice in children:

during the winter

that patients get Pneumonia, viral:

in midwinter and spring, when influenza may reach epidemic proportions, which is due in

part to "population closeness"
of infection with Rotavirus:

during the cooler months of the year

...TISSUES involved with:

Toxocara canis:

lungs, heart, liver, skeletal muscle, brain, and eyes

...VALVE AFFECTED BY BACTERIAL ENDOCARDITIS:
the mitral valve

...VEINS AFFECTED BY PHLEBOTHROMBOSIS:
deep leg veins

...VENEREAL DISEASE in the US and western Europe, diagnosed:

Chlamydia trachomatis, N. Gonorrhoeae

...VIRUSES WHICH CAUSE ACUTE ENCEPHALITIS:
herpes simplex virus, arboviruses, and enteroviruses

...TOGAVIRUSES IN THE UNITED STATES:
the alphaviruses

MEDICAL ISSUES

...HOSPITAL DISCHARGE DIAGNOSES (by groups):
diseases of the circulatory system and digestive system; complications of pregnancy; accidents, poisoning and violence; and problems of the genitourinary and respiratory systems.

...MEDICAL PROBLEMS:

Acute: upper respiratory conditions, influenza, and injuries

in Young Women:

The Most Common
OTHERS:
dysmenorrhea

...MEDICAL SPECIALISTS:

surgical subspecialists, internal medicine subspecialists, general practitioners, general internists and general surgeons.

...REASONS FOR OFFICE VISITS:

general examination, routine prenatal examination, throat problems, diagnosis and management of hypertension, postoperative visits, cough, head cold, upper respiratory infection, back symptoms, skin rash and gynecologic examination.

...REFERENCE BOOK CONSULTED IN MANY PUBLIC LIBRARIES:

the *Physicians' Desk Reference*

MUSCULOSKELETAL AND CONNECTIVE TISSUE

...BONES AFFECTED IN MULTIPLE MYELOMA:

skull, spine, ribs, pelvis, and femur

...BONE FRACTURED DURING CHILDBIRTH:

the clavicle

...CHEST WALL DEFORMITY:

an exceedingly depressed sternum (pectus excavatum - funnel chest)

...COMPLAINT:

in Clostridial myositis and cellulitis (gas gangrene):

severe pain at the site of injury

...CONNECTIVE TISSUE DISORDER:

Systemic Lupus Erythematosus, primary Sjogren's disease

280

The Most Common
OTHERS:

...DISEASE:
> of Connective tissue, heritable:
>> Marfan syndrome, Ehler-Danlos syndrome, and osteogenesis imperfecta

...DISORDER:
> Connective Tissue:
>> Systemic Lupus Erythematosus, primary Sjogren's disease

...DRUGS:
> Used to treat:
>> Necrotizing fasciitis:
>>> penicillin and an aminoglycoside

...DYSTONIAS, adult onset, not-inherited:
>> torticollis

...EYE MUSCLE involved in Grave's Disease:
>> Inferior Rectus

...FINDING:
> in Cardiac involvement in Systemic Lupus Erythematosus:
>> pericarditis, although all layers of the heart may be involved
> in Osteoarthritis (primary):
>> Heberden's nodes

...JOINT AFFECTED BY JUVENILE RHEUMATOID ARTHRITIS, in pauciarticular JRA:
> the knee

...MUSCLE GROUP AFFECTED BY:
> Dystonic Reactions (a form of Extra-Pyramidal Side Effects of Antipsychotic therapy):
>> those of the face, neck, and tongue
> Trichinosis larvae in cysts:
>> muscles of the limbs, diaphragm, tongue, jaw, larynx, ribs, and eye. Larvae in other organs,

The Most Common
OTHERS:

including the heart and brain, cause edema, necrosis, and focal infiltration of neutrophils, eosinophils, and lymphocytes, but they do not encyst

...MUSCULAR DYSTROPHY:

Duchenne's muscular dystrophy

...MYOPATHY:

Hereditary: muscular dystrophies, myotonic muscle disorders, metabolic myopathies, congenital myopathies

...ORGAN AFFECTED BY:

Scleroderma (progressive systemic sclerosis):

the skin and blood vessels. Also the gastrointestinal tract, lungs, kidneys, and heart.

...ORGANISM:

which Produces:

Myotoxin in Clostridial Myonecrosis (Gas Gangrene):

C. perfringens Type A (80-90% of cases), but myotoxin may also come from *C. novyi*, *C. septicum*, and rarely from three other species

Toxin (myotoxin) in Clostridial Myonecrosis (Gas Gangrene):

C. perfringens Type A (80-90% of cases), but myotoxin may also come from *C. novyi*, *C. septicum*, and rarely from three other species

...PROCEDURE PERFORMED FOR:

Osteogenic sarcoma:

amputation

...SYMPTOM:

of Osteomyelitis in older children:

fever and localized bone tenderness. Local swelling, redness, warmth, and suppuration may occur subsequently

282

<u>NEOPLASTIC</u>

...AGE OF MALES PRESENTING WITH SERTOLI-LEYDIG
TUMORS OF THE TESTICLE:

30 to 45 years of age

...ATRIUM AFFECTED BY CARDIAC MYXOMA:

left > right

...BONES AFFECTED IN MULTIPLE MYELOMA:

skull, spine, ribs, pelvis, and femur

...CARCINOMA OF THE BREAST:

infiltrating adenocarcinoma of ductal origin

...CARCINOMA OF THE GASTROINTESTINAL TRACT AS-
SOCIATED WITH ACANTHOSIS NIGRI-
CANS:

tumors of the stomach

...CARCINOMA METASTATIC TO THE KIDNEYS:

bronchogenic, often oat cell

...CARDIAC TUMOR:

direct extension of bronchogenic carcinoma

...COMPLAINT:
associated with Carcinoma of the Gallbladder:

right upper quadrant pain

...DEGENERATIVE CHANGE of leiomyoma:

hyalinization, cystic degeneration, calcification (most commonly in postmenopausal
women)

...DISEASE:
in Children:
Malignant:

The Most Common
OTHERS:

acute leukemia

...EFFECTS OF:
   Oat cell carcinoma, bronchial carcinoid:

humoral effects of circulating polypeptide
substances

...EXTRACRANIAL SOLID TUMOR OF CHILDHOOD:

neuroblastoma

...FATAL CANCER IN MEN AND WOMEN:

carcinoma of the lung

...FINDING:
   on Pelvic examination of a patient with myomata uteri:

uterine enlargement

   in Renal cell carcinoma (clear cell carcinoma, Grawitz's tumor, renal adenocarcinoma, hypernephroma):

hematuria

...GASTROINTESTINAL CARCINOMA ASSOCIATED WITH
      ACANTHOSIS NIGRICANS:

tumors of the stomach

...GLIOMA of spinal cord in adults:

ependymoma

...HISTOLOGIC PATTERN SEEN IN:
   Bronchial adenoma:

carcinoid

   Ovarian cancers of childhood:

endodermal sinus tumor

...IMMUNOPHENOTYPE OF CELLS IN CHILDREN WITH
      ACUTE LYMPHOCYTIC LEUKEMIA
      (ALL):
   CALLA-positive non-T, non-B cell ALL >
   CALLA-negative non-T, non-B cell ALL (3
   to 4 times)

The Most Common

OTHERS:

...LYMPH NODES INVOLVED IN METASTASES OF HYPO-
PHARYNGEAL CARCINOMAS:

the upper, mid, and lower jugular chain nodes;
the retropharyngeal nodes of Rouviere; and,
less frequently, the nodes along the spinal accessory nerve in the posterior triangle

...MASSES OF:

Mediastinum:

Anterosuperior mediastinum:

thyroid, thymus, teratoma, lymphoma, lipo-
matosis

Middle mediastinum:

aneurysm, lymphoma, metastases, esophageal
tumor, duplication cysts

Posterior mediastinum:

neurogenic tumor, aneurysm, duplication
cysts, metastases, infection

Uterine origin:uterine leiomyomas

...METAPLASIA seen:

squamous metaplasia of bronchial epithelium

...MODE OF:

spread of Colon cancer:

lymphatic spread

Discovery of tubular adenomas of the colon:

as incidental lesions at autopsy, or during endoscopic or barium enema studies performed
for investigation of some other intestinal problem. Occasionally, however, they come to
clinical attention because of bleeding. Rarely,
large pedunculated lesions may be the leading
point of an intussusception

...NODES INVOLVED IN METASTASES OF HYPOPHARYN-
GEAL CARCINOMAS:

285

The Most Common

OTHERS:

the upper, mid, and lower jugular chain nodes; the retropharyngeal nodes of Rouviere; and, less frequently, the nodes along the spinal accessory nerve in the posterior triangle

...OUTCOME FOR CHILDREN WITH ACUTE LYMPHOCYTIC LEUKEMIA (ALL):

continuous complete remission

...PHENOTYPE IN CHILDREN WITH ACUTE LYMPHOCYTIC LEUKEMIA (ALL):

early pre-B-cell type

...POLYPS OF THE COLON:

adenomatous polyp (aka: polypoid adenoma, tubular adenoma)

...PRESENTING COMPLAINT:
in Wilm's tumor (nephroblastoma):

abdominal mass

...PRESENTING SYMPTOMS:
in Symptomatic Small Bowel Tumors:

bleeding, perforation, or obstruction

...PRIMARY NEOPLASMS WHICH METASTASIZE TO THE:
Heart: lung breast, lymphoma, leukemia, melanoma

...PROCEDURE PERFORMED FOR:
Osteogenic sarcoma:

amputation

...RISK FACTORS for:
Cancer:

Endometrial:

unopposed endogenous or exogenous estrogen exposure, polycystic ovary disease (particularly in those under 40), obesity, late menopause (due to longer, chronic estrogen levels), estrogen - secreting tumors, nulliparity, family his-

The Most Common

OTHERS:

tory, menstrual irregularities (chronic, unopposed estrogen), concurrent malignancies of the ovaries, breast, or colon

...SIGNS OF:

Breast cancer: breast lump, then spontaneous nipple discharge. Other presenting manifestations include skin changes, axillary lymphadenopathy, or signs of locally advanced or disseminated disease.

...SIGNS OF:

Wilms' tumor:

Physical findings:

a palpable abdominal mass. Hypertension is rare

...SITUATION IN WHICH:

Brachytherapy is employed:

gynecologic and head and neck tumors, usually in combination with external beam radiation

...SITUATION IN WHICH:

Lymphangiosarcoma is seen:

after a mastectomy that is complicated by lymphedema of the arm

...SIZE OF ADENOMATOUS POLYPS OF THE COLON:

smaller than 1 cm in diameter

...SIZE OF CARCINOMAS OF THE STOMACH AT THE TIME OF DISCOVERY:

between 2 and 10 cm in diameter (80%) > less than 2 cm (~10%)

...STAGE OF PROSTATE ADENOCARCINOMA AT DETECTION:

Stage C

287

The Most Common

OTHERS:

...SURGICAL PROCEDURE PERFORMED FOR:

Osteogenic sarcoma:

amputation

...SYMPTOM:

of Brain tumor:

headaches, irritability, vomiting, and gait abnormalities. Morning headaches are most characteristic, but drowsiness and abnormal behavior are also quite common. Symptoms may be intermittent, particularly in very young children, who have open fontanelles

of Cancer of the pancreas:

pain

of invasive Carcinoma of the Cervix:

postcoital or irregular bleeding

of Endometrial Carcinoma:

irregular menses or postmenopausal bleeding

of Pancreatic cancer:

pain

of Squamous cell carcinoma of the vagina:

vaginal discharge, which is often bloody

of Testicular cancer:

a painless enlargement usually noticed during bathing or after a minor trauma. Painful enlargement of the testis occurs in 30 to 50% of patients and may be the result of bleeding or

infarction in the tumor.

of Wilms' tumor:

enlarged abdomen, abdominal pain, and painless hematuria

...TARGET ORGANS FOR METASTATIC DISEASE:

lung, liver, bone, and brain

...TIME:
> that Carneous degeneration of uterine leiomyomas occurs:
>> during pregnancy

...VISCERAL CANCER IN THE UNITED STATES:
>> carcinoma of the colon and rectum

NEUROLOGIC

...BACTERIA:
> involved in Brain abscess:
>> *Streptococci* (may be in combination with other anaerobes [*Bacteroides* and *Propionibacterium*] or enterobacteriaceae [*E. coli* and *Proteus*]), *Staphylococci*

...CONGENITAL ANOMALY:
> of the Nervous system:
>> myelomeningocele

...COROLLARY OF CHRONIC ALCOHOLISM:
>> atrophy of the Purkinje and granular cells of the cerebellum

...DEMYELINATING DISEASE:
>> multiple sclerosis

...DISEASE:
> of Peripheral nerves:
>> Presumed autoimmune, postinfectious:
>>> Guillain-Barre syndrome. Others include some cases of Bell's palsy and sixth nerve palsy. Gradenigo syndrome (sixth nerve palsy associated with pain in the distribution of the fifth cranial nerve) is secondary to osteomyelitis of the petrous ridge of the sphenoid bone. Brachial plexus neuropathies have been asso-

289

The Most Common
OTHERS:

...DISORDER:
                                 ciated with influenza vaccination

...DISORDER:
    Neurologic, of newborns:
                asphyxial brain injury, seizures, pericranial and intracranial hemorrhage, hydrocephalus, hypotonia, myelomeningocele
    Neurologic motor, in the neonatal period:
                hypotonia

...GLIOMA of spinal cord in adults:
                ependymoma

...GROUP OF NEUROLOGIC DISEASES:
                epilepsy

...NEUROECTODERMAL DEFECT involved in bacterial meningitis:
                congenital sinus tract

...NEUROLOGICAL DISORDERS:
                stroke, epilepsy, Parkinson's Disease
    in the Neonatal period:
                asphyxial brain injury
        Motor disorder:
                hypotonia
    in Newborns: asphyxial brain injury, seizures, pericranial and intracranial hemorrhage, hydrocephalus, hypotonia, myelomeningocele

...NEUROPATHY:
    Compressive: carpal tunnel syndrome, ulnar nerve injury, peroneal nerve (usually fibular head)
    Peripheral: hereditary sensory and motor neuropathy (HSMN), Guillain-Barre syndrome and other postinfectious, presumably autoimmune, neuropathies. Less common causes include bra-

OTHERS:

chial and lumbar plexus neuropathies, hereditary sensory neuropathies, giant cell neuropathy, Leber's optic atrophy, and neuroaxonal
dystrophy

...NEUROTRANSMITTERS IN THE SYNAPSES IN THE HU-
MAN BRAIN:

gamma-aminobutyric acid (GABA) and gly-
cine

...PERIPHERAL NEUROPATHIES:

hereditary sensory and motor neuropathy
(HSMN), Guillain-Barre syndrome and other
postinfectious, presumably autoimmune, neuropathies. Less common causes include brachial and lumbar plexus neuropathies, hereditary sensory neuropathies, giant cell
neuropathy, Leber's optic atrophy, and neuroaxonal dystrophy

...SEIZURE in:

Neonate: focal clonic

Adult: tonic clonic (grand mal)

...SYMPTOM:

of Brain tumor:

headaches, irritability, vomiting, and gait abnormalities. Morning headaches are most
characteristic, but drowsiness and abnormal
behavior are also quite common. Symptoms
may be intermittent, particularly in very
young children, who have open fontanelles

...VIRUSES WHICH CAUSE ACUTE ENCEPHALITIS:

herpes simplex virus, arboviruses, and enteroviruses

The Most Common
OTHERS:
NUTRITIONAL AND METABOLIC

...AMINO ACID DISORDER:

>>> PKU (phenylketonuria)

...CONGENITAL ENZYME DEFICIENCY:

>>> combined deficiency of sucrase and isomaltase. Congenital lactase deficiency is much less common, but a transient lactase deficiency frequently follows an episode of infectious

>> gastroenteritis

...DISORDER:

> of Amino acid metabolism:

>>> PKU (phenylketonuria)

> of Eating:
>> in Children:

>>> anorexia nervosa, then bulimia

> Metabolic, of red blood cells:

>>> G6PD deficiency

> Nutritional:
>> in the Industrialized countries:

>>> obesity

...EATING DISORDER OF CHILDREN:

>>> anorexia nervosa, then bulimia

...ENDOCRINE-METABOLIC DISEASE OF CHILDHOOD:

>>> insulin-dependent diabetes mellitus (IDDM),

>>> type I

...ENZYMES WHICH CAUSE ENZYMOPATHIC HEMOLYTIC ANEMIAS:

> Glycolytic enzymes:

>>> pyruvate kinase (PK)

> Hexose monophosphate shunt enzymes:

>>> glucose-6-phosphate dehydrogenase (G6PD)

The Most Common
OTHERS:

...FOODS:

which cause Allergic reactions:

> milk, eggs, shellfish, peanuts and other nuts, cereal grains (gluten), citrus fruits, and the preservatives (metabisulfite) and dyes (yellow food dye no. 5) added to foods

Contaminated with *Clostridium botulinum* toxin:

> most commonly present in vegetables or other foods that have been improperly home-canned and stored without refrigeration, conditions that provide suitable anaerobic conditions for growth of the vegetative cells that elaborate the neurotoxins (A-G)

...GENETIC HYPERLIPIDEMIA IN CHILDHOOD:

> familial hypercholesterolemia

...HYPERLIPIDEMIA IN CHILDHOOD:

Genetic: familial hypercholesterolemia

...INTRACELLULAR STORAGE PARTICLES:

> fat, pigments and dust(carbon dust particles, lipofuscin, iron, melanin, bilirubin)

...METABOLIC DISORDER OF RED BLOOD CELLS:

> G6PD deficiency

...NUTRITIONAL DISORDER IN THE INDUSTRIALIZED COUNTRIES:

> obesity

...ORGAN AFFECTED BY:

Mucopolysaccharidoses (MPSs):

> the liver and spleen (hepatosplenomegaly), skeleton (skeletal dysplasia, dwarfism, and joint contractures), brain (megalencephaly and mental retardation), heart (aortic and mitral valve incompetence), and respiratory system

293

The Most Common
OTHERS:

(tracheal stenosis)

...RED BLOOD CELL METABOLIC DISORDER:

G6PD deficiency

...SURGICAL PROCEDURE PERFORMED FOR:

Morbid obesity:

vertical banded gastroplasty; then stomach bypass with Roux en Y

OBSTETRICS AND GYNECOLOGY

...ANOMALY:

Congenital:

of the Uterus:

Rokitansky-Kuster-Hauser syndrome

...β2-ADRENERGIC AGENTS USED FOR PREMATURE LABOR:

ritodrine and terbutaline

...BONE FRACTURED DURING CHILDBIRTH:

the clavicle

...BREECH PRESENTATION during childbirth:

Frank type (feet by face)

...CARCINOMA OF THE BREAST:

infiltrating adenocarcinoma of ductal origin

...CARDIAC DISEASE (form of):

Preexisting, in pregnancy:

rheumatic heart disease

...CHARACTERISTIC associated with myomata uteri:

abnormal menstrual bleeding

...CHROMOSOMAL ABNORMALITY:

in Maternal age over 35 years of age:

OTHERS:

Trisomy 21. Others include other autosomal trisomies (i.e., 13 and 18) and sex chromosomal abnormalities

...COAGULATION ABNORMALITY in women with PIH (pregnancy-induced hypertension):

thrombocytopenia

...COMPLAINT:

in Endometriosis:

pelvic pain, dysmenorrhea, dyspareunia

in a Gynecologic Practice:

pelvic pain and abdominal pain

...CONGENITAL ANOMALY:

of the Uterus: Rokitansky-Kuster-Hauser syndrome

...CONGENITAL MALFORMATION:

In diabetes (maternal) during pregnancy:

caudal regression, situs inversus, renal anomalies (ureter duplex, agenesis, cystic kidney), heart anomalies (transposition of the great vessels, ventricular septal defect, atrial septal defect), CNS defects (anencephaly, spina bifida, hydrocephalus), anal/rectal atresia

...CONSEQUENCES:

of Prenatal rubella infection:

cataracts, deafness, congenital heart disease, brain damage (sometimes including microcephaly), and secondary retardation. Some cases of early infantile autism have also been associated with prenatal rubella

of Toxic exposure at the preimplantation stage of embryonic development:

embryonic death

...CONTRAINDICATIONS for:

Pregnancy: Eisenmenger's syndrome, primary pulmonary

The Most Common

OTHERS:

> hypertension, congestive cardiomyopathy, inoperable cyanotic congenital heart disease, congestive cardiac failure despite adequate medical treatment

...DIAGNOSIS:

in self-referred Female Clinic Patients with sexually transmitted disease:

> vaginitis

...DRUGS:

Abused during pregnancy:

> alcohol, cocaine (Beck)

Used to treat:

Preeclampsia, severe:

> $MgSO_4$

...EVENT ASSOCIATED WITH THE ONSET OF ACUTE PELVIC INFLAMMATORY DISEASE:

> a recent menstrual flow

...FINDING:

in Nipple discharge, unilateral:

> an intraductal area of papillomatosis or a single intraductal papilloma, but 30% of patients will have cancer (from Stillman)

on Pelvic examination of a patient with myomata uteri:

> uterine enlargement

...FREQUENCY USED IN OBSTETRIC ULTRASOUND:

> 3.5 mHz and 5 mHz

...HISTOLOGIC PATTERN SEEN IN:

Ovarian cancers of childhood:

> endodermal sinus tumor

...INCISION employed in Cesarean Section:

> Kerr (low transverse)

296

...INDICATIONS:

for Cesarean section:

>fetal distress, dystocia, abnormal presentation, hemorrhagic complications, metabolic complications, previous cesarean section

for Hospitalizing pregnant diabetic patients:

>uncontrolled hyperglycemia, ketoacidosis, persistent ketonuria, proteinuria, hypertension, deterioration in renal function, pyelonephritis, excessive weight gain, preterm labor

for Ultrasound in obstetric patients:

>pregnancy dating, diagnosis of multiple pregnancy, fetal growth, placental localization, presentation, position and lie of the fetus, amniocentesis for prior knowledge of placental site and position of fetal parts, and detection of congenital anomalies

...INFECTION:

Maternal, which causes congenital anomalies and mental retardation:

>cytomegalic inclusion body disease, rubella

Natal and Prenatal, resulting in mental retardation:

>cytomegalic inclusion disease, rubella, herpes simplex, toxoplasmosis, and syphilis

associated with a Papovavirus:

>skin warts (verrucae)

Trichomonas vaginalis:

>vaginal infections

in Women ages 16-25 years of age (most common serious infection):

>acute PID (pelvic inflammatory disease)

...LAPAROSCOPIC FINDINGS in patients with false-positive

The Most Common
OTHERS:

clinical diagnosis of acute pelvic inflammatory disease (PID) with pelvic disorders other than PID:

acute appendicitis, endometriosis, corpus luteum bleeding, ectopic pregnancy, pelvic adhesions only, benign ovarian tumor, chronic salpingitis, miscellaneous

...LAPAROSCOPY AND LAPAROTOMY DIAGNOSES in patients with false-negative clinical diagnosis of Acute Pelvic Inflammatory Disease (PID) by laparoscopy:

ovarian tumor, acute appendicitis, ectopic pregnancy, chronic salpingitis, acute peritonitis, endometriosis, uterine myoma, uncharacteristic pelvic pain, miscellaneous

...MASSES OF UTERINE ORIGIN:

uterine leiomyomas

...MATERNAL INFECTION WHICH CAUSES RETARDATION:

cytomegalic inclusion body disease

...MATERNAL INFECTION WHICH CAUSES CONGENITAL ANOMALIES AND MENTAL RETARDATION:

not available. Rubella #2 according to Gregory.

...MEDICAL PROBLEMS:
in Young Women:

dysmenorrhea

...METHOD OF:
Antepartum Monitoring:

non-stress testing

Contraception in industrialized countries:

oral contraceptives

298

The Most Common

OTHERS:

...NATAL AND PRENATAL INFECTIONS RESULTING IN
MENTAL RETARDATION:

cytomegalic inclusion disease, rubella, herpes
simplex, toxoplasmosis, and syphilis

...OPERATION IN OBSTETRICS:

episiotomy

...ORGAN AFFECTED BY:

Birth injury: the head, skeleton, liver, and peripheral nerves

...ORGANISM:

which Causes:

Puerperal Mastitis:

Staphylococcus aureus from the infant's nose
and throat

...PROBLEMS:

of Infants of diabetic mothers:

hypoglycemia, hypocalcemia, polycythemia,
hyperbilirubinemia, and neonatal macrosomia

of the Preterm Neonate:

respiratory distress syndrome

Medical:

in Young Women:

dysmenorrhea

...REASONS THAT MANY TEENAGERS STOP USING
ORAL CONTRACEPTIVES:

bleeding between menstrual periods

...RENAL PROBLEM SEEN BY OBSTETRICIANS:

symptomatic bacteriuria

...RISK FACTORS for:

Cancer:

Endometrial:

unopposed endogenous or exogenous estrogen
exposure, polycystic ovary disease (particular-

The Most Common
OTHERS:

ly in those under 40), obesity, late menopause (due to longer, chronic estrogen levels), estrogen - secreting tumors, nulliparity, family history, menstrual irregularities (chronic, unopposed estrogen), concurrent malignancies of the ovaries, breast, or colon

Gestational diabetes:

family history of Diabetes mellitus (including distant relatives), history of glycosuria, history of diabetic tendency or glucose intolerance, obesity (over 120% of ideal body weight), patient's own birthweight over 9 lbs., poor obstetric history (including habitual abortions, large baby or suspected large for gestational age [LGA] in present pregnancy, unexplained stillbirths, congenital anomalies, history of toxemia, polyhydramnios [past or present], pyelonephritis or recurrent urinary tract infections)

Preterm labor: previous preterm labor or delivery, anomalous uterus (DES daughter, uterine surgery), second trimester abortion (≥ 2, SAB or TAB), incompetent cervix, cone biopsy, large fibroids, multiple gestation, pyelonephritis, recurrent urinary tract infections, cervical dilation or effacement (≤ 36 weeks), uterine "irritability" (≤ 36 weeks), placenta previa, oligo-polyhydramnios

Uteroplacental insufficiency:

preeclampsia/ eclampsia, chronic hypertension, collagen vascular disease, diabetes mellitus, renal disease, anemia, Rh sensitization,

The Most Common

OTHERS:
hyperthyroidism, advanced maternal age, cyanotic heart disease, prolonged pregnancy, isoimmunization, adolescent pregnancy, drug abuse, AIDS ·

...SEXUALLY TRANSMITTED DISEASE:
Chlamydial infection - Chlamydial cervicitis and urethritis (since *Chlamydia trachomatis* is hard to isolate and since the infection is not a reportable disease at this time, exact figures about its prevalence are not available)

Non-gonococcal:
Chlamydia trachomatis

Reported in the United States:
Neisseria gonorrhoeae (since *Chlamydia trachomatis* is hard to isolate and since the infection is not a *reportable* disease at this time, exact figures about its prevalence are not available)

...SEXUALLY TRANSMITTED PROTOZOAL INFECTION:
Trichomonas vaginalis

...SIDE EFFECT:
in Women using oral contraceptives:
break-through bleeding and weight gain

...SIGNS OF:
Breast cancer: breast lump, then spontaneous nipple discharge. Other presenting manifestations include skin changes, axillary lymphadenopathy, or signs of locally advanced or

disseminated disease.

...SURGICAL PROCEDURE PERFORMED FOR:
Stress Urinary Incontinence:
vaginal cystourethropexy

301

The Most Common
OTHERS:

...SYMPTOM:

    of invasive Carcinoma of the Cervix:

        postcoital or irregular bleeding

    of Ectopic Pregnancy:

        abnormal uterine bleeding or spotting, which usually begins 7-14 days after the missed menstrual period. Then unilateral pelvic pain, which may be knife-like and stabbing or dull and less well-defined.

    of Endometrial Carcinoma:

        irregular menses or postmenopausal bleeding

    of Premenstrual Syndrome:

        abdominal bloating, anxiety, breast tenderness, crying spells, depression, fatigue, irritability, weight gain

    of Squamous cell carcinoma of the vagina:

        vaginal discharge, which is often bloody

    of Vulvar Hyperplastic Dystrophy:

        constant pruritus

    of Vulvar Lichen Sclerosus:

        chronic soreness associated with "vulvar dysuria", pruritus

    of Vulvovaginitis:

        Vulvar symptoms:

            burning, inching, odor

...TERATOGEN (major teratogen) TO WHICH A FETUS MAY BE EXPOSED:

        alcohol

...TIME:

    of Anovulation:

        during the 2 years after menarche (i.e., the first menses) and the 3 years before meno-

The Most Common
OTHERS:

pause
that Carneous degeneration of uterine leiomyomas occurs:

during pregnancy
during which Inversion of the Uterus occurs:

immediately following delivery
for Miscarriage:

first trimester pregnancy
that Nausea and vomiting, distaste for food, and queasiness
occur during the first 3 months of pregnancy:
most often noted upon rising (therefore called

"morning sickness")

...TREATMENT:
for Ectopic Pregnancy:

salpingectomy

...TUMORS:

of Breast:
Palpable:
in Patients under 30 years of age:
fibroadenoma, papillomatosis, breast abscess,
cystosarcoma phyllodes, and mesothelial neoplasms
in Patients over 30 years of age:
breast cysts, fibrocystic disease, breast cancer,
breast abscess, fat necrosis, or cystosarcoma
phyllodes
...VENEREAL DISEASE in the US and western Europe, diagnosed:

Chlamydia trachomatis, N. Gonorrhoeae

The Most Common
OTHERS:
OPHTHALMOLOGY

...ABNORMALITY:
>   of Extrinsic ocular muscles in patients with Grave's disease:
>> upper rotation. Lateral rotation is frequent too

...EYE MUSCLE involved in Grave's Disease:
>> Inferior Rectus

...LESION:
>   Ocular, in children afflicted with herpes simplex:
>> keratoconjunctivitis

OTOLARYNGOLOGY

...LANGUAGE DISORDER:
>> developmental language disorder

...METHOD OF:
>   Diagnosing:
>> acute Sinusitis:
>>> radiography

...ORGANISM:
>   which Causes:
>> Sinusitis: *S. pneumoniae*, unencapsulated strains of *H. influenzae*, and *B. catarrhalis*

...SYMPTOM:
>   of Sinusitis in younger children:
>> fever, purulent nasal discharge, and daytime cough that persists longer than 10 days. Suggestive signs of acute sinusitis include periorbital swelling, localized tenderness to pressure, and malodorous breath

304

PANCREAS

...ANATOMICAL RELATIONSHIP:
  between the Common bile duct and the pancreatic duct:
> the ducts most commonly unite outside the
> duodenum and traverse the duodenal wall and
> papilla as a single duct, the ducts join the du-
> odenal wall and have a short common chan-
> nel, least commonly they enter the duodenum
> independently

...INDICATION:
  for Surgical Intervention in chronic pancreatitis:
> unrelenting pain

...METHOD OF:
  Diagnosing:
    Pseudocysts:
> ultrasound or CT scan

...RAPID NONINVASIVE TEST USED FOR DIAGNOSING
        CHOLELITHIASIS, DILATATION OF
        BILE DUCTS, OR ENLARGEMENT OF
        THE PANCREAS:
> ultrasonography

...SITUATION IN WHICH:
  Pancreas is removed for benign disease:
> surgical therapy for chronic pancreatitis

...SYMPTOM:
  of Cancer of the pancreas:
> pain
  of Pancreatic cancer:
> pain

The Most Common
OTHERS:

<u>PEDIATRICS</u>

...BONE FRACTURED DURING CHILDBIRTH:

        the clavicle

...CARDIAC DISEASE (form of):

  in young Children:

        congenital heart disease

...CHRONIC DISEASE:

  in Children: chronic lung disease; asthma is the most com-

        mon of the chronic lung diseases

...CHRONIC LUNG DISEASE OF CHILDREN:

        asthma

...DISEASE:

  in Children:

    Chronic: chronic lung disease; asthma is the most com-

        mon of the chronic lung diseases

    Malignant:

        acute leukemia

    Endocrine-metabolic, in childhood:

        insulin-dependent diabetes mellitus (IDDM),

        type I

...DISORDER:

  Clinically important, in Caucasian children:

    Autosomal recessive:

        cystic fibrosis

  of Eating:

    in Children:

        anorexia nervosa, then bulimia

  of primary Esophageal motility in children:

        gastroesophageal reflux. Others are rare, most

306

commonly achalasia

Neurologic, of newborns:

asphyxial brain injury, seizures, pericranial and intracranial hemorrhage, hydrocephalus, hypotonia, myelomeningocele

Neurologic motor, in the neonatal period:

hypotonia

...DRUGS:

Abused by American teenagers:

alcohol

...EATING DISORDER OF CHILDREN:

anorexia nervosa, then bulimia

...EMERGENCY IN NEONATES, acquired:

Gastrointestinal:

necrotizing enterocolitis

...ENDOCRINE-METABOLIC DISEASE OF CHILDHOOD:

insulin-dependent diabetes mellitus (IDDM), type I

...EXTRACRANIAL SOLID TUMOR OF CHILDHOOD:

neuroblastoma

...FATAL CONGENITAL HEART LESION IN NEWBORNS:

hypoplastic left heart syndrome

...GASTROINTESTINAL EMERGENCY IN NEONATES, acquired:

necrotizing enterocolitis

...GENERAL SURGICAL PROCEDURE in the child:

repair of an inguinal hernia

...GENETIC HYPERLIPIDEMIA IN CHILDHOOD:

familial hypercholesterolemia

...HISTOLOGIC PATTERN SEEN IN:

The Most Common
OTHERS:

Ovarian cancers of childhood:

endodermal sinus tumor

...HYPERLIPIDEMIA IN CHILDHOOD:

Genetic: familial hypercholesterolemia

...IMMUNOPHENOTYPE OF CELLS IN CHILDREN WITH ACUTE LYMPHOCYTIC LEUKEMIA (ALL):

CALLA-positive non-T, non-B cell ALL > CALLA-negative non-T, non-B cell ALL (3 to 4 times)

...INDICATIONS:

for Acute Abdominal surgery in childhood:

appendicitis

...INDICATION:

of a Genetic problem that is recognized in the school-aged child:

mental retardation

...INFECTION:

Adenovirus:

in Children:

pharyngoconjunctivitis

...INJURY:

Resulting in an emergency ward visit by children:

that due to a fall

Treated in emergency departments for all children under 16 years of age:

poisoning #3

...LANGUAGE DISORDER:

developmental language disorder

...LUNG DISEASE OF CHILDREN, chronic:

asthma

...MICROBES in:
>Stools:
>>of Bottle fed infants:
>>>*Lactobacillus acidophilus*, gram-negative enteric rods, enterococci, and anaerobic rods such as *Clostridium* sp.
>>of Breast fed infants:
>>>*Lactobacillus bifidus*, enteric rods, enterococci, and staphylococci

...MODE OF:
>Suicide among teenagers:
>>drug overdose

...NEUROLOGICAL DISORDERS:
>in the Neonatal period:
>>asphyxial brain injury
>Motor disorder:
>>hypotonia

>in Newborns: asphyxial brain injury, seizures, pericranial and intracranial hemorrhage, hydrocephalus, hypotonia, myelomeningocele

...ORGAN AFFECTED BY:
>Birth injury: the head, skeleton, liver, and peripheral nerves

...ORGANISM:
>which Causes:
>>Fungal infections of the skin in adolescents:
>>>*Microsporum*, *Trichophyton*, *Epidermophyton*, and *Pityrosporum*

...ORIGIN OF BACTERIAL INFECTION AND NEONATAL SEPSIS:
>acquired via the birth canal or nosocomially. The infection almost always is bacteremic (often with seeding of the meninges via the

OTHERS:

blood) and associated with systemic symptoms

...OUTCOME FOR CHILDREN WITH ACUTE LYMPHOCYTIC LEUKEMIA (ALL):

continuous complete remission

...PATHOGEN OF CHILDHOOD DIARRHEA in developed countries:

rotavirus

...PHENOTYPE IN CHILDREN WITH ACUTE LYMPHOCYTIC LEUKEMIA (ALL):

early pre-B-cell type

...PRESENTING COMPLAINT:
   in Wilm's tumor (nephroblastoma):

abdominal mass

...PROBLEMS:
   Esophageal:
      in Infants:

gastroesophageal reflux

   of Infants of diabetic mothers:

hypoglycemia, hypocalcemia, polycythemia, hyperbilirubinemia, and neonatal macrosomia

   of the Preterm Neonate:
      respiratory distress syndrome

   Medical:
      in Young Women:

dysmenorrhea

...PULMONARY FUNCTION TESTS USED IN CHILDREN:
      spirometry, flow-volume curves, and lung volumes. Tests less commonly used in children include maximal voluntary ventilation (MVV), diffusing capacity of the lung (DL_{CO}), and closing volume (CV).

...REASONS THAT ADOLESCENTS DO NOT USE BIRTH
CONTROL:

> denial of the ability to get pregnant and the
> unexpected nature of the intercourse

...REASONS THAT MANY TEENAGERS STOP USING
ORAL CONTRACEPTIVES:

> bleeding between menstrual periods

...SEIZURE in:

Neonate: focal clonic

...SIGNS OF:

Wilms' tumor:

Physical findings:

> a palpable abdominal mass. Hypertension is
> rare

...SITUATION IN WHICH:

Incest between siblings occurs:

> in families in which children share the same
> bedroom

...SKIN PROBLEM IN ADOLESCENTS:

> acne, fungal infections

...SUBSTANCE ABUSED BY ADOLESCENTS:

> alcohol

...SURGICAL PROCEDURE PERFORMED FOR:

Gastroesophageal reflux in children:

> Nissen fundoplication

...SYMPTOM:

of Celiac disease in children:

> diarrhea. Failure to thrive is frequently seen.
> Vomiting is more common in younger pa-
> tients. There may be abdominal distention
> and irritability. Short-stature, iron-resistant
> anemia, and rickets may be seen in older chil-

The Most Common
OTHERS:

dren
of Cow's milk and soy protein intolerance in children:
vomiting and diarrhea. Rectal bleeding may
be seen if colitis is present. Edema secondary
to excessive enteric protein loss may be dramatic and is often associated with anemia.
Rhinorrhea, wheezing, and eczema may occasionally be seen and are frequently accompanied by eosinophilia and an elevated serum
immunoglobulin E (IgE) level. Anaphylaxis

rarely is observed but may be life threatening
of Gastroesophageal reflux in children:

vomiting
of Osteomyelitis in older children:
fever and localized bone tenderness. Local
swelling, redness, warmth, and suppuration

may occur subsequently
of Sinusitis in younger children:
fever, purulent nasal discharge, and daytime
cough that persists longer than 10 days. Suggestive signs of acute sinusitis include periorbital swelling, localized tenderness to pres-

sure, and malodorous breath
of Wilms' tumor:
enlarged abdomen, abdominal pain, and pain-

less hematuria
...SYSTEMS AFFECTED BY CYSTIC FIBROSIS:

the gastrointestinal and respiratory systems
...THERAPEUTIC AGENTS USED TO TREAT CHILDHOOD
HYPERTENSION:
Thiazide diuretics (Chlorothiazide, hydrochlo-
rothiazide); Vasodilators (hydralazine); β-
adrenergic antagonists [β - blockers] (propran-

312

olol, metoprolol); central sympatholytics (methyldopa). Other agents, including newer β- blockers, prazosin, minoxidil, clonidine, guanabenz, and captopril are proving to be effective and well tolerated but are not officially

approved for use in children

...THERAPY EMPLOYED FOR CHILDHOOD AUTOIMMUNE HEMOLYTIC ANEMIA:

supportive care and judicious use of transfusions and corticosteroids

...THYROID CONDITION IN CHILDHOOD AND ADOLESCENCE:

chronic lymphocytic thyroiditis (CLT) (commonly referred to as Hashimoto's thyroiditis)

...TIME:

during which Brain Dysfunction/Hyperactivity/Attention Deficit Disorder usually presents:

the school aged child (age 7-10)

of infestation with Head lice in children:

during the winter

of Presentation of:

Insulin-dependent diabetes mellitus (IDDM) in children:

in early adolescence

Necrotizing enterocolitis in preterm infants:

within the first week of feeding

that Umbilical hernias close by:

closure by the age of 2 years

...TRACHEOESOPHAGEAL FISTULA pattern:

distal segment of esophagus (connected to stomach) forms a connection to the bronchus near the carina. The proximal segment ends as a blind pouch in the midthorax.

313

The Most Common
OTHERS:

<u>CLINICAL PHARMACOLOGY</u>

...AGENTS USED FOR INDUCTION OF GENERAL ANES-
      THESIA OR SEDATION FOR REGIONAL
      ANESTHESIA:

    the benzodiazepines and droperidol

...ANOMALY:
   secondary to in utero exposure to Anticonvulsants:

    oral clefts and congenital heart defects

...ANTIBIOTICS:
   Implicated in pseudomembranous colitis:

    ampicillin, clindamycin, and cephalosporins.
    Then penicillins other than ampicillin, eryth-
    romycin, and sulfur drugs. Rarely tetracy-
    cline, cloramphenicol, and enterally adminis-

    tered aminoglycosides

   Used to treat:
    Clostridial infections other than tetanus:

      penicillin is most often used, although many
      antibiotics have prevented gas gangrene in la-
      boratory animals

    Diverticulitis:

      ampicillin

...ANTIHISTAMINES PRESCRIBED AS ANTIANXIETY
        DRUGS:
      diphenhydramine (Benadryl) and hydroxyzine

      (Atarax or Vistaril)

...ANTIHYPERTENSIVE AGENTS USED:

      thiazides

...ANTIPSYCHOTIC ASSOCIATED WITH EJACULATORY
        DYSFUNCTIONS:

314

thioridazine

...β2-ADRENERGIC AGENTS USED FOR PREMATURE LA-
BOR:

ritodrine and terbutaline

...CATHARTICS USED IN TREATMENT OF POISONING:

magnesium sulfate administered at 250 mg/
kg, sodium sulfate administered at 250 mg/kg,
and magnesium citrate administered at 4 ml/
kg

...CONSEQUENCES:

of Toxic exposure at the preimplantation stage of embryonic
development:

embryonic death

...COROLLARY OF CHRONIC ALCOHOLISM:

atrophy of the Purkinje and granular cells of
the cerebellum

...DEPRESSANTS ABUSED IN SUBSTANCE ABUSE:

barbiturates, methaqualone, and tranquilizers

...DIGITALIS GLYCOSIDE USED:

digoxin

...DOPAMINERGIC AGONIST USED TO TREAT PARKIN-
SON'S DISEASE:

levodopa, usually in combination with carbidopa

...DRUGS:

Abused by American teenagers:

alcohol

Abused during pregnancy:

alcohol, cocaine (Beck)

involved in Malignant Hyperthermia:

halothane and succinylcholine, but may occur

315

The Most Common
OTHERS:
with all anesthetic agents

associated with Raynaud's Phenomenon:

nicotine, propranolol, and the ergot derivatives

Used to treat:

Gilles de la Tourette Syndrome:

haloperidol

Leprosy: dapsone

Necrotizing fasciitis:

penicillin and an aminoglycoside

Preeclampsia, severe:

$MgSO_4$

Seizures:

Generalized tonic-clonic seizures:

carbamazepine (Tegretol), phenytoin (Dilantin), valproate (Depakene, Depakote), phenobarbital (Luminal), primidone (Mysoline)

Partial seizures:

carbamazepine (Tegretol), phenytoin (Dilantin), phenobarbital (Luminal), primidone (Mysoline)

Absence (petit mal) seizures:

ethosuximide (Zarontin), valproate (Depakene, Depakote), clonazepam (Klonopin)

Upper gastrointestinal tract infections after gastrointestinal surgery:

a cephalosporin or a penicillin-aminoglycoside combination

...HALLUCINOGENIC AGENTS available on the street and abused:

LSD (lysergic acid diethylamide), mescaline, psilocybin, and phencyclidine (PCP)

which people Overdose on:

PCP
...INHALANTS ABUSED:

toluene (found in glue), trichloroethylene, gasoline, and fluorinated hydrocarbons and nitrous oxide (found in aerosol sprays)

...INHALATION ANESTHETIC AGENTS used today:

nitrous oxide, then halothane

...MACROLIDE ANTIBIOTIC in use:

erythromycin

...MALFORMATION ASSOCIATED WITH THE USE OF:

Streptomycin: ototoxicity

Synthetic progestins:

hypospadias

Thalidomide: limb reduction

...METHOD OF:

Contraception in industrialized countries:

oral contraceptives

...MUSCLE GROUP AFFECTED BY DYSTONIC REACTIONS (a form of Extra-Pyramidal Side Effects of Antipsychotic therapy):

those of the face, neck, and tongue

...MUSCLE RELAXANT USED IN ANESTHESIA:

Depolarizing agent:

succinylcholine

...NARCOTICS ABUSED:

heroin, methadone, meperidine, and propoxyphene

...ORGAN AFFECTED BY:

Thalidomide exposure:

ears (microtia and anotia) and the heart

...REASONS THAT MANY TEENAGERS STOP USING ORAL CONTRACEPTIVES:

The Most Common
OTHERS:
bleeding between menstrual periods

...RESULT OF HYPERTENSION SECONDARY TO TYRA-
MINE INGESTION WHEN ON MAO IN-
HIBITORS:
an intense, throbbing headache accompanied
by other unpleasant sensations; cerebrovascular accidents, hyperpyrexia, and death have infrequently occurred

...ROUTE OF ADMINISTRATION OF COCAINE among experienced users:
intravenously or intranasally (inhaling through
a straw or rolled paper); occasionally it may
be sprinkled on the genitalia

...SIDE EFFECT:
Endocrine and Endocrine-like:
of antipsychotic and non-MAO inhibitor anti-depressant
therapy:
weight gain. Others include amenorrhea or
other menstrual changes, inappropriate lactation in females and galactorrhea in males,
breast enlargement in either sex, alterations of
glucose metabolism, peripheral edema due to
fluid retention, alterations in various laboratory tests
of Indomethacin (Indocin):
gastrointestinal distress and headaches
of MAO inhibitors:
drowsiness or stimulation (short lived), insomnia, giddiness, dizziness, dry mouth, impotence, orthostatic hypotension, constipation,
and weight gain. They also can precipitate a
manic or schizoaffective attack. Occasional
patients develop hepatotoxicity. The most serious (but infrequent) side effect is hyperten-

318

sion (hypertensive crisis, cerebrovascular bleeding) and hyperpyrexia in response to ingested tyramine (or other pressor amines)

of Smallpox vaccination:

eczema vaccinatum (eczema resulting from vaccinia virus infection)

in Women using oral contraceptives:

break-through bleeding and weight gain

...SITUATION IN WHICH:

Low dose heparin therapy fails:

following operations that greatly stimulate thrombosis, such as hip replacement; in patients with an active thrombotic process, or; when poor absorption or clearance of heparin results in inadequate therapeutic levels

...STIMULANTS USED IN SUBSTANCE ABUSE:

amphetamines and cocaine

...SUBSTANCE ABUSED BY ADOLESCENTS:

alcohol

...TERATOGEN (major teratogen) TO WHICH A FETUS MAY BE EXPOSED:

alcohol

...THERAPEUTIC AGENTS USED TO TREAT CHILDHOOD HYPERTENSION:

Thiazide diuretics (Chlorothiazide, hydrochlorothiazide); Vasodilators (hydralazine); β−adrenergic antagonists [β - blockers] (propranolol, metoprolol); central sympatholytics (methyldopa). Other agents, including newer β- blockers, prazosin, minoxidil, clonidine, guanabenz, and captopril are proving to be effective and well tolerated but are not officially approved for use in children

319

The Most Common
OTHERS:

...THERAPY EMPLOYED FOR CHILDHOOD AUTOIM-
MUNE HEMOLYTIC ANEMIA:
supportive care and judicious use of transfusions and corticosteroids

...TIME:
that Akathisia appears during antipsychotic therapy:
between the second and tenth weeks of therapy

that Jaundice secondary to antipsychotics and non-MAO inhibitor anti-depressants occurs:
between the second and fourth weeks of therapy

that Pseudoparkinsonism appears during antipsychotic therapy:
between the second and tenth weeks of therapy

...TREATMENT:
for Hypothyroidism:
L-Thyroxine

...UNTOWARD EFFECT OF BARBITURATES:
sedation

...USED AND ABUSED SUBSTANCE:
alcohol

PHYSICAL AGENTS

...AGENT RESPONSIBLE FOR INJURY IN MOTOR VEHI-
CLE ACCIDENTS:
kinetic energy

...EFFECTS OF:

320

Exposure to nickel: dermatitis ("nickel itch")

...HALOGEN PRESENT IN BIOLOGIC SYSTEMS:

chlorine

...INDUCERS OF DNA MUTATIONS:

chemical mutagens

...INHALANTS ABUSED:

toluene (found in glue), trichloroethylene, gasoline, and fluorinated hydrocarbons and nitrous oxide (found in aerosol sprays)

...ORGANIC DUSTS which cause hypersensitivity pneumonitis:
thermophilic actinomycetes, fungi, and avian proteins

...POLLENS WHICH CAUSE ALLERGIC RHINITIS:
ragweed, other weeds, grasses, and trees

PSYCHIATRIC

...ANTIHISTAMINES PRESCRIBED AS ANTIANXIETY DRUGS:
diphenhydramine (Benadryl) and hydroxyzine (Atarax or Vistaril)

...ANTIPSYCHOTIC ASSOCIATED WITH EJACULATORY DYSFUNCTIONS:

thioridazine

...CHANGES AFTER A COMPLETE COURSE OF ELECTRO-CONVULSIVE THERAPY (ECT):
weight gain (in comparison with pretreatment weight), EEG changes that persist for several months, amenorrhea, and memory impairment that gradually normalizes. The permeability of the blood-brain barrier is temporarily in-

The Most Common
OTHERS:

creased, which may significantly alter the effects of certain drugs. Rare changes include prolonged memory impairment and spontaneous seizures.

...DEFENSE MECHANISM EXPERIENCED EARLY IN THE COURSE OF HOSPITALIZATION:

regression

...DIAGNOSIS:
associated with Suicide:

depression

...DISTURBANCE OF PERCEPTION IN SCHIZOPHRENIA:
hallucinations, usually auditory but also visual, olfactory, and tactile. The auditory hallucinations are most often voices - one or several

...DOPAMINERGIC AGONIST USED TO TREAT PARKINSON'S DISEASE:
levodopa, usually in combination with carbidopa

...DRUG USED TO TREAT GILLES DE LA TOURETTE SYNDROME:
haloperidol

...EVENT WHICH PRECIPITATES SUICIDE:
a conflict with parents. Others include a breakup with a girlfriend or boyfriend, a conflict with peers, pregnancy, etc.

...METHOD OF:
committing Suicide in the United States:
firearms, hanging, and drug overdose

Women: drug overdose

...MODE OF:
Suicide among teenagers:

drug overdose

...MUSCLE GROUP AFFECTED BY DYSTONIC REAC-
TIONS (a form of Extra-Pyramidal Side Effects of Antipsychotic therapy):

those of the face, neck, and tongue

...PEOPLE WHO ATTEMPT SUICIDE:

females > males

Successfully:

by Age: Ages 75-84 > ages 65-74 > ages 85 and over
> ages 55-64 > ages 45-54 > ages 25-34 >
ages 35-44 > ages 15-24 > ages 5-15

by Intelligence:

higher intelligence > lower intelligence

by Race and Sex:

white males > white, both sexes > nonwhite
males > nonwhite, both sexes > white females
> nonwhite females

by Sex: males > females

by Socioeconomic Status:

higher socioeconomic status > lower socioeconomic status

Unsuccessfully:

females > males

...PSYCHIATRIC PROBLEM in elderly:

depression, dementia

...PSYCHOTIC DISORDER:

schizophrenia

...RETROSPECTIVE PSYCHIATRIC DIAGNOSIS in some series of suicides:

severe depression, alcoholism

...RESULT OF HYPERTENSION SECONDARY TO TYRA-
MINE INGESTION WHEN ON MAO IN-
HIBITORS:

an intense, throbbing headache accompanied

323

The Most Common
OTHERS:

by other unpleasant sensations; cerebrovascular accidents, hyperpyrexia, and death have infrequently occurred

...SIDE EFFECT:

following Electroconvulsive Therapy (ECT):

headaches of several hours' duration; transient centrally mediated changes in blood pressure and cardiac rhythm; increased appetite (often a therapeutic benefit); brief euphoria; and postconvulsive confusion and amnesia. Rare side effects and complications that may occur during or immediately following a single treatment include: cardiac arrest; prolonged apnea; dental fractures and tongue biting; minor hemorrhages from nose, ears, or poorly healed abrasions; aspiration of gastric contents; and significant cardiac arrhythmias

Endocrine and Endocrine-like:

of antipsychotic and non-MAO inhibitor anti-depressant therapy:

weight gain. Others include amenorrhea or other menstrual changes, inappropriate lactation in females and galactorrhea in males, breast enlargement in either sex, alterations of glucose metabolism, peripheral edema due to fluid retention, alterations in various laboratory tests

...SIGNS AND SYMPTOMS OF MOOD DISORDERS:

Depression:

Signs: stooped and slow moving, tearful and sad facies, dry mouth and skin, constipation

Symptoms:

Cognitive features:

self-criticism, <u>sense of worthlessness</u>, guilt,

324

OTHERS:

pessimism, <u>hopelessness</u>, despair, distractible, <u>poor concentration</u>, uncertain and indecisive, variable obsessions, somatic complaints (<u>particularly in the elderly</u>), memory impairment, delusions and hallucinations

Emotional features:

<u>depressed</u> mood,"blue", <u>irritability</u>, anxiety, <u>anhedonia</u>, <u>loss of interest</u>, loss of zest, diminished emotional bonds, interpersonal withdrawal, preoccupation with death

Vegetative features:

<u>fatigability</u>, no energy, <u>insomnia</u> or hypersomnia, anorexia or hyperrexia, weight loss or gain, psychomotor retardation, psychomotor agitation, impaired libido, frequent diurnal variation

Mania:

Signs: psychomotor agitation

Symptoms:

Cognitive features:

elevated self-esteem, <u>grandiosity</u>, speech disturbances (loud, word rhyming [clanging], pressure of speech, flight of ideas, progression to incoherence), <u>poor judgement</u>, disorganization, paranoia, delusions and hallucinations

Emotional features:

excited, elevated mood, euphoria, emotional <u>lability</u>, rapid temporary shifts to acute depression, <u>irritability</u>, low frustration tolerance, demanding, egocentric

Physiological features:

boundless energy, insomnia, <u>little need for sleep</u>, decreased appetite

...SITUATION IN WHICH:

325

The Most Common
OTHERS:
Incest between siblings occurs:

in families in which children share the same bedroom

...TIME:

that Akathisia appears during antipsychotic therapy:

between the second and tenth weeks of therapy

during which Brain Dysfunction/Hyperactivity/Attention Deficit Disorder usually presents:

the school aged child (age 7-10)

that Pseudoparkinsonism appears during antipsychotic therapy:

between the second and tenth weeks of therapy

...USE OF:

Hypnosis within the field of somatic medicine:

for the relief of various painful states, especially during childbirth and in dentistry

PULMONARY

...BACTERIA:

Causing:

Empyema:

streptococci, pneumococci, and staphylococci

...CHRONIC LUNG DISEASE OF CHILDREN:

asthma

...CONDITION ASSOCIATED PLEURAL EFFUSIONS:

Exudate: infection, infarction, or neoplasm

Transudate: congestive heart failure, cirrhosis, or renal disease

326

OTHERS:

...HISTOLOGIC PATTERN SEEN IN:
Bronchial adenoma:

carcinoid

...LUNG DISEASE OF CHILDREN, chronic:

asthma

...METHOD OF:
Introducing pathogens into the respiratory tract:

inhalation of aerosolized microorganisms

...ORGANIC DUSTS which cause hypersensitivity pneumonitis:
thermophilic actinomycetes, fungi, and avian

proteins

...ORGANISM:
which Causes:
Bronchopulmonary infections (recurrent bronchitis, bronchiectasis, and bronchopneumonia) in patients with Cystic fibrosis:

Staphylococcus aureus and a mucoid form of

Pseudomonas aeruginosa

...PEOPLE SEEN WITH GIANT CELL PNEUMONITIS SECONDARY TO MEASLES:

Hosts unable to form antibody

...PNEUMONIA IN ADULTS:

influenza A virus pneumonia

...PREDISPOSING CONDITIONS for:
Deep-vein thrombosis and pulmonary embolism:

surgery, childbirth

...PULMONARY COMPLICATION FOLLOWING SURGERY:
atelectasis

...PULMONARY DISEASE CAUSING PULMONARY HYPERTENSION:
obstructive emphysema

...PULMONARY FUNCTION TESTS PERFORMED:

The Most Common
OTHERS:

              spirometry

in Children: spirometry, flow-volume curves, and lung volumes. Tests less commonly used in children include maximal voluntary ventilation (MVV), diffusing capacity of the lung (DL_{CO}), and closing volume (CV)

...TIME:

that patients get Pneumonia, viral:

in midwinter and spring, when influenza may reach epidemic proportions, which is due in part to "population closeness"

...TRACHEOESOPHAGEAL FISTULA pattern:

distal segment of esophagus (connected to stomach) forms a connection to the bronchus near the carina. The proximal segment ends as a blind pouch in the midthorax.

...TRIGGERS FOR ASTHMA ATTACKS:

a respiratory viral infection is the most common trigger in young children. Common agents include rhinovirus, respiratory syncytial virus, and parainfluenza virus. Air pollutants, especially ozone, sulfur dioxide, or cigarette smoke, are also common triggers. Allergens include animal danders, molds, pollens of ragweed and other grasses, and house dust. Foods are seldom a cause but, when implicated, include chocolate, shellfish, nuts, and (very rarely) milk. Exercise-induced symptoms are very common. Emotions play a major role in asthma. They can trigger attacks; also, symptoms are frequently exacerbated by laughing or crying.

328

The Most Common
OTHERS:

RADIOLOGY

...CHEST RADIOGRAPHIC FINDINGS OF NONDISSECTING
ANEURYSM OF THE THORACIC AORTA:
mediastinal widening or a focal bulge of the
aortic contour. Displacement of the trachea or
esophagus frequently occurs. Curvilinear cal-
cifications are frequently seen in the wall of
the aneurysm. The presence of a pleural effusion raises the possibility of leakage from the
aneurysm

...ROENTGENOGRAPHIC FINDINGS IN PATIENTS WITH
LACTOSE INTOLERANCE AND MALAB-
SORPTION:
the most commonly reported findings are rapid dilution of the barium in the small and large
bowel; rapid transit time, i.e., barium reaching
the ascending and transverse colon within 30
to 60 minutes; and dilation of the small bowel
loops

RENAL AND ELECTROLYTES

...ACID-BASE DISORDER:
metabolic alkalosis > respiratory alkalosis >
respiratory acidosis > metabolic acidosis
in traumatized, postoperative, and Critically ill patients who
have not deteriorated to serious renal, circulatory, or pulmonary dysfunction:
alkalosis
in severely injured and Critically ill patients who have suf-
fered renal, pulmonary, or circulatory dysfunction:

329

The Most Common
OTHERS:

acidosis

...CARCINOMA METASTATIC TO THE KIDNEYS:

bronchogenic, often oat cell

...CLINICAL FEATURE seen in kidneys in congestive heart failure:

mild to moderate proteinuria

...COMPOSITION OF URINARY CALCULI
(in descending order of occurrence)

calcium oxalate and calcium phosphate, calcium oxalate, struvite (magnesium ammonium phosphate), calcium phosphate, uric acid, cystine

...FINDING IN RENAL CELL CARCINOMA (clear cell carcinoma, Grawitz's tumor, renal adenocarcinoma, hypernephroma):

hematuria

...ELECTROLYTE ABNORMALITY IN HOSPITALIZED PATIENTS:

hyponatremia, which has an incidence of 1%

...LONG-TERM SEQUELA OF RECURRENT PYELONEPHRITIS:

hypertension

...MECHANISM FOR HYPONATREMIA IN SURGICAL PATIENTS:

the administration of hypotonic fluids.

...PREOPERATIVE DISORDER OF FLUID IMBALANCE:

intravascular volume depletion, usually a result of disease process, such as from hemorrhage, vomiting, or diarrhea.

...ROUTE FOR NONRENAL LOSS OF POTASSIUM:

the gastrointestinal tract (i.e. vomiting, diarrhea [especially the watery-diarrhea syndrome], laxative abuse, and villous adenoma

330

of the colon)
...SITUATION IN WHICH:
    Hyperkalemia arises:

        during acute acidosis
...TIME:
    of Presentation of:
        adult Polycystic Kidney:
            in the fifth decade

SEXUALLY RELATED

...ANTIPSYCHOTIC ASSOCIATED WITH EJACULATORY
                    DYSFUNCTIONS:

        thioridazine
...GENOTYPE OF TRUE HERMAPHRODITES:
        46,XX

SURGICAL

...ADRENAL CORTICAL ABNORMALITY PRESENT IN
            THE PERIOPERATIVE SETTING:
            a relative hypoadrenalism referred to as secon-
            dary adrenal insufficiency, due to glandular
            suppression in patients taking daily exogenous
            glucocorticoids.
...AGENTS USED FOR INDUCTION OF GENERAL ANES-
            THESIA OR SEDATION FOR REGIONAL
            ANESTHESIA:

        the benzodiazepines and droperidol
...ANATOMICAL RELATIONSHIP:
    between the Common bile duct and the pancreatic duct:

The Most Common
OTHERS:

the ducts most commonly unite outside the duodenum and traverse the duodenal wall and papilla as a single duct, the ducts join the duodenal wall and have a short common channel, least commonly they enter the duodenum independently

of the Cystic artery:

nearly always a branch of the right hepatic artery that passes behind the cystic duct

between the Cystic duct and the hepatic duct:

an acute angle

...BACTERIA:

in wound Infections after surgery on the colon:

E. coli

...DRUGS:

Used to treat:

Upper gastrointestinal tract infections after gastrointestinal surgery:

a cephalosporin or a penicillin-

aminoglycoside combination

...ENDOCRINE AUTOGRAFT used:

parathyroid autotransplantation

...FATAL EVENT following the more usual surgical procedures such as herniorrhaphy and cholecystectomy:

pulmonary embolism

...GENERAL SURGICAL PROCEDURE in the child:

repair of an inguinal hernia

...INCISION employed in Cesarean Section:

Kerr (low transverse)

...INDICATIONS:

for Acute Abdominal surgery in childhood:

appendicitis

for Cardiac transplantation:

>ischemic heart disease and cardiomyopathy

for Cesarean section:

>fetal distress, dystocia, abnormal presentation, hemorrhagic complications, metabolic complications, previous cesarean section

for Cholecystectomy:

>chronic cholecystitis

for Coronary artery bypass surgery:

>disabling angina pectoris refractory to medical management. Other clinical indications for surgery include post-myocardial infarction angina (ischemic chest pain at rest occurs within days or weeks of acute myocardial infarction and is refractory to medical therapy); myocardial ischemia not accompanied by angina pectoris; precocious ischemic heart disease (e.g., one or more myocardial infarctions occurring in patients ≤ 45 years of age); and angina pectoris in patients undergoing other cardiac surgery such as valve replacement

for Elective Surgery in Crohn's disease:

>failure of symptoms to respond to medical management

for Emergency Laparotomy in Hong Kong:

>#1 not available. Oriental cholangiohepatitis (recurrent pyogenic cholangitis) is the third most common indication

for Intra-Aortic Balloon Pump (IABP) in the CCU:

>cardiogenic shock complicating acute myocardial infarction. Patients with a surgically correctable mechanical defect (acute ventricular septal defect, papillary muscle rupture, or ventricular aneurysm) are most likely to benefit.

The Most Common
OTHERS:

An IABP may also be helpful in stabilizing patients with severe, reversible myocardial stunning following reperfusion with a thrombolytic agent or coronary angioplasty

for Surgery after plombage therapy for tuberculosis:

pleural infection (pyogenic or tuberculous) and migration of the plombage material, causing pain or compression of other organs. Following pulmonary resection, tuberculous empyema may develop in the postpneumonectomy space, sometimes associated with a bronchopleural fistula or bony sequestration. Persistent bronchopleural fistula after chemotherapy and closed tube drainage may require direct operative closure

for Surgical Intervention in chronic pancreatitis:

unrelenting pain

...MECHANISM FOR HYPONATREMIA IN SURGICAL PATIENTS:

the administration of hypotonic fluids.

...METHOD OF:

Bypassing severe occlusive disease in the aorta and iliac arteries:

aortoiliac or aortofemoral grafting using artificial graft material

Managing anal fissures:

surgical excision

...MODE OF:

development of Anorectal abscess:

extension of a local traumatic abscess within the anorectal canal

...NON-BILIARY SURGERIES ASSOCIATED WITH POST-OPERATIVE ACUTE ACALCULOUS

CHOLECYSTITIS:
Major cardiac and aortic surgery or renal transplantation

...NONSELECTIVE PORTAL-SYSTEMIC SHUNT PERFORMED:
end-to-side portacaval shunt, followed by the mesocaval (mesenteric-caval) shunt and the side-to-side portacaval shunt

...ORGANS INVOLVED IN HERNIAS:
incarcerated hernia:
small intestine and omentum are the most commonly incarcerated tissues
Epigastric hernias:
the falciform ligament and omentum
Richter's hernia:
it most commonly involves the antimesenteric border of the small intestine

...ORGANISM CULTURED FROM ANAL RECTAL ABSCESS FISTULAS:
E. Coli

...PORTAL-SYSTEMIC SHUNT PERFORMED:
Nonselective: end-to-side portacaval shunt, followed by the mesocaval (mesenteric-caval) shunt and the side-to-side portacaval shunt

Selective: the distal splenorenal (Warren) shunt

...PREOPERATIVE DISORDER OF FLUID IMBALANCE:
intravascular volume depletion, usually a result of disease process, such as from hemorrhage, vomiting, or diarrhea.

...PROCEDURE PERFORMED FOR:
Osteogenic sarcoma:
amputation
emergency Portacaval shunting:

The Most Common
OTHERS:

an end-to-side portacaval shunt or a mesocaval shunt

...SELECTIVE PORTAL-SYSTEMIC SHUNT PERFORMED:

the distal splenorenal (Warren) shunt

...SHUNT PERFORMED:

Portal-systemic:

Nonselective:

end-to-side portacaval shunt, followed by the mesocaval (mesenteric-caval) shunt and the side-to-side portacaval shunt

Selective: the distal splenorenal (Warren) shunt

Tetralogy of Fallot:

Blalock-Taussig operation (i.e., anastomosis of the subclavian artery to a pulmonary artery branch) and the modified Blalock-Taussig operation (i.e., interposition of a tubular graft between the subclavian and pulmonary arteries)

...SITUATION IN WHICH:

Bench surgery is utilized:

kidney surgery such as heminephrectomy, resection of distal renal artery aneurysms, or repair of a traumatic injury

Pancreas is removed for benign disease:

surgical therapy for chronic pancreatitis

...SURGICAL PROCEDURES PERFORMED:

diagnostic dilatation and curettage ("D and C") of the uterus, hysterectomy, tonsillectomy, sterilization of women, hernia repair, oophorectomy (removal of one or both ovaries), Cesarean section, gallbladder removal, muscle surgery and setting of fractures.

in people over Age 65:

Cataract surgery

336

OTHERS:

for Broncholithiasis:

> lobectomy. Bronchoesophageal fistula may require only fistula repair

as Drainage procedure along with truncal vagotomy for peptic ulcer:

> pyloroplasty (Heineke-Mikulicz procedure). Gastrojejunostomy is used less often

for Gastroesophageal reflux in children:

> Nissen fundoplication

for Impotence: penile prosthesis insertion

for Morbid obesity:

> vertical banded gastroplasty; then stomach bypass with Roux en Y

for Osteogenic sarcoma:

> amputation

for Stress Urinary Incontinence:

> vaginal cystourethropexy

...TIME:

for Dehiscence of postoperative wounds:

> although it may occur at any time following wound closure, it is most commonly observed between the fifth and eighth postoperative days, when the strength of the wound is at a minimum

that Myocardial infarction, perioperative, occurs:

> during the first 3 postoperative days. The remainder occur during the next 3 days.

that Perioperative myocardial infarction occurs:

> during the first 3 postoperative days. The remainder occur during the next 3 days.

that Postcardiotomy delirium occurs:

> the symptoms most often appear after the third postoperative day

that Postoperative Atelectasis occurs:

The Most Common
OTHERS:

most frequently in the first 48 hours after operation

that Postoperative Intussusception of the small bowel occurs:
90% occur during the first 2 postoperative weeks, and more than half are in the first week. They most often follow retroperitoneal and pelvic operations

that Postoperative Pancreatitis occurs:
it occurs most often after operations performed in the vicinity of the pancreas and os observed in 2-4% of those patients. Pancreatitis is occasionally observed following cardiopulmonary bypass, parathyroid surgery, and renal transplantation

References

Banov, CH, MD. Treating the itch that persists. *Patient care.* 15 October 1989,.p. 79.

Beck, WW: *Obstetrics and Gynecology.* (The National Medical Series for Independent Study). New York, John Wiley & Sons, Inc., 1989.

Benson, RC: *Handbook of Obstetrics and Gynecology.* Los Altos, Lange Medical Publications, 1983.

Braunstein, H: *Outlines and Review of Pathology.* St. Louis, C.V. Mosby Company, 1987.

Braunwald, E, ed: *Harrison's Principles of Internal Medicine,* 11th ed.. New York, McGraw-Hill Book Company, 1987.

Casciato, DA, ed: *Manual of Clinical Oncology,* 2nd ed. Boston, Little, Brown and Company, 1988.

Chandrasoma, P: *Key Facts in Pathology.* New York, Churchill

Livingstone, Inc., 1986.

Creighton University Lecture Series, Introduction to Clinical Medicine course, Pathology course, Pharmacology course, 1988-89.

Creighton University Lecture Series, Department of OB/GYN, Department of Surgery, 1989-90.

Dworkin, PH: *Pediatrics* (The National Medical Series for Independent Study). New York, John Wiley & Sons, Inc., 1987.

Evans, MI: *Obstetrics and Gynecology* (Pre-Test Series). New York, McGraw Hill, Inc., 1989.

Gregory, I: *Psychiatry*. Boston, Little, Brown and Company, Inc., 1983.

Hiyama, DT, ed.: *The Mont Reid Surgical Handbook* St. Louis, Mosby Year Book, 1990.

Jacob, LS: *Pharmacology* (The National Medical Series for Independent Study). Media, Harwal Publishing Company, 1984.

Jarrell, BE: *Surgery* (The National Medical Series for Independent Study). Media, Harwal Publishing Company, 1986.

Kingsbury, DT, ed.: *Microbiology* (The National Medical Series for Independent Study). Media, Harwal Publishing Company, 1985.

Kraushar, MF: Medical Malpractice Litigation in Cataract Surgery. *Arch Ophthalmol* 1987;105:1339-43.

Krug, RS: *Behavioral Sciences* (Oklahoma Notes Series). New York, Springer-Verlag, 1987.

LiVolsi, VA, ed: *Pathology* (The National Medical Series for Independent Study). Media, Harwal Publishing Company, 1984.

Myers, AR, ed.: *Medicine* (The National Medical Series for Independent Study). Media, Harwal Publishing Company, 1986.

Purdy, RE.: *Handbook of Cardiac Drugs.* Boston, Little, Brown and Company, 1988.

Rich, MW, ed.: *Coronary Care for the House Officer.* Baltimore, Williams & Wilkins, 1989.

Robbins, SL: *Pathologic Basis of Disease.* Philadelphia, W.B.

The Most Common
OTHERS:

Saunders Company, 1984.

Rubin, E, ed.: *Pathology*. Philadelphia, J.B. Lippincott Company, 1988.

Sabiston, DC: *Sabiston's Essentials of Surgery*. Philadelphia, W.B. Saunders Company, 1987.

Schwartz, SI: *Principles of Surgery*. New York, McGraw-Hill Book Company, 1989.

Sierles, FS: *Behavioral Science for the Boreds*. Miami, MedMaster, Inc., 1987.

Stillman, RM: *Surgery Diagnosis and Therapy*. East Norwalk, Appleton and Lange, 1989.

Straub, WH, ed.: *Manual of Diagnostic Imaging*, 2nd ed. Boston, Little, Brown and Company, 1989.

Tomb, DA: *Psychiatry for the House Officer*. Baltimore, Williams & Wilkins, 1988.

Walzer, PD, MD. *Pneumocystic carinii* pneumonia. *Infections in Medicine*. March, 1987, p. 110.

Way, LW: *Current Surgical Diagnosis and Treatment*. Norwalk, Appleton and Lange, 1988.

The Most Common

People Affected or Infected By...

...ABSENCE OF THE KIDNEYS (Congenital), Bilateral:

males > females

...ABSCESS:

Hepatic:

Amebic: male adults

Psoas:

Primary: children and young adults. These abscesses are more common in underdeveloped countries

Secondary:

the most common cause is Crohn's disease; these patients will have the highest incidence

Retropharyngeal:

infants or young children

Spinal epidural:

usually occurs in a patient with an underlying infection, either remote (e.g., a furuncle or dental abscess) or contiguous (e.g., vertebral osteomyelitis, decubitus ulcer, or retroperitoneal abscess). About 1/3 of cases, however, arise spontaneously

...ACCIDENTAL POISONING:

toddlers aged 1 1/2 to 3

...ACUTE CHOLECYSTITIS:

women > men

...ACUTE EPIDIDYMITIS:

young males. The disease is less common in older males

...ACUTE LEUKEMIA:

male predilection only in the very young and the elderly

Lymphoblastic leukemia:

children (80%)

Lymphocytic leukemia (ALL):

white children > black children; males > fe-

The Most Common
PEOPLE AFFECTED OR INFECTED BY:

males (1.2 to 1.3 times)

Myelogenous leukemia (AML):

adults (90%)

Nonlymphocytic leukemia (ANLL):

males > females; black children > white children

...ACUTE PARANOID DISORDER:

persons who have experienced drastic changes in their environment, such as immigrants, refugees, inductees into military service, or prisoners of war

...ACUTE SPASMOTIC LARYNGITIS:

children between 1 and 3 years old

...ACUTE STAPHYLOCOCCAL OSTEOMYELITIS:

boys between 3 and 10 years of age, most of whom have a history of infection or trauma

...ACUTE URETHRITIS:

Gonococcal: blacks > whites

Chlamydial: whites > blacks

...ADENOCARCINOMA:

of the Esophagus:

patients with Barrett's esophagus

of the Kidney (hypernephroma, renal cell carcinoma):

men > women (3:1); usually occurs in the sixth or seventh decade of life

of the Pancreas:

men > women; people aged 50 to 70

...ADENOVIRUS PHARYNGOCONJUNCTIVITIS:

children and infants

...ADRENAL CARCINOMA:

women (two-thirds) > men

...ADYNAMIC COLONIC ILEUS (pseudo-obstruction):

the seriously ill patient with multisystem pathology

...AFFECTIVE DISORDERS:

344

females > males

...AGORAPHOBIA:

women > men (2:1)

...ALCOHOL USE AND ABUSE:

males > females

...ALCOHOL WITHDRAWAL DELIRIUM (DELIRIUM TREMENS):

chronic alcoholics following a brief episode of
sharply increased alcohol consumption
("binge"), even when this is followed by a return to the previous level and not by total abstinence. It may also be provoked by acute illness, injury, or surgery in alcoholics

...ALCOHOLIC PANCREATITIS:

men who have ingested large amounts of alcohol over a period of at least 10 years

...ALCOHOLISM: men > women

...ALPORT'S SYNDROME (hereditary nephritis):

males

...AMNESIA, psychogenic:

women in their teens or 20's, or in men during
the stress of war

...ANALGESIC NEPHROPATHY:

women with a history of chronic headaches,
arthritis, or muscular pain

...ANENCEPHALY:

people in Ireland and Wales; female fetuses >
males (2:1)

...ANEURYSMS:

Intracranial:

Saccular: women are affected slightly more often than
men

of the Splenic artery:

women > men (4:1)

of the Thoracic aorta:

345

The Most Common
PEOPLE AFFECTED
OR INFECTED BY:

Posttraumatic:

these occur more frequently in a younger age group and may not be detected until years after the chest trauma

...**ANGIOMYOLIPOMA OF THE KIDNEY:**

this is seen most often in adults with tuberous sclerosis (adenoma sebaceum, epilepsy, and mental retardation). It is often detected following spontaneous retroperitoneal hemorrhage

...**ANGIOSARCOMA (malignant hemangioendothelioma):**

males > females

...**ANOREXIA NERVOSA:**

this disorder usually develops in adolescence (teenage girls); females > males (10:1)

...**ANTISOCIAL PERSONALITY (DISORDER):**

males > females (3-10:1)

...**ANXIETY DISORDERS:**

women > men

...**AORTIC DISSECTION ("Dissecting Aneurysm"):**

males > females

...**AORTIC STENOSIS:**

aortic stenosis may appear at any stage of adulthood, and there is no clear distinction between the congenital and acquired forms of the disease. It is more common in men than in women

...**AORTOILIAC OCCLUSIVE DISEASE:**

limited to the Aortic bifurcation and common iliac arteries:
female > male

extends from the aorta to include Femoral and distal vessels:
males > females

...**APPENDICITIS:** children between 10 and 15 years of age. Less than 10% of patients are under 5 years old

346

Acute: young adults

...ARCUS SENILIS (Gerontoxon):

it is more frequently observed in the aged, and in men

...ARTERIOVENOUS (AV) MALFORMATIONS BLEEDING:

Cerebral circulation:

the peak incidence for bleeding is between the ages of 15 and 30 years. The majority of AV malformation hemorrhages occur before age 40

...ARTHRITIS:

Rheumatoid: more frequent among women than among men, and also tends to be familial

Juvenile: girls > boys; it begins before age 16 years, most commonly between ages 1 and 4 years

...ASCITES, chylous:

most patients are adults - many of them adult women - with occult cancer, often a lymphoma or adenocarcinoma (of the pancreas or stomach), causing lymphatic obstruction. About 15% of cases occur in young children (usually less than 1 year old) with congenital lymphatic anomalies

...ASTHMA: asthma may begin at any age but most often begins within the first 5 years of life. Before puberty, twice as many boys are affected, but at puberty the incidence of asthma in girls increases

...ASYMPTOMATIC BACTERIURIA of pregnancy:

black multiparas with sickle cell trait

...ATELECTASIS, postoperative:

it affects 25% of patients who have abdominal surgery. It is more common in patients who are elderly or overweight and in those who smoke or have symptoms of respiratory dis-

The Most Common
PEOPLE AFFECTED
OR INFECTED BY:
ease

...ATRIAL SEPTAL DEFECTS:
> females > males (2:1)

...ATROPHIC VAGINITIS:
> postmenopausal women. Also may be found in surgically castrated young women and in women who are breast-feeding (lactating)

...ATTENTION DEFICIT DISORDER:
> males > females

...AUTISM: boys > girls

...AUTOIMMUNE DISEASES:
> females > males

...AUTOIMMUNE HEMOLYTIC ANEMIA:
> women > men, and most commonly those < 50 years old

...BACTERIAL ENDOCARDITIS:
> individuals 50 years of age or older; men > women

...BASAL CELL CARCINOMA:
> predominantly in whites

...BENIGN FEBRILE CONVULSIONS:
> children between 6 months and 3 years of age

...BILATERAL ABSENCE OF THE KIDNEYS (Congenital):
> males > females

...BIPOLAR DISORDER:
> women > men

...BLEEDING OF ARTERIOVENOUS (AV) MALFORMA-
> TIONS:

Cerebral circulation:
> the peak incidence for bleeding is between the ages of 15 and 30 years. The majority of AV malformation hemorrhages occur before age 40

...BLUE VALVE (myxomatous transformation of valve and mi-tral valve prolapse):

females > males

...BRAIN CANCER, primary:

males > females (3:2)

...BRIQUET'S SYNDROME:

women > men

...BRONCHIAL ADENOMAS:

women > men (2:1)

...BRONCHIECTASIS:

patients with cystic fibrosis. Other underlying diseases include foreign body aspiration, immotile cilia syndrome, measles, immunodeficiency syndrome. Other etiologies include dysautonomia, gastroesophageal reflux, tuberculosis, sarcoidosis, and neoplasms

...BRONCHIOLITIS:

this occurs most often during the first 6 months of life, primarily during cold weather months; second and third attacks are rare

...BUERGER'S DISEASE (Thromboangiitis obliterans):

males under 35 years of age, younger than diabetic patients, and are addicted to cigarette smoking

...BULIMIA: females > males (10-20:1)

...CANCER OF:

the Anus: women > men; patients over 50 years old

the Colon: women > men (5:4)

the Colon and Rectum:

people in the United States. The incidence is greater than in Japan, India, Africa, and Latin America

the Esophagus:

males > females (3:1)

of the Gallbladder:

women > men

the Head and neck:

349

The Most Common
PEOPLE AFFECTED
OR INFECTED BY:

                        men aged 50-70 years old.
the Liver and biliary tract:
                        males = females
the Pancreas: males > females (5:4)
the Prostate: the tumor is more prevalent in black males
                 than any other group in the USA. The tumor
                 rarely occurs before age 50, and the incidence
                 increases with age such that in the eighth dec-
                 ade, more than 60% of men have prostate can-
                 cer. In most of these older men, however, the
                 disease is not clinically apparent; only 10% of
                 men over age 65 develop clinical evidence
the Rectum: males > females (4:3)
the Small bowel:
                 males = females
the Stomach: males > females (3:2); Japanese people. A
                 high incidence has also been observed in Lat-
                 in American countries, particularly Chile.
                 Stomach cancer is also common in Iceland
                 and Eastern Europe
Carcinoma of:
    Colon and Rectum:
                 patients who are 60-70 years of age
    Gallbladder:
                 women > men (2:1)
    Large Bowel:
        Proximal to the rectum:
                 no sex predominance
        Rectal:
                 males > females (2:1)
    Stomach: men over 50 years of age
    Thyroid:
        Follicular:
                 females > males (3:1)
        Papillary:

females > males

Ureter:

Transitional cell carcinoma:

men > women (2:1). These lesions develop in persons age 60-70

Vulva: women between the age of 60 and 79 years of age. Fewer are under the age of 40

...CANCERS ATTRIBUTED TO SUN EXPOSURE (namely basal cell carcinoma, squamous carcinoma, and melanoma):

predominantly in whites

...CANDIDIASIS OF THE URINARY TRACT:

women > men (4:1)

...CARBUNCLES ON THE BACK OF THE NECK:

diabetic patients

...CARDIAC MYXOMA:

individuals 30 to 60 years of age

...CARPAL TUNNEL SYNDROME:

this condition primarily afflicts people between 30 and 65 years of age. It is more common in women than in men (2-3:1)

...CAT SCRATCH DISEASE:

children (80%) > adults, and there may be clustering when a stray cat or kittens joins a family

...CEREBROVASCULAR ACCIDENTS (CVA; stroke):

it has a higher incidence with increasing age (25% of CVA's occur in individuals in the 40- to 55-year old age-group; 50% occur in the 65- to 79-year-old group). Men are more susceptible than women. In addition, occurrence of CVA is higher when there is evidence of generalized atherosclerosis

...CHANCROID (*Hemophilus ducreyi*):

young sexually active men who visit prosti-

The Most Common
PEOPLE AFFECTED
OR INFECTED BY:

tutes; people in tropical and subtropical regions and especially in the Far East; it is more frequent in men than women and is associated with promiscuity and poor personal hygiene

...CHEYNE-STOKES RESPIRATION:

patients with cerebral atherosclerosis and other cerebral lesions, but the prolongation of the circulation time from the lung to the brain which occurs in heart failure, particularly in patients with hypertension and coronary artery disease and associated cerebral vascular disease, also appears to precipitate this form of breathing

...CHILD ABUSE:

Abused: although child abuse can affect children of any age, children under 5 are affected most commonly (Sierles); Woods indicates that children less than 3 years of age are affected most frequently and most severely

Abusers: mothers, more often than fathers, are the abusers. Abusing parents commonly were abused when they were children, and families in which child abuse occurs can be found in all socioeconomic strata

...CHILDHOOD PULMONARY DISEASES:

males > females

...*CHLAMYDIA TRACHOMATIS* in women:

young adults, especially those in the lower socioeconomic population and those with multiple sexual partners

...CHOLANGIOCARCINOMA:

people aged 60 -70 years old; men > women

...CHOLECYSTITIS:

Acute: women > men

Emphysematous:

352

males > females (3:1), and 20% of all patients have diabetes mellitus

Postoperative: males (75%) > females (25%)

...CHONDROBLASTOMA:

males > females (2:1); people between the ages of 5 and 25 years of age (90%)

...CHONDROMALACIA PATELLAE:

women

...CHONDROSARCOMA:

people in the middle ages of life (fourth to sixth decades); men > women (2:1)

...CHROMOSOMAL ABERRATIONS:

children born to older women > those born to younger mothers

...CHRONIC GRANULOCYTIC LEUKEMIA:

people in the fourth decade, although children and older adults are also affected

...CHRONIC LYMPHOCYTIC LEUKEMIA:

people > 50 years of age (90%); men > women (2.5:1.0)

...CHRONIC LYMPHOCYTIC (Hashimoto's) THYROIDITIS:

this occurs almost exclusively in women

...CHRONIC MYELOMONOCYTIC LEUKEMIA:

the elderly

...CHYLOUS ASCITES:

most patients are adults - many of them adult women - with occult cancer, often a lymphoma or adenocarcinoma (of the pancreas or stomach), causing lymphatic obstruction.
About 15% of cases occur in young children (usually less than 1 year old) with congenital lymphatic anomalies

...CLEAR CELL CARCINOMA OF THE KIDNEY (Grawitz's tumor, renal adenocarcinoma, hypernephroma, renal cell carcinoma):

353

The Most Common
PEOPLE AFFECTED
OR INFECTED BY:

men > women (3:1); usually occurs in the fifth, sixth or seventh decade of life

...CLEFT LIP WITH OR WITHOUT CLEFT PALATE:

boys (60-80%) > girls; white children (1:1000) > black American children (0.4:1000); Oriental and American Indians > blacks

...CLEFT PALATE (isolated):

girls > boys

...COARCTATION OF THE AORTA:

males > females (2:1). Kravath indicates that coarctation of the aorta occurs most frequently in individuals who have Turner's syndrome

...COARSE BRAIN DISEASES:

men > women

..."COIN LESIONS" OF THE LUNG (Solitary Pulmonary Nodules):

males > females (3-9:1)

...COLORECTAL CARCINOMA:

patients who are 60-70 years of age

...CONGENITAL DISLOCATION OF THE HIP:

girls > boys

...CONGENITAL HYPOTHYROIDISM:

boys = girls

...CONJUNCTIVITIS, vernal:

boys > girls

...CONSTITUTIONAL DELAY OF PUBERTY (growth and development):

boys > girls

...CONVULSIONS, benign febrile:

children between 6 months and 3 years of age

...CORONARY ARTERY DISEASE:

males > females (4:1)

...CORTICAL RENAL NECROSIS, bilateral:

pregnant women, especially after placenta abruptio

...COXA PLANA (Legg-Calve-Perthes disease):

boys between the ages of 4 and 10 years

...CRYPTOCOCCOSIS:

patients with Hodgkin's disease and other forms of malignant lymphoma as well as renal allograft recipients

...CVA (cerebrovascular accidents; stroke):

it has a higher incidence with increasing age (25% of CVA's occur in individuals in the 40- to 55-year old age-group; 50% occur in the 65- to 79-year-old group). Men are more susceptible than women. In addition, occurrence of CVA is higher when there is evidence of generalized atherosclerosis

...CYCLOTHYMIA:

females > males (2:1)

...CYSTIC ADVENTITIAL DEGENERATION OF THE POPLITEAL ARTERY:

young men

...CYSTIC FIBROSIS:

whites (95%) > blacks, and almost never in Orientals

...CYSTITIS: females > males

...D-TRANSPOSITION OF THE GREAT ARTERIES:

males > females

...DEHISCENCE OF POSTOPERATIVE WOUNDS:

it is rare in patients under age 30 but affects about 5% of patients over age 60 having laparotomy. It is more common in patients over age 60 having laparotomy. It is more common in patients with diabetes mellitus, uremia, immunosuppression, jaundice, and cancer; in obese patients; and in those receiving

355

The Most Common
PEOPLE AFFECTED
OR INFECTED BY:

corticosteroids

...DELIRIUM TREMENS:

    chronic alcoholics following a brief episode of sharply increased alcohol consumption ("binge"), even when this is followed by a return to the previous level and not by total abstinence. It may also be provoked by acute illness, injury, or surgery in alcoholics

...DEMENTIA, senile:

    women > men

...DEPENDENT PERSONALITY DISORDER:

    women > men

...DEPRESSION: women > men

...DESMOID TUMORS of the abdominal wall:

    women > men; seem to be more frequent in postpartum women

...DEVELOPMENTAL DISORDERS:

Pervasive:	more frequent among the mentally retarded
Specific:	boys > girls

...DIPHTHERIA:

Cutaneous:	adults living in the tropics
Pharyngeal:	children between 5 and 14 years of age

...DIROFILARIASIS, pulmonary:

    originally reported from Japan and Australia, pulmonary dirofilariasis is most common in the southern and eastern United States

...DISSECTING ANEURYSM OF THE AORTA (Aortic Dissection):

    males > females

...DISTURBANCES OF MEIOTIC DIVISION:

    individuals with structurally abnormal chromosomes

...DIVERTICULUM OF THE BLADDER:

    men > women, most occur in middle age

...DROWNING: males > females; blacks > whites

356

...DRUG DEPENDENCE:

     males > females

...DUODENAL ULCERS:

     males > females (~4:1); duodenal ulcers may occur in any age group but are most common in the young and middle-aged (20-45 years). They are 10 times more common than gastric ulcers in young patients, but in the older age groups the frequency is about equal

...DYSGERMINOMA of the ovary:

     women under the age of 30 (children and adolescents)

...DYSTHYMIA: women > men (3-4:1)

...DYSTONIC REACTIONS (form of Extra-Pyramidal Side Effects of Antipsychotic therapy):

     men > women; almost all cases occur in young persons

...ELECTIVE MUTISM:

     girls > boys

...ELECTRICAL BURNS:

     children under 5 years of age

...EMPHYSEMA, centrilobular:

     men > women

...EMPHYSEMATOUS CHOLECYSTITIS:

     males > females (3:1), and 20% of all patients have diabetes mellitus

...ENDOCARDIAL FIBROELASTOSIS:

     infants and children

  Secondary form:

     adults

...ENDOCARDITIS:

     people over 30 years of age

...EOSINOPHILIC GRANULOMA:

     young adults

The Most Common
PEOPLE AFFECTED
OR INFECTED BY:

...EPIDIDYMITIS, Acute:

young males. The disease is less common in older males

...EPIGASTRIC HERNIAS:

males > females

...ESOPHAGEAL CARCINOMA:

men over the age of 50 years

...ESOPHAGITIS, acute corrosive:

children under the age of 6 years

...EWING'S SARCOMA:

adolescents (two-thirds occur in patients younger than 20 years of age); males > females (1.5 -2:1); rarely seen in blacks

...EXTRA-PYRAMIDAL SIDE EFFECTS OF ANTIPSYCHOT-IC THERAPY:

Dystonic reactions:

men > women; almost all cases occur in young persons

Non-dystonic reactions:

women > men

...FALLS: boys > girls; people in urban areas > people in suburban and rural areas

...FAMILIAL DYSAUTONOMIA (Riley-Day syndrome):

Ashkenazi Jews

...FEBRILE CONVULSIONS, benign:

children between 6 months and 3 years of age

...FECAL IMPACTION:

the elderly, the mentally ill, and the bedridden patient

...FEMORAL HERNIAS:

females > males

...FIBROADENOMA OF THE BREAST, female:

women under 30 years of age

...FIBROMUSCULAR MEDIAL HYPERPLASIA of the renal

358

arteries:
young adults and older children

...FIBROPLASIA OF THE RENAL ARTERIES:
Intimal: males, generally young
Medial: middle-aged women
Subadventitial: young females

...FIRST TRIMESTER MISCARRIAGE:
women over 40 years > women under 30

...FLOPPY VALVE (myxomatous transformation of valve and mitral valve prolapse):
females > males

...FOCAL NODULAR HYPERPLASIA OF THE LIVER:
women > men

...FOLLICULAR CARCINOMA OF THE THYROID:
females > males

...FURUNCLES: furunculosis usually occurs in young adults and is associated with hormonal changes resulting in impaired skin function

...FUSOSPIROCHETOSIS (Vincent's disease; Necrotizing ulcerative gingivitis; trench mouth;):
seen most frequently in young adults. May also occur in children

...GALLSTONE ILEUS:
women > men, and the average age is about 70. However, gallstone ileus may occur in any age group where cholesterol stones are found

...GALLSTONES:
Cholesterol: the incidence of cholesterol gallstone disease is highest in American Indians, lower in Caucasians, and lowest in blacks, with a 2-fold gradient from one group to the next. More than 75% of American Indian women over age 40 are affected. Before puberty, the disease is rare but of equal frequency in both sex-

The Most Common
PEOPLE AFFECTED
OR INFECTED BY:

es. Thereafter, women are more commonly affected than men until after menopause, when the discrepancy lessens

Pigment: pigment stones account for 25% of gallstones in the USA and 60% of those in Japan. The incidence is similar in men and women and in blacks and whites. Pigment stones are rare in American Indians

...GANGRENE, wet or infected:
        diabetics

...GASTRIC ULCERS:
        the peak incidence of gastric ulcer is in patients aged 40-60 years, or about 10 years older than those with duodenal ulcer; men > women; elderly; and in the lower socioeconomic classes

...GASTRITIS, hypertrophic (Menetrier's Disease):
        men over 40 to 60 years of age

...GAUCHER'S DISEASE:
        Jewish children

...GERMINOMA OF THE TESTICLE:
        males before age 45

...GERONTOXON (Arcus Senilis):
        it is more frequently observed in the aged, and in men

...GIANT CELL TUMORS OF BONE:
        people in the middle ages of life

...GOOD MENTAL HEALTH:
        most frequent among those with parents of superior socioeconomic status, and also tends to be associated with high occupational stability or upward mobility

...GRAVE'S DISEASE:
        females > males, including girls > boys (4:1)

...GRAWITZ'S TUMOR (renal adenocarcinoma, clear cell carci-

noma, hypernephroma, renal cell carcinoma):
men > women (3:1); usually occurs in the
fifth, sixth or seventh decade of life

...HAIRY-CELL LEUKEMIA:
men > women (5:1); older people (people less
than 30 years of age are unusual)

...HAMARTOMA OF THE LUNG:
men > women (2:1)

...HASHIMOTO'S DISEASE (lymphadenoid goiter):
women > men, including girls > boys (> 2:1)

...HASHIMOTO'S (Chronic Lymphocytic) THYROIDITIS:
this occurs almost exclusively in women

...HEADACHE, Post Dural-Puncture, after spinal anesthesia:
young women

...HEMANGIOMA:
Hepatic: women > men

...HEMANGIOPERICYTOMA:
adults of all ages

...*HEMOPHILUS DUCREYI* (Chancroid):
young sexually active men who visit prostitutes

...HEPATIC ABSCESS:
Amebic: male adults

...HEPATIC HEMANGIOMA:
women > men

...HEPATOCELLULAR ADENOMA:
women, especially those on oral contraceptives

...HEPATOCELLULAR CARCINOMA (hepatoma):
males > females

...HEPATOMA (hepatocellular carcinoma):
males > females

...HEREDITARY NEPHRITIS (Alport's syndrome):
males

The Most Common
PEOPLE AFFECTED
OR INFECTED BY:

...HERNIAS:

Epigastric:	males > females
Femoral:	females > males (according to Schrock, Jarrell and other sources). Sabiston is the only source reviewed which contradicts this data, citing that femoral hernias are much more common in males than females
Inguinal:	males > females
in Children:	
	males > females (6:1)
Indirect:	males > females
Parastomal:	more common in obese patients and in those in whom a colostomy is placed lateral to the rectus muscle or through the incision of the initial operation
Umbilical:	females > males; black children > white children

...HERPES GENITALIS:

Primary:	teenage girls and unmarried women

...HIGH-ALTITUDE SYSTEMIC EDEMA:

women > men (2:1)

...HIRSCHSPRUNG'S DISEASE:

male infants > females (4:1), except when the entire colon is involved. In that situation, the frequency ratio is reversed, with females predominating

...HISTOPLASMOSIS:

in the United States:

people who reside in Ohio, Indiana, Kentucky, Tennessee, Arkansas, Missouri, and the southern part of Illinois

...HODGKIN'S DISEASE in the developed Western countries:

young adults (except in Japan, a developed country where young adult disease is distinctly uncommon)

362

Adults: the NS subtype of Hodgkin's disease shows a
slight female predominance, whereas the other
histologic subtypes are more common in
males

Children: males (~85%) > females

...HUMAN IMMUNODEFICIENCY VIRUS (HIV):
men > women

...HYPERACTIVITY/MBD SYNDROME:
boys > girls

...HYPEREOSINOPHILIC SYNDROME:
men (> 90%) > women; whites (>80%). Most
patients are in the fifth decade of life, but pediatric and elderly patients have been described

...HYPERNEPHROMA (renal cell carcinoma, renal adenocarcinoma, clear cell carcinoma, Grawitz's tumor):
men > women (3:1); usually occurs in the
fifth, sixth or seventh decade of life

...HYPERPARATHYROIDISM, primary:
more frequent in women (women:men ratio 2-
3:1), especially after the menopause, reflect-
ing the efficacy of estrogens as inhibitors of
PTH-mediated osteolysis

...HYPERSPLENISM, primary:
females > males

...HYPERTENSION:
it is more frequent (and severe) in blacks than
whites

...HYPERTHYROIDISM:
women > men (6:1)

...HYPERTROPHIC SCARS:
blacks, Orientals, and dark-skinned white patients, and are more common in younger patients

...HYPOCALCEMIA:

The Most Common
PEOPLE AFFECTED OR INFECTED BY:

hypoalbuminemic patients, with normal ionized fraction

...HYPOTHYROIDISM:

Congenital: boys = girls

Juvenile: girls > boys

Spontaneous: females > males

...IDIOPATHIC AUTOIMMUNE HEMOLYTIC ANEMIA:

people over the age of 50; women > men

...IDIOPATHIC CONGESTIVE CARDIOMYOPATHY:

adults

...IDIOPATHIC THROMBOCYTOPENIC PURPURA, chronic:

adults; women > men

...ILEUS, gallstone:

women > men, and the average age is about 70. However, gallstone ileus may occur in any age group where cholesterol stones are found

...ILLUSIONS: illusions are most common in delirium but may also occur in functional psychoses

...IMPERFORATE ANUS:

males > females (2:1)

...INCEST: daughters and father (usually stepfather), and may also often occur between siblings

...INDIRECT INGUINAL HERNIAS:

males > females

...INFECTIONS OF THE RESPIRATORY TRACT, Staphylococcal:

infants less than 2 years of age, and especially those under 2 months

...INFECTIOUS MONONUCLEOSIS:

adolescents and young adults

...INGUINAL HERNIAS:

males > females

in Children: males > females (6:1)

364

...INSULINOMA:
    Malignant: males > females
...INTERSTITIAL CYSTITIS:
    middle-aged females
...INTIMAL FIBROPLASIA of the renal arteries:
    males, generally young
...INTUSSUSCEPTION:
    children from 6 months to 2 years of age
...IRON DEFICIENCY IN CHILDHOOD:
    children between 6 and 24 months of age
...ISCHEMIC COLITIS:
    patients over 50
...ISCHEMIC HEART DISEASE:
    individuals from 35 to 64 years of age; men >
    women, whites > blacks
...ISOLATED CLEFT PALATE:
    girls > boys
...JUVENILE HYPOTHYROIDISM:
    girls > boys
...JUVENILE RHEUMATOID ARTHRITIS:
    girls > boys; it begins before age 16 years,
    most commonly between ages 1 and 4 years
...JUXTACORTICAL OSTEOSARCOMA (osteogenic sarcoma):
    women > men
...KAPOSI'S SARCOMA:
    men > women
...*KLEBSIELLA* PNEUMONIA:
    males over 50 years of age with gross dental
    and oral sepsis.
...LARGE BOWEL OBSTRUCTION:
    people after the age of 50 (males = females)
...LARYNGITIS, acute spasmotic:
    children between 1 and 3 years old
...LEGG-CALVE-PERTHES DISEASE (Coxa Plana):
    boys between the ages of 4 and 10 years

The Most Common
PEOPLE AFFECTED
OR INFECTED BY:

...LENTIGO MALIGNA MELANOMA:

> men = women

...A LESION OF THE MEDIAL LONGITUDINAL FASCICU-
LUS:

> multiple sclerosis patients

...LEUKEMIA:

in Childhood:

Acute lymphocytic leukemia (ALL):

> white children > black children; males > fe-
males (1.2 to 1.3 times)

Acute nonlymphocytic leukemia (ANLL):

> males > females; black children > white chil-
dren

Acute leukemia:

> male predilection only in the very young and
the elderly

Acute lymphoblastic leukemia:

> children (80%)

Acute myelogenous leukemia:

> adults (90%)

Chronic granulocytic leukemia:

> people in the fourth decade, although children
and older adults are also affected

Chronic lymphocytic leukemia:

> people > 50 years of age (90%); men > wom-
en (2.5:1.0)

Chronic myelomonocytic leukemia:

> the elderly

Hairy-cell leukemia:

> men > women (5:1); older people (people less
than 30 years of age are unusual)

...LINGUAL THYROID:

> females > males

...LIPOID NEPHROSIS (minimal change disease or nil lesion):

> children between ages 2 and 5 years

366

...LISTERIOSIS, Septicemic:

    in Adults: immunodeficient patients

...LUNG TUMORS:

    Benign: these may occur at almost any age
       Hamartomas:

                men > women (2:1)

    Malignant: about 95% of lung cancers occur in patients who are more than 40 years of age. Seventy-five percent of all lung carcinomas are related to smoking; affected individuals usually have a history of smoking 1 or more packs of cigarettes daily for 20 years

...LYMPHADENOID GOITER (Hashimoto's disease):

                women > men

...LYMPHEDEMA PRAECOX:

                females > males

...LYMPHOGRANULOMA VENEREUM:

                men > women (it is diagnosed more frequently in men than in women, a situation that probably reflects underdiagnosis and asymptomatic disease in women)

...LYMPHOMA:

    Non-Hodgkin's:

                white men, people over 50 years of age

...MALIGNANT EXOPHTHALMOS in Grave's disease:

                males > females

...MALIGNANT HEMANGIOENDOTHELIOMA (ANGIOSARCOMA):

                males > females

...MALIGNANT HYPERTHERMIA:

                children > adults (1:15,000 : 1:50,000) - highest incidence in young, athletic males. A genetic predisposition exists

...MALIGNANT MASTOCYTOSIS:

                Israelis and light-skinned whites (most fre-

The Most Common
PEOPLE AFFECTED
OR INFECTED BY:

quently reported in these people)

...MALIGNANT OTITIS EXTERNA:
    diabetics

...MALLORY-WEISS SYNDROME:
    the majority of patients are alcoholics, but the tear may appear after severe retching for any reason. Several cases have been reported following closed chest cardiac compression

...MASTOCYTOSIS:
  Malignant: Israelis and light-skinned whites (most frequently reported in these people)

...MEASLES:
  in the United States:
    teenagers and young adults who did not receive the live vaccine

...MEATAL STENOSIS (of the urethra):
  in Children: in the child with hypospadias

...MECONIUM ASPIRATION SYNDROME:
    post-term infants and infants who are small for gestational age due to intrauterine growth retardation

...MEDIAL FIBROPLASIA of the renal arteries:
    middle-aged women

...MELANOMA: predominantly in whites
  Lentigo maligna:
    men = women
  Nodular: men > women
  Superficial spreading:
    women > men

...MENTAL RETARDATION:
    men > women; boys > girls

...MESOTHELIOMA OF THE PERITONEUM:
    men over age 50 years (and is associated with asbestos exposure)

...MINIMAL CHANGE DISEASE (lipoid nephrosis or nil le-

sion):
children between ages 2 and 5 years

...MITRAL STENOSIS:
women

...MIXED CONNECTIVE TISSUE DISEASES:
female > male; most are adults

...MONONUCLEOSIS, infectious:
adolescents and young adults

...MUCINOUS DEGENERATION (myxomatous transformation of valve and mitral valve prolapse):
females > males

...MULTIPLE MYELOMA:
older patients (average age, 64 years); men > women (2:1)

...MULTIPLE PERSONALITY DISORDER:
females > males (3-9:1)

...MUTISM, elective:
girls > boys

...MYCOPLASMA PNEUMONIA:
children and adolescents

...MYOPATHY of thyrotoxicosis:
men > women

...MYXOMATOUS TRANSFORMATION OF VALVE AND MITRAL VALVE PROLAPSE:
females > males

...NARCOLEPSY: males > females

...NECROTIZING ULCERATIVE GINGIVITIS (Vincent's disease; trench mouth; Fusospirochetosis):
most frequently young adults; also in children

...NEONATAL NECROTIZING ENTEROCOLITIS:
premature and asphyxiated infants, usually suffering from other medical problems. Necrotizing enterocolitis rarely is observed in healthy term infants

...NEPHRITIS, hereditary (Alport's syndrome):

369

The Most Common
PEOPLE AFFECTED
OR INFECTED BY:
males

...NEPHROBLASTOMA:

infants and young children

...NEPHROPATHY, analgesic:

women with a history of chronic headaches, arthritis, or muscular pain

...NEUROGENIC TUMORS OF THE POSTERIOR MEDIASTINUM:

Seventy-five percent of these neurogenic tumors occur in children under 4 years of age

...NEUROTIC PERSONALITY (DISORDERS):

females > males (~3:2)

...NIL LESION (lipoid nephrosis or minimal change disease):

children between ages 2 and 5 years

...NODULAR MELANOMA:

men > women

...NON-A, NON-B HEPATITIS:

intravenous drug addicts and hemophiliacs in the United States.

...NON-HODGKIN'S LYMPHOMA:

white men; people who are over 50 years of age

...NOSEBLEEDS:

Anterior (originating in Kiesselbach's plexus [Little's area]): children

Posterior: the incidence of posterior bleeds rises sharply in patients over age 50 years

...NOSOCOMIAL PNEUMONIA:

elderly patients with underlying chronic disease

...NUTRITIONAL DEPRIVATION IN PATIENTS WITH NEOPLASIA:

patients who have head and neck and upper gastrointestinal tract cancers

...OBESITY: obesity is *inversely* related to socioeconomic

370

status, with overweight being about six times more frequent at the lower than at the upper socioeconomic levels. Overweight is also more than twice as frequent at age 50 as it is at age 20. In addition, there is probably a larger hereditary component than is generally recognized

...OBSTRUCTION OF THE DISTAL SMALL BOWEL CAUSED BY INTUSSUSCEPTION:
　　　　male infants less than 2 years of age
...OBSTRUCTION OF THE LARGE BOWEL:
　　　　people after the age of 50 (males = females)
...ORCHITIS, chronic infectious granulomatous:
　　　　young adults
...OSGOOD-SCHLATTER DISEASE:
　　　　males who are active in sports
...OSTEOARTHRITIS:
　　of the Hip:　　men
　　of the Interphalangeal joints:
　　　　middle aged women
　　Primary, generalized:
　　　　middle aged women
...OSTEOCHONDRITIS DISSECANS:
　　　　males > females
...OSTEOGENIC SARCOMA (osteosarcoma):
　　　　children and adolescents (persons between the ages of 10 and 20 years); males > females
　　Juxtacortical:　women > men
...OSTEOID OSTEOMA:
　　　　males > females (3:1)
...OSTEOMYELITIS, Staphylococcal:
　　Acute:　　boys between 3 and 10 years of age, most of whom have a history of infection or trauma
...OSTEOPOROSIS:
　　　　white women > black women

The Most Common
PEOPLE AFFECTED
OR INFECTED BY:

...OSTEOSARCOMAS (osteogenic sarcoma):

> children and adolescents (persons between the ages of 10 and 20 years); males > females

...OTITIS EXTERNA

Malignant: diabetics

...OVARIAN TUMORS:

Benign: these occur mostly in young women between the ages of 20 and 45 years

Epithelial tumors:

Brenner tumors:

> the age of affected patients ranges from 6 years to 81 years, with a mean age at diagnosis of 50 years

Clear cell carcinomas:

> the average age of affected patients is 50-55 years

Endometrioid carcinomas:

> the mean age of affected patients is 53 years

Mixed mesodermal tumors:

> these occur predominantly in postmenopausal women; the median age is from 53 to 65 years

Mucinous tumors:

> these occur principally in middle adult life (third through sixth decades of life) and are rare before puberty and after menopause

Serous tumors:

> these occur at any age, but are most common between the ages of 20 and 50 (Robbins) or 30 and 60 (LiVolsi), the malignant forms being seen later in life. They are quite uncommon before puberty

Germ Cell tumors:

> they occur primarily in children and young women

Benign dermoid cyst (benign cystic teratoma):

usually occurs during the reproductive years

Immature teratomas:

usually occur in young females; the median age of onset is 18 years

Malignant dysgerminoma:

occurs predominantly in children and women under 30 years of age

Gonadal - Stromal tumors:

these can occur at any age

Malignant:

these are more common in older age groups, between 40 and 65

...PANCREATIC ADENOCARCINOMA:

men > women; people aged 50 to 70

...PANCREATITIS:

Alcoholic:

men who have ingested large amounts of alcohol over a period of at least 10 years

...PAPILLARY CARCINOMA OF THE THYROID:

females > males

...PARACOCCIDIOIDOMYCOSIS:

although positive skin tests are equally distributed in men and women, the male to female ratio of patients with clinically significant infection is 9:1

...PARANOID DISORDER, acute:

persons who have experienced drastic changes in their environment, such as immigrants, refugees, inductees into military service, or prisoners of war

...PELVIC INFLAMMATORY DISEASE (PID):

women ages 15 to 24 years

...PEPTIC ULCER DISEASE:

men > women (3:1); duodenal ulcers are 10 times more common than gastric ulcers in young patients, but in the older age groups the frequency is about equal

373

The Most Common
PEOPLE AFFECTED OR INFECTED BY:

in Children older than age 6 years:

> boys > girls

in Children younger than 6 years of age:

> boys = girls

Duodenal ulcers:

> males > females (~4:1); duodenal ulcers may occur in any age group but are most common in the young and middle-aged (20-45 years). They are 10 times more common than gastric ulcers in young patients, but in the older age groups the frequency is about equal

Gastric ulcers: the peak incidence of gastric ulcer is in patients aged 40-60 years, or about 10 years older than those with duodenal ulcer; men > women; elderly; and in the lower socioeconomic classes

...PERINATAL DEATH:

> children born before 33 weeks gestation (~ 50%)

...PERITONITIS, primary ("spontaneous"):

> it occurs mostly in patients with cirrhosis or the nephrotic syndrome. It may also occur with systemic lupus erythematosus or after splenectomy during childhood

...PERITONSILLAR ABSCESSES:

> common in young adults but rare in children

...PERVASIVE DEVELOPMENTAL DISORDERS:

> more frequent among the mentally retarded

...PHOBIAS, simple:

> more frequent among women

...PHOTOTOXICITY SECONDARY TO ANTIPSYCHOTICS AND NON-MAO ANTIDEPRESSANTS:

> young women

...PHYTOBEZOARS:

> older males

374

...PICA: children in the second year, but pica may rarely persist to adulthood

...PITUITARY TUMORS:

FSH- and/or LH-secreting tumors:
usually detected in men between 45 and 65 years of age

Growth-hormone (GH)-secreting adenomas:
they are usually found in patients between 10 and 40 years of age and are slightly more prevalent in women than men

Nonsecreting adenomas:
when diagnosed, they are generally found in patients between 30 and 60 years of age with an equal frequency in men and women

Prolactin-hormone (PH)-secreting adenomas:
these are most frequently diagnosed in women of childbearing age who present with amenorrhea, galactorrhea, and/or headaches. In men, impotence, decreased libido, headaches, and/or gynecomastia are typical presenting complaints; the average age of men at diagnosis is 35 years

...PLACENTA PREVIA:
multiparous women > primigravidas; women over 35, regardless of parity > women under 25

...PLEOMORPHIC ADENOMAS OF THE SALIVARY GLANDS:
women > men

...*PNEUMOCYSTIS CARINII*:
patients receiving cancer chemotherapy, in immunosuppressed organ transplant recipients, and in homosexual men with acquired immune deficiency syndrome (AIDS)

375

The Most Common
PEOPLE AFFECTED
OR INFECTED BY:

...PNEUMONIA:

Nosocomial: elderly patients with underlying chronic disease

Pneumococcal:

the very young, the elderly, and individuals whose immunologic defenses are compromised. Patients who have trouble handling upper respiratory tract secretions because of increased volume of the secretions or poor laryngeal reflexes during sleep also are more susceptible to infection

...POLYMYOSITIS/DERMATOMYOSITIS:

women > men

...POSTDATISM: the young and elderly primigravidas and in the grandmultiparas

...POST DURAL-PUNCTURE HEADACHE, after spinal anesthesia:

young women

...POSTTRAUMATIC ANEURYSMS OF THE THORACIC AORTA:

these occur more frequently in a younger age group and may not be detected until years after the chest trauma

...PRECOCIOUS PUBERTY:

Central (gonadotropin-dependent):

girls > boys (in girls there is rarely underlying CNS disease and it is, therefore, considered "idiopathic." There is a significant incidence of CNS pathology, especially tumors, in males with central precocious puberty)

secondary to a Tumor of the central nervous system:

boys > girls (in girls there is rarely underlying CNS disease and it is, therefore, considered "idiopathic." There is a significant incidence of CNS pathology, especially tumors, in males

376

with central precocious puberty)

...PREECLAMPSIA:

> primigravidas (and nulliparous females), particularly those in the extremes of reproductive life, that is, teenagers and women over 35 years of age; multiple pregnancies; molar degeneration; other factors complicating (diabetes mellitus, hypertension, etc.)

...PREMATURITY:

> boys > girls

...PRIMARY HERPES GENITALIS:

> teenage girls and unmarried women

...PRIMARY HYPERSPLENISM:

> females > males

...PRIMARY TUBERCULOSIS, progressive:

in Adults: patients with suppressed or defective immunity

...PROGRESSIVE PRIMARY TUBERCULOSIS:

in Adults: patients with suppressed or defective immunity

...PROSTATE CANCER:

> the tumor is more prevalent in black males than any other group in the USA. The tumor rarely occurs before age 50, and the incidence increases with age such that in the eighth decade, more than 60% of men have prostate cancer. In most of these older men, however, the disease is not clinically apparent; only 10% of men over age 65 develop clinical evidence

...*PSEUDOMONAS AERUGINOSA* PNEUMONIA:

> Hospitalized debilitated or otherwise compromised patients, especially those requiring mechanical ventilation

...PSEUDO-OBSTRUCTION (adynamic colonic ileus):

> the seriously ill patient with multisystem pa-

The Most Common
PEOPLE AFFECTED
OR INFECTED BY:
thology

...PSYCHIATRIC DISORDERS:
based on Marital status:
the divorced > the single > the widowed > the married

...PSYCHIATRIC IMPAIRMENT:
most frequent among those with parents of low socioeconomic status, and also among those with downward occupational mobility

...PSYCHOGENIC AMNESIA:
women in their teens or 20's, or in men during the stress of war

...PULMONARY DISEASES:
Childhood: males > females

...PULSELESS DISEASE (Takayasu disease):
young women

...PYELONEPHRITIS:
Xanthogranulomatous pyelonephritis:
middle aged diabetic women; women > men

...PYLORIC STENOSIS:
males > females (4:1); whites > blacks. Pyloric stenosis occurs early in life, usually between the ages of 2 weeks and 2 months

...RAYNAUD'S PHENOMENON:
young women

...REBLEEDING FROM UPPER GASTROINTESTINAL HEMORRHAGE:
patients with varices, peptic ulcer, anemia, or shock. About 10-15% of patients require surgery to control bleeding, and most of these patients have bleeding ulcers or, less commonly, esophageal varices

...RECTAL PROLAPSE:
inactive elderly or institutionalized patients

...RECURRENCE OF ULCER AFTER SURGERY FOR PEP-

TIC ULCER:

after vagotomy, ulcers recur most often in patients whose preoperative maximal acid output is greater than 40-45 meq/h, where the reduction in secretion following the procedure (60%) may be insufficient. Acid output is decreased even more by subtotal gastrectomy or antrectomy and vagotomy (80%), and recurrences after these procedures are correspondingly less common

...RENAL ADENOCARCINOMA (clear cell carcinoma, Grawitz's tumor, hypernephroma, renal cell carcinoma):

men > women (3:1); usually occurs in the fifth, sixth or seventh decade of life

...RENAL ARTERY ANEURYSMS:

women > men (slightly)

...RENAL ARTERY ATHEROSCLEROSIS:

men > women (2:1)

...RENAL CANCER:

men > women (2:1)

...RENAL CELL CARCINOMA (clear cell carcinoma, Grawitz's tumor, hypernephroma, renal adenocarcinoma):

men > women (3:1); usually occurs in the fifth, sixth or seventh decade of life

...RENAL CYSTS, solitary:

older adults

...RESPIRATORY TRACT INFECTIONS, Staphylococcal:

infants less than 2 years of age, and especially those under 2 months

...RETINOBLASTOMA:

Asians > whites (4:1)

...RETROPERITONEAL FIBROSIS:

most patients are men over age 50 who

The Most Common
PEOPLE AFFECTED
OR INFECTED BY:

present with renal failure of obstructive uropathy

...RHABDOMYOMA:

infants and children

...RHEUMATIC FEVER:

children aged 5 to 15 years; blacks; uncommon in adults

...RHEUMATIC FEVER AND RHEUMATIC HEART DISEASE:

children aged 5 to 15 years; blacks; uncommon in adults

...RHEUMATIC HEART DISEASE:

children aged 5 to 15 years; blacks; uncommon in adults

...RHEUMATOID ARTHRITIS:

more frequent among women than among men, and also tends to be familial

Juvenile: girls > boys; it begins before age 16 years, most commonly between ages 1 and 4 years

...RHINOSCLEROMA:

women (slightly) > men

...RIEDEL'S (STRUMA) THYROIDITIS:

women > men

...RILEY-DAY SYNDROME (Familial Dysautonomia):

Ashkenazi Jews

...SARCOIDOSIS: the highest incidence is reported in Scandinavia, England, and the USA. The incidence in blacks is 10-17 times that in whites. Half of patients are ages 20 to 40 years, with women more frequently affected than men

...SARCOMA BOTRYOIDES of the genitourinary tract in infancy:

males > females

...SARCOMA OF THE PROSTATE:

half of cases occur in boys under age 5

380

The Most Common
PEOPLE AFFECTED
OR INFECTED BY:

...SCHISTOSOMIASIS:

> people in the Far East and Africa

...SCHIZOID DISORDER OF CHILDHOOD OR ADOLES-
CENCE:

> boys > girls

...SCHIZOPHRENIA:

> men > women. It occurs more frequently in urban populations and in lower socioeconomic groups - probably due to a "downward drift" (e.g., poorly functional, unemployable persons end up in marginal settings)

...SCOLIOSIS:

of Adolescent onset:

> women > men

Idiopathic: adolescent girls

...SEASONAL AFFECTIVE DISORDER:

> females > males (3-4:1)

...SEMINOMA OF THE MEDIASTINUM:

> 20 to 30 year old men

...SENILE DEMENTIA:

> women > men

...SEPTICEMIC LISTERIOSIS:

in Adults: immunodeficient patients

...SERTOLI-LEYDIG TUMORS OF THE TESTICLE:

> infants and children

...SEVERE PROLIFERATIVE GLOMERULONEPHRITIS:

> children

...SEXUAL DEVIATION:

> males > females

...SEXUALLY TRANSMITTED DISEASE:

> adolescents and young adults (ages 15 to 24 years)

due to Neisseria gonorrhoeae:

> 15 to 29 year old people

The Most Common
PEOPLE AFFECTED
OR INFECTED BY:

...SIDS (Sudden Infant Death Syndrome):

> it is more common among the poor, in blacks, in premature infants, in the winter, and at night. It predominantly affects infants between 1 and 5 months of age, and peaks around 3 months

...SIGMOVESICULAR FISTULA in diverticulitis:

> men > women, women who have had a hysterectomy.

...SIMPLE PHOBIAS:

> more frequent among women

...SLIPPED CAPITAL FEMORAL EPIPHYSIS:

> males > females; occurs typically in adolescents; most common among obese boys

...SOCIOPATHY: men > women

...SOLITARY NODULES (of the Lung); ("Coin lesions"):

> males > females (3-9:1)

...SOLITARY RENAL CYSTS:

> older adults

...SPECIFIC DEVELOPMENTAL DISORDERS:

> boys > girls

...SPLENIC ARTERY ANEURYSMS:

> women > men (4:1)

...SPONTANEOUS HYPOTHYROIDISM:

> females > males

...SQUAMOUS CARCINOMA:

> predominantly in whites

...STAPHYLOCOCCAL INFECTIONS OF THE RESPIRATORY TRACT:

> infants less than 2 years of age, and especially those under 2 months

...STAPHYLOCOCCAL OSTEOMYELITIS, acute:

> boys between 3 and 10 years of age, most of whom have a history of infection or trauma

...STOMACH CANCER:

Japanese. A high incidence has also been observed in Latin American countries, particularly Chile. Stomach cancer is also common
in Iceland and Eastern Europe

...*STREPTOCOCCUS*, Group A:

children 5 to 15 years of age

...STRESS URINARY INCONTINENCE:

white parous women. Rarely in nulliparous
women. Infrequent in black and Oriental
women. Unknown in men

...STROKE (CVA; cerebrovascular accident):

it has a higher incidence with increasing age
(25% of CVA's occur in individuals in the 40-
to 55-year old age-group; 50% occur in the
65- to 79-year-old group). Men are more susceptible than women. In addition, occurrence
of CVA is higher when there is evidence of
generalized atherosclerosis

...SUBACUTE THYROIDITIS:

females > males

...SUBADVENTITIAL FIBROPLASIA of the renal arteries:

young females

...SUBLUXATION OF THE HEAD OF THE RADIUS:

children who are two to five years of age and
have been jerked forcibly by the hand

...SUDDEN INFANT DEATH SYNDROME (SIDS):

it is more common among the poor, in blacks,
in premature infants, in the winter, and at
night. It predominantly affects infants between 1 and 5 months of age, and peaks
around 3 months

...SUICIDE:

Attempts:	females > males (3:1)
Successes:	males > females (3:1)

...SUPERFICIAL SPREADING MELANOMA:

The Most Common
PEOPLE AFFECTED
OR INFECTED BY:
women > men

...SYSTEMIC LUPUS ERYTHEMATOSUS:
females > males; females between the ages of 12 and 40

...TAKAYASU DISEASE (pulseless disease):
young women

...TAY-SACHS DISEASE:
Ashkenazi Jews and French Canadian populations

...TERATOMAS OF THE MEDIASTINUM:
adolescents

...TESTICLE TUMORS:
whites > blacks (6:1) (cancerous tumor). Orientals also have a lower incidence than whites

Germinomas: males before age 45

Sertoli-Leydig group:
infants and children

...THROMBOANGIITIS OBLITERANS (Buerger's Disease):
men under 35 years of age, younger than diabetic patients, and are addicted to cigarette smoking

...THYMIC TUMORS:
Males and females are equally affected. They are most common in the fifth and sixth decades of life. Some 40-50% of patients with thymomas have associated myasthenia gravis

...THYROID CANCER:
women > men (3:2)

...THYROIDITIS:
Chronic Lymphocytic (Hashimoto's):
this occurs almost exclusively in women

Hashimoto's (Chronic Lymphocytic):
this occurs almost exclusively in women

Subacute: females > males

384

...TIC DISORDERS:

    Transient: boys > girls, and they run in families

...TORSION OF THE SPERMATIC CORD (intravaginal torsion):

    adolescent boys

...TOXIC ADENOMA OF THE THYROID:

    people in their thirties to forties

...TRANSIENT TACHYPNEA OF THE NEWBORN:

    infants born near term by cesarean section, without preceding labor

...TRANSIENT TIC DISORDERS:

    boys > girls, and they run in families

...TRANSPOSITION OF THE GREAT ARTERIES:

    males > females

    D-Transposition:

    males > females

...TRANSSEXUALISM:

    males predominate

...TRENCH MOUTH (Necrotizing ulcerative gingivitis; Vincent's disease; Fusospirochetosis):

    seen most frequently in young adults. May also occur in children

...TRICHINOSIS: this infection by the nematode *Trichinella spiralis* is cosmopolitan but is most common in eastern and central Europe, North America, and Central and South America

...TRICHOBEZOARS:

    young, neurotic women.

...TUBERCULOSIS, primary, progressive:

    in Adults: patients with suppressed or defective immunity

...TUMORS OF:

    Bladder: males > females (2:1)

    Kidney:

The Most Common
PEOPLE AFFECTED
OR INFECTED BY:

Angiomyolipoma:

this is seen most often in adults with tuberous sclerosis (adenoma sebaceum, epilepsy, and mental retardation). It is often detected following spontaneous retroperitoneal hemorrhage

Urethra:

Malignant:

females > males

...ULCERATIVE COLITIS:

the age at onset has a bimodal distribution, with the first peak in young adults in the second to fourth decade of life (ages 15 to 30 years), and a second, lower peak in the sixth to eighth decade; females > males; Caucasians > blacks; Jews > non-Jews

...ULCERS, duodenal:

males > females (~4:1)

...UMBILICAL HERNIAS:

females > males; black children > white children

...UPPER GASTROINTESTINAL HEMORRHAGE REBLEEDING:

patients with varices, peptic ulcer, anemia, or shock. About 10-15% of patients require surgery to control bleeding, and most of these patients have bleeding ulcers or, less commonly, esophageal varices

...URETEROCELE:

it is most common in females with ureteral duplication

...URETHRAL CANCER:

women > men (3:1)

...URETHRITIS: men > women

Acute:

> Gonococcal:
>> blacks > whites
>
> Chlamydial:
>> whites > blacks

...URINARY TRACT INFECTIONS:
(by age group)

Childhood: females > males

Newborns: males > females. This is due to the greater frequency of congenital urological anomalies in male infants

Ages between newborn and adulthood:
> females > males (from 10:1 to 50:1 ratio)

Adults over age 50:
> men > women. This is due to the development of prostatism in men

Candidiasis: women > men (4:1)

...UROTHELIAL TUMORS (transitional cell):
> males > females

...VAGINITIS, atrophic:
> postmenopausal women. Also may be found in surgically castrated young women and in women who are breast-feeding (lactating)

...VERNAL CONJUNCTIVITIS:

> boys > girls

...VINCENT'S DISEASE (Necrotizing ulcerative gingivitis; trench mouth; Fusospirochetosis):
> seen most frequently in young adults. May also occur in children

...VITAMIN D INTOXICATION:
> dialysis patients or women undergoing treatment for osteomalacia

...VULVAR CARCINOMA:
> women between the age of 60 and 79 years of

The Most Common
PEOPLE AFFECTED
OR INFECTED BY:
age, fewer are under the age of 40
...VULVAR DYSTROPHIES:
postmenopausal women
...WHIPPLE'S DISEASE:
middle-aged men
...WILMS' TUMOR:
children between 1 and 5 years of age, and rarely those more than 8 years of age; nearly two-thirds of the tumors present in children under 3 years of age; males = females

References

Beck, WW: *Obstetrics and Gynecology*. (The National Medical Series for Independent Study). New York, John Wiley & Sons, Inc., 1989.

Braunstein, H: *Outlines and Review of Pathology*. St. Louis, C.V. Mosby Company, 1987.

Braunwald, E, ed: *Harrison's Principles of Internal Medicine*, 11th ed.. New York, McGraw-Hill Book Company, 1987.

Casciato, DA, ed: *Manual of Clinical Oncology*, 2nd ed. Boston, Little, Brown and Company, 1988.

Chandrasoma, P: *Key Facts in Pathology*. New York, Churchill Livingstone, Inc., 1986.

Creighton University Lecture Series, Microbiology course, 1988-89.

Day, AL, MD. Subarachnoid hemorrhage. *AFP*. 1989;40:95.

388

The Most Common
PEOPLE AFFECTED
OR INFECTED BY:

Dworkin, PH: *Pediatrics* (The National Medical Series for Independent Study). New York, John Wiley & Sons, Inc., 1987.

Goldberg, S: *Clinical Neuroanatomy Made Ridiculously Simple*, Miami, MedMaster, Inc., 1986.

Gregory, I: *Psychiatry*. Boston, Little, Brown and Company, Inc., 1983.

Hiyama, DT, ed.: *The Mont Reid Surgical Handbook* St. Louis, Mosby Year Book, 1990.

Jarrell, BE: *Surgery* (The National Medical Series for Independent Study). Media, Harwal Publishing Company, 1986.

Kingsbury, DT, ed.: *Microbiology* (The National Medical Series for Independent Study). Media, Harwal Publishing Company, 1985.

Kravath, RE, ed.: *Pediatrics* (Pre-Test Series). New York, McGraw Hill Book Company, 1987.

LiVolsi, VA, ed: *Pathology* (The National Medical Series for Independent Study). Media, Harwal Publishing Company, 1984.

Macaraeg, PV, Jr., MD. Arcus Not So Senilis. *Annals of Internal Medicine*. 1968;68:345.

McCue, RW, MD. Carpal Tunnel Syndrome: Etiology and Therapy. *Medical Student*. 1989;16:4.

Medical Student. Epistaxis: Diagnosis and Treatment. *Medical Student*. November/December, 1990, p. 20.

The Merck Manual of Diagnosis and Therapy. Rahway, Merck Sharp & Dohme Research Laboratories, 1987.

Myers, AR, ed.: *Medicine* (The National Medical Series for Independent Study). Media, Harwal Publishing Company, 1986.

Nelson, WE, ed.: *Nelson Textbook of Pediatrics*, 13th ed. Philadelphia, W.B. Saunders Company, 1987.

Robbins, SL: *Pathologic Basis of Disease*. Philadelphia, W.B. Saunders Company, 1984.

Rubin, E, ed.: *Pathology*. Philadelphia, J.B. Lippincott Company, 1988.

The Most Common
PEOPLE AFFECTED
OR INFECTED BY:

Rudolph, AM, ed.: *Pediatrics*, 18th ed. Norwalk, Appleton & Lange, 1987.

Sabiston, DC: *Sabiston's Essentials of Surgery*. Philadelphia, W.B. Saunders Company, 1987.

Schrock, TR, ed.: *Handbook of Surgery*, 9th ed. Greenbrae, Jones Medical Publications, 1989.

Schwartz, SI: *Principles of Surgery*. New York, McGraw-Hill Book Company, 1989.

Sierles, FS: *Behavioral Science for the Boreds*. Miami, MedMaster, Inc., 1987.

Stillman, RM: *Surgery Diagnosis and Therapy*. East Norwalk, Appleton and Lange, 1989.

Straub, WH, ed.: *Manual of Diagnostic Imaging*, 2nd ed. Boston, Little, Brown and Company, 1989.

Tisher, CC, ed.: *Nephrology for the House Officer*. Baltimore, Williams & Wilkins, 1989.

Tomb, DA: *Psychiatry for the House Officer*. Baltimore, Williams & Wilkins, 1988.

Way, LW: *Current Surgical Diagnosis and Treatment*. Norwalk, Appleton and Lange, 1988.

Woods, SM, ed.: *Psychiatry*, 5th ed. (Pre-Test Series). New York, McGraw Hill Inc., 1989.

The Most Common

Presentation Of...

The Most Common
PRESENTATION OF:

...ACQUIRED IMMUNE DEFICIENCY SYNDROME (AIDS):

infection with *Pneumocystis carinii* (pneumonia) (PCP). The radiographic findings are usually diffuse symmetric increased interstitial lung markings predominantly in the perihilar and lower lobe regions. A large number of patients will have an atypical presentation, including small nodules, alveolar disease, asymmetric distribution upper lobe predominance, or a miliary nodular pattern. Pleural effusions and intrathoracic lymph node enlargement is rare. Cytomegalovirus (CMV) pneumonia occurs less commonly than PCP

...ACUTE CYSTITIS:

pain or burning urination, gross blood in urine

...ACUTE TUBULOINTERSTITIAL NEPHRITIS, drug-induced:

Laboratory findings:

hematuria (95%), eosinopilia (80%), sterile pyuria, low grade proteinuria, eosinophiluria, white blood cell casts

Signs and Symptoms:

fever (85-100%), maculopapular rash (25-50%), arthralgias, uremic symptoms

...ADENOMATOUS POLYPS OF THE COLON:

asymptomatic, although they may present as rectal bleeding

...ADOLESCENTS:

Gynecologic: dysmenorrhea

...ADULT POLYCYSTIC KIDNEY:

hematuria, hypertension, proteinuria, renal failure; most commonly in the fifth decade

...AIDS (Acquired immune deficiency syndrome):

infection with *Pneumocystis carinii* (pneumonia) (PCP). The radiographic findings are usually diffuse symmetric increased interstitial lung markings predominantly in the perihilar and lower lobe regions. A large number of patients will have an atypical presentation, including small nodules, alveolar disease, asymmetric distribution upper lobe predominance, or a miliary nodular pattern. Pleural effusions and intrathoracic lymph node enlargement is rare. Cytomegalovirus (CMV) pneumonia occurs less commonly than PCP

...ALPORT SYNDROME (hereditary nephritis):

in Childhood: asymptomatic hematuria. Hypertension is also common. Renal insufficiency usually does not begin until the second decade

...ARTERIOVENOUS MALFORMATIONS (AVMs) OF THE BRAIN:

seizure

...B-CELL (non-lymphoblastic) LYMPHOMA:

abdominal masses. Peripheral lymph node enlargement can be seen. Less common presentations include obstructing nasopharyngeal tumor, bone tumor, skin tumor

...BENIGN PAROTID TUMOR:

freely mobile, non-tender mass which is located just in front of or below the auricle. There are no other associated physical findings

...BLADDER INFLAMMATION:

pain or burning urination, gross blood in the urine

...BREAST CANCER:

breast lump, then spontaneous nipple discharge. Other presenting manifestations include skin changes, axillary lymphadenopathy, or signs of locally advanced or

394

disseminated disease

...CARCINOMA:

of the Gallbladder:

the most common presenting complaint is of right upper quadrant pain similar to previous episodes of biliary colic but more persistent. Obstruction of the cystic duct by tumor sometimes initiates an attack of acute cholecystitis. Other cases present with obstructive jaundice and, occasionally, cholangitis due to secondary involvement of the common duct

of the Hypopharynx:

Squamous carcinoma:

infiltrating ulcers with indurated borders

...CHRONIC LYMPHOCYTIC THYROIDITIS (Hashimoto's thyroiditis):

asymptomatic thyroid enlargement (goiter)

...CYSTITIS, acute:

pain or burning urination, gross blood in urine

...DIPHTHERIA: pharyngeal diphtheria. After an incubation period of 1 to 7 days, during which the corynebacteria proliferate at the site of implantation, the patient experiences fever, sore throat, malaise, and sometimes nausea and vomiting

...EWING'S SARCOMA:

pain and localized swelling

...FACTITIOUS DISORDER WITH PHYSICAL SYMPTOMS (Munchausen syndrome):

abdominal pain (may have an abdomen "like a railroad yard"); heart (Complains of pain. May induce arrhythmias with digitalis or produce tachycardia with amphetamines or thyroid.); bleeding (patient may take anticoagulants or add blood from a scratch to lab samples); neurological (weakness, seizures,

The Most Common
PRESENTATION OF:

unconsciousness - difficult to differentiate from conversion symptoms); fever (produced by manipulating the thermometer [e.g., hot coffee in the mouth]); skin (look for lesions in a linear pattern in areas the patient can reach)

...FOCAL NODULAR HYPERPLASIA OF THE LIVER:
asymptomatic, and is discovered as an incidental finding

...HASHIMOTO'S THYROIDITIS (chronic lymphocytic thyroiditis):
asymptomatic thyroid enlargement (goiter)

...HEAD AND NECK TUMORS:
pain, bleeding, obstruction, and a mass

...HEPATIC ARTERY ANEURYSMS:
rupture of the aneurysm into the peritoneal cavity, biliary tree, or a nearby viscus

...HEPATIC HEMANGIOMA:
asymptomatic. Most commonly it is discovered as a calcification on an abdominal roentgenogram

...HEPATOCELLULAR CARCINOMA:
a dull aching pain in the right upper quadrant; malaise, fever, and jaundice may be present

...HEREDITARY NEPHRITIS (Alport syndrome):
in Childhood: asymptomatic hematuria. Hypertension is also common. Renal insufficiency usually does not begin until the second decade

...HERNIA:
Inguinal: a mass in the groin which is present with straining or exercise and reduces upon assuming the supine position. Physical activity may cause mild pain

...HODGKIN'S DISEASE:
localized adenopathy, especially in the cervical region

396

The Most Common
PRESENTATION OF:

...IgM NEPHROPATHY (mesangial proliferative glomerulonephritis):
recurrent or persistent hematuria or as frequently relapsing or steroid-resistant nephrotic
syndrome

...INGUINAL HERNIA:
a mass in the groin which is present with
straining or exercise and reduces upon assuming the supine position. Physical activity may
cause mild pain

...INTERNAL HEMORRHOIDS:
painless blood-streaked stool

...LARGE BOWEL OBSTRUCTION:
left colon obstruction secondary to cancer

...LYMPHOBLASTIC (T-cell) LYMPHOMA:
anterior mediastinal masses, sometimes associated with pleural effusions. Peripheral
lymph node enlargement can be seen. Less
common presentations include obstructing nasopharyngeal tumor, bone tumor, skin tumor

...LYMPHOMA:
B-cell, or nonlymphoblastic:
abdominal masses. Peripheral lymph node enlargement can be seen. Less common presentations include obstructing nasopharyngeal tumor, bone tumor, skin tumor

Non-Hodgkin's:
painless adenopathy. Any node may be involved, and multiple areas of involvement are
characteristic

T-cell, or lymphoblastic:
anterior mediastinal masses, sometimes associated with pleural effusions. Peripheral
lymph node enlargement can be seen. Less
common presentations include obstructing na-

397

The Most Common
PRESENTATION OF:

sopharyngeal tumor, bone tumor, skin tumor

...MALIGNANT MELANOMA OF THE ANAL CANAL:

rectal bleeding

...MALIGNANT SMALL BOWEL TUMORS:

bleeding, perforation, or obstruction (which may be due to intussusception)

...MALROTATION OF THE INTESTINE in infants:

bilious vomiting

...MESANGIAL PROLIFERATIVE GLOMERULONEPHRITIS (IgM nephropathy):

recurrent or persistent hematuria or as frequently relapsing or steroid-resistant nephrotic syndrome

...MUNCHAUSEN SYNDROME (factitious disorder with physical symptoms):

abdominal pain (may have an abdomen "like a railroad yard"); heart (Complains of pain. May induce arrhythmias with digitalis or produce tachycardia with amphetamines or thyroid.); bleeding (patient may take anticoagulants or add blood from a scratch to lab samples); neurological (weakness, seizures, unconsciousness - difficult to differentiate from conversion symptoms); fever (produced by manipulating the thermometer [e.g., hot coffee in the mouth]); skin (look for lesions in a linear pattern in areas the patient can reach)

...NEPHRITIS, hereditary (Alport syndrome):

in Childhood: asymptomatic hematuria. Hypertension is also common. Renal insufficiency usually does not begin until the second decade

...NEUROBLASTOMA:

abdominal tumors (accounting for 70% of the cases). Presenting features are abdominal mass which often displaces the kidneys ante-

398

rolaterally and inferiorly, abdominal pain, systemic hypertension if there is compression of the renal vasculature; Thoracic tumors are the next most common presentation and are located in the posterior mediastinum. Presenting features are respiratory distress and incidental finding on a chest x-ray that was obtained for unrelated symptoms; Head and neck tumors present as palpable tumors sometimes with Horner syndrome, epidural tumors arise from the posterior growth in dumbbell fashion of abdominal or thoracic tumors, producing back pain and symptoms of cord compression

...NON-HODGKIN'S LYMPHOMA:

painless adenopathy. Any node may be involved, and multiple areas of involvement are characteristic

...NON-LYMPHOBLASTIC (B-cell) LYMPHOMA:

abdominal masses. Peripheral lymph node enlargement can be seen. Less common presentations include obstructing nasopharyngeal tumor, bone tumor, skin tumor

...POLYCYSTIC KIDNEY, adult:

hematuria, hypertension, proteinuria, renal failure; most commonly in the fifth decade

...PROSTATE ADENOCARCINOMA:

at least Stage C when detected

...PULMONARY INVOLVEMENT IN RHEUMATOID ARTHRITIS:

a pleural effusion

...RECTAL CARCINOMA:

blood in the stool. Obstruction is uncommon

...RHABDOMYOSARCOMA:

a painless, enlarging mass. Hematuria and urinary tract obstruction is seen with primary

The Most Common
PRESENTATION OF:

tumors of the genitourinary tract. The painless swelling is often noticed after minor trauma that calls attention to the enlarging mass

...SQUAMOUS CARCINOMA OF THE HYPOPHARYNX:

infiltrating ulcers with indurated borders

...T-CELL (lymphoblastic) LYMPHOMA:

anterior mediastinal masses, sometimes associated with pleural effusions

...TRANSIENT HYPOGAMMAGLOBULINEMIA OF INFANCY:

diarrhea or recurrent upper respiratory tract infections and otitis media

...VAGINAL CANCER:

vaginal discharge and bleeding

...WILMS' TUMOR:

abdominal mass. Abdominal pain, especially with hemorrhage into the tumor, is also seen. There may be associated fever and anemia; Hematuria is not common but, when present, is more often microscopic than gross; Hypertension is seen in approximately one-fourth of all patients and may be related to elaboration of renin by tumor cells or, less frequently, to compression of the renal vasculature by the tumor; Genetic and nongenetic abnormalities; Associated abnormalities that occur in a few patients include hemihypertrophy, aniridia, genitourinary tract abnormalities, mental retardation

The Most Common
PRESENTATION OF:

References

Braunstein, H: *Outlines and Review of Pathology*. St. Louis, C.V. Mosby Company, 1987.

Casciato, DA, ed: *Manual of Clinical Oncology*, 2nd ed. Boston, Little, Brown and Company, 1988.

Dworkin, PH: *Pediatrics* (The National Medical Series for Independent Study). New York, John Wiley & Sons, Inc., 1987.

Jarrell, BE: *Surgery* (The National Medical Series for Independent Study). Media, Harwal Publishing Company, 1986.

Myers, AR, ed.: *Medicine* (The National Medical Series for Independent Study). Media, Harwal Publishing Company, 1986.

Rubin, E, ed.: *Pathology*. Philadelphia, J.B. Lippincott Company, 1988.

Stillman, RM: *Surgery Diagnosis and Therapy*. East Norwalk, Appleton and Lange, 1989.

Straub, WH, ed.: *Manual of Diagnostic Imaging*, 2nd ed. Boston, Little, Brown and Company, 1989.

Tisher, CC, ed.: *Nephrology for the House Officer*. Baltimore, Williams & Wilkins, 1989.

Tomb, DA: *Psychiatry for the House Officer*. Baltimore, Williams & Wilkins, 1988.

Way, LW: *Current Surgical Diagnosis and Treatment*. Norwalk, Appleton and Lange, 1988.

The Most Common

Site Of...

The Most Common
SITE OF:

...ABDOMINAL HERNIAS:

inguinal (75-80%). Then incisional ventral hernias (8-10%), and umbilical hernias (3-8%)

...ABSCESSES:

in Dirofilariasis, subcutaneous:

the subcutaneous tissue of the trunk, but the conjunctiva, eyelid, scrotum, and breast can also be affected

Intra-abdominal:

Intraperitoneal:

the most common abscess sites are in the lower quadrants, followed by the pelvic, and the subphrenic (subhepatic and subdiaphragmatic) spaces. Others include the lateral gutters along the posterior peritoneal cavity, periappendiceal or pericolonic areas

due to Septicemic Melioidosis:

Acute: in the lungs, liver, spleen, lymph nodes, and bone marrow, but any organ may be involved

Chronic: usually localized to a single organ, most often the lung

...ACCESSORY SPLEENS:

in the tail of the pancreas. Less frequently in the mesentery

...ADENOCARCINOMA:

of the Lung: peripheral (75%) > central (25%)

of the Pancreas:

in the head of the pancreas (two thirds) > in the body or tail (one third)

of the Small Intestine:

in the proximal jejunum, but in Crohn's disease it may be distal

...ADENOID CYSTIC CARCINOMA:

salivary glands or the large airways

...ADENOMATOUS POLYPS OF THE COLON:

The Most Common
SITE OF:

the rectosigmoid colon

Tubular: in the left colon, including the rectum (75%). About 50 to 60% arise in the rectosigmoid

Villous: rectum (50-55%), sigmoid (30%), descending colon (10%). The remainder are distributed throughout the more proximal levels of the large bowel

...AMELOBLASTOMA:

in the mandible (80%) (70 percent in the molar areas). The remaining 20% of histologically similar tumors arise in other bones and, occasionally, soft tissues

...ANAL FISSURE:

midline, more often posterior than anterior

...ANEURYSM:

Atherosclerotic:

the abdominal aorta, especially distal (iliac bifurcation), the popliteal artery, the common femoral artery, the arch and descending portions of the thoracic aorta, the carotid arteries, and other peripheral arteries

Cerebral:

Arteriosclerotic:

these most commonly originate from long segments of the internal carotid or basilar arteries and produce a fusiform enlargement of that vessel

Saccular: most arise at branch points within the circle of Willis. 80-85% occur within the carotid circulation; the remainder arise from branches of the vertebrobasilar system

Men:

the anterior cerebral-anterior communicating artery junction is the most common location for saccular aneurysms

406

The Most Common
SITE OF:

Women:

the internal carotid-posterior communicating artery bifurcation is the most frequent location

Intra-abdominal:

abdominal aorta, the splenic artery

Peripheral arterial:

the popliteal artery (70%). The next most common is the femoral artery, but this is unusual

Syphilitic:

the arch and ascending aorta, especially about the right innominate artery

of the Thoracic aorta:

Posttraumatic:

the descending thoracic aorta, just distal to the origin of the left subclavian artery (Straub). Scialabba indicates the aortic isthmus is the most common site. The arch and ascending aorta are next in frequency

...ARTERIAL OCCLUSION OF THE LEG:

the superficial femoral artery. Then iliac and popliteal arteries and the aortic bifurcation

...ARTHRITIS:

in Inflammatory bowel disease:

the knees and ankles, although any joint may be affected

...ASPERGILLOSIS:

the lung, but any organ may be invaded, as well as virtually any orifice or surface, including the ear, nose, nasal sinuses, eye, skin, and intestine

Acute and disseminated infection:

A. fumigatus

...ASPIRATION: Superior segment of lower lobes or posterior segments of upper lobes of the lungs
...ASTROCYTIC TUMORS in:(see GLIOMAS)

The Most Common
SITE OF:
Children: optic nerve, walls of the third ventricle, midbrain, pons, and cerebellum

Young adults: spinal cord (predominantly thoracic and cervical segments)

Adults and elderly:

cerebral hemispheres

...ATHEROSCLEROTIC ANEURYSMS:

the abdominal aorta, especially distal (iliac bifurcation), the popliteal artery, the common femoral artery, the arch and descending portions of the thoracic aorta, the carotid arteries, and other peripheral arteries

...BENIGN HYPERPLASIA OF THE PROSTATE:

median lobe and lateral lobes. Location is limited to inner glands (contrast with carcinoma), outer glands are atrophic, compressed against capsule

...BILIARY-ENTERIC FISTULA:

the duodenum, but the colon or any other intra-abdominal or intrathoracic viscera may be penetrated

...BIRTH INJURY:

the head, skeleton, liver, and peripheral nerves

... BLASTOMYCOSIS:

Disseminated: the skin, bone, urogenital organs, and less commonly, the brain

Local: the lung

...BRAIN TUMOR:

Age < 1 year: supratentorial

Age between 2 and 12 years:

infratentorial (85%)

Age after 12 years:

the relative incidence of supratentorial tumors increases (refer to above age groups)

...CNS TUMORS: intracranially (90%) and within the spinal canal (10%); 70% of childhood brain tumors originate in the cerebellar hemisphere; 90% of adult brain tumors are supratentorial

...CAFE AU LAIT SPOTS IN NEUROFIBROMATOSIS (von Recklinghausen's disease):

in the crease areas of the body; over the trunk

...CANDIDIASIS, systemic:

the urinary tract

...CANCER:

in Adenoma of the colon:

in the tip of the adenoma

which causes Death:

in Men (years of age):

Less than 15:

leukemia, CNS, lymphoma, connective tissue, bone

15-34:

leukemia, CNS, lymphoma, skin, Hodgkin's

33-54:

lung, bowel, CNS, pancreatic adenocarcinoma, leukemia

55-74:

lung, bowel, prostate, pancreas, stomach

More than 75:

lung, prostate, bowel, pancreas, bladder

All ages:

lung, bowel, prostate, pancreas, leukemia

in Women (years of age):

Less than 15:

leukemia, CNS, connective tissue, bone, kidney

15-34:

breast, leukemia, uterus, CNS, Hodgkin's

35-54:

The Most Common
SITE OF:
> breast, lung, bowel, ovary, uterus

55-74:
> lung, breast, bowel, ovary, pancreas

More than 75:
> bowel, breast, lung, pancreas, uterus

All ages:
> lung, breast, bowel (colon), ovary, pancreas
> (1988 data: lung ↑ to #1 in women)

of the Esophagus:
> lower third (50%) > middle third (40%) >
> upper third (10%)

which Metastasizes to the bone:
> the vertebral column

in Multiple myeloma:
> skull, spine, ribs, pelvis, and femur

of the Stomach:
> pylorus and antrum (50%) > lesser curvature
> (20%) > body (20%) > cardia (7%) > greater
> curvature (3%)

of the Vagina: on the anterior wall of the upper and middle
third of the vagina. If the cervix is involved,
the disease is defined as cervical, rather than
vaginal, cancer. If the vulva is involved, the
disease is defined as vulvar cancer

of the Vulva: labia majora, labia minora, clitoris, and peri-
neum

...CARCINOID TUMOR:
> appendix, then small bowel (usually the ile-
> um), then rectum. Other sites are uncommon.

of the Lung: centrally located in the main stem or lobar
bronchi (90-95%) > peripherally (5-10%)

...CARCINOMA:
Adenoid cystic:
> salivary glands or the large airways

410

Colorectum: the rectum, rectosigmoid, or sigmoid colon (70-75%). The remainder are fairly evenly distributed all the way back to the cecum

Esophagus:
  Squamous cell carcinoma:
    in the middle third (50%) > in the lower third (30%) > in the upper third of the esophagus (20%)(LiVolsi reports that the distal third is the most common)

Hypopharynx: the piriform sinus (60%), the postcricoid region (25%), and the posterior pharyngeal wall (15%).

Lung:
  Adenocarcinoma:
    peripheral (75%) > central (25%)
  Oat cell carcinoma:
    centrally located (80%) > peripherally located (20%)
  Squamous cell carcinoma:
    centrally near the hilum (two-thirds) > peripherally (one-third)

Nasal cavity and paranasal sinuses:
  Squamous cell carcinoma:
    the maxillary antrum; primary malignant neoplasms of the nasal cavity are rare

Stomach: pyloric antrum

...CARDIAC MYXOMA:
  atria (most commonly the left atrium)

...CENTRAL NERVOUS SYSTEM TUMORS:
  intracranially (90%) and within the spinal canal (10%); 70% of childhood brain tumors originate in the cerebellar hemisphere; 90% of adult brain tumors are supratentorial

...CHANCRE in Syphilis:
  in Men: on glans or prepuce of penis; shaft less fre-

411

The Most Common
SITE OF:

...CHANCROID:

quently affected

in Men: on glans or prepuce of penis; shaft less frequently affected

...CHEMODECTOMA (PARAGANGLIOMA):

carotid body (neck mass) or glomus jugulare (petrous bone)

...CLEFT LIP: the left side > the right side

...COLITIS CYSTICA PROFUNDA:

rectum

...COLON CANCER:

rectosigmoid region

...COLON RUPTURE:

the cecum

...COLONIC PERFORATION IN ULCERATIVE COLITIS:

the sigmoid colon and the splenic flexure

...COLORECTAL CANCER:

the rectum, rectosigmoid, or sigmoid colon (70-75%). The remainder are fairly evenly distributed all the way back to the cecum

...CONGENITAL LUNG CYSTS:

these may occur anywhere in the lungs but involve the lower lobes twice as often as other sites

...CROHN'S DISEASE involvement:

the distal ileum

in Children: ileocolic, the small intestine only, and the colon only

...CSF OBSTRUCTIVE CONGENITAL MALFORMATION:

the aqueduct of Sylvius

...CUTANEOUS ANTHRAX:

hands, forearms, neck, scalp, and other exposed areas

...CYSTIC HYGROMAS:

in the neck. Also in the groin, axilla, and

412

mediastinum

...DESMOID TUMORS OF THE ABDOMINAL WALL:
> at sites of abdominal wall injury such as surgical incisions

...DIAPHRAGMATIC HERNIA:
> left side > right

through the foramen of Bochdalek:
> left side > right

through the foramen of Morgani:
> right > left

...DIVERTICULOSIS:
> lower descending and rectosigmoidal colon

...DIVERTICULUM OF THE BLADDER:
> adjacent to the ureters

...DROWNING IN THE FIRST YEAR OF LIFE:
> bathtubs

...DRUG HYPERSENSITIVITY REACTIONS:
> the skin

...DUCT CELL ADENOCARCINOMA OF THE PANCREAS:
> in the head of the pancreas (two thirds) > in the body or tail (one third)

...DUODENAL DIVERTICULA:
> opposite the ampulla of Vater

...DUODENAL ULCER:
> about 95% are situated within 2 cm of the pylorus, in the duodenal bulb

...DUODENAL ULCER PERFORATION:
> ulcers on the anterior surface of the duodenum. Occasionally, ulcers can perforate posteriorly into the lesser sac

...DYSPLASIA: in hyperplastic squamous epithelium, and in areas of squamous metaplasia, sites other than squamous epithelium such as dysplastic changes in the mucosal cells

The Most Common
SITE OF:

...ECHINOCOCCUS CYSTS:
> most commonly in the liver. These can also involve the lung and, less commonly, the brain, kidney, spleen, muscle, soft tissues, and bone

Pastoral echinococcus:
> liver, lungs

Sylvatic echinococcus:
> lungs, liver

...ECTOPIC KIDNEY:
> in the pelvis

...ECTOPIC PREGNANCY:
> the fallopian tube. It can also occur in the ovary, cervix, or abdominal cavity

...ENDOCARDITIS:
> heart valves (mitral, aortic, tricuspid, pulmonic)

...ENDODERMAL SINUS TUMOR OF THE OVARY:
> the right ovary > the left ovary

...ENDOMETRIOSIS:
> ovary, the pouch of Douglas (including the uterosacral ligaments and the rectovaginal septum), the pelvic peritoneal surfaces, the round ligament, oviduct, lower bowel, pelvic lymph nodes, appendix, cecum, cervix, vulva, vagina, small intestine, umbilicus, bladder, ureter, laparotomy scars, episiotomy scars, hernial sacs, tubal stumps, arm, leg, pleura, lung, diaphragm, kidney, spleen, gall bladder, nasal mucous membranes, stomach, and breast

...EPENDYMOMAS:
> fourth ventricle, intramedullary (of the lumbosacral spinal cord), lateral ventricles

414

in Children: fourth ventricle

...ESOPHAGITIS, acute corrosive:

level of the tracheal bifurcation

...EWING'S SARCOMA:

in the midshaft of the humerus, femur, tibia, or fibula, but also occur in the ribs, scapula, or pelvis. It has been described as an extraosseous tumor (these behave more like rhabdomyosarcoma)

...FATTY INVASION (lipomatosis) OF THE HEART:

the right ventricular wall

...FIBROPLASIA OF THE RENAL ARTERIES:

Subadventitial: right > left

...FILARIASIS, Bancroftian and Malayan:

the adult worms (*Wuchereria bancrofti* and *Brugia malayi*, respectively) inhabit lymphatic vessels, most frequently those in the lymph nodes, testis, and epididymis

...FISTULA in:

Crohn's Disease:

ileoileal, ileosigmoid, and ileocecal

Diverticulitis: between the sigmoid colon and the bladder

...FORAMEN OF BOCHDALEK:

it occurs most often in the left hemidiaphragm. It is bilateral in fewer than 10% of infants

...FOREIGN BODY INJURY:

in Children under 1 year of age:

the larynx

in Children 1 to 4 years of age:

the trachea and bronchi

...GASTRIC ULCERS:

95% of gastric ulcers are located on the lesser curvature, and 60% of these are within 6 cm of the pylorus

The Most Common
SITE OF:

Type I ulcers: 95% are on the lesser curvature, usually near the incisure angularis. They are usually located within 2 cm of the boundary between parietal cell and pyloric mucosa, but always in the latter

Type II ulcers: these are usually located close to the pylorus

Type III ulcers: these occur in the antrum

...GASTRINOMA IN ZOLLINGER-ELLISON SYNDROME: most occur in the pancreas. Others are found submucosally in the duodenum and rarely in the antrum or ovary

...GASTROINTESTINAL LYMPHOMAS: the stomach and small intestine. The next most favored sites are the ileum, large intestine, and appendix

...GLIOMAS of:

Childhood: brain stem and cerebellum

Adult: cerebrum

...GLOMANGIOMA (glomus tumor): fingers. Some are found in viscera (stomach, lung)

...GLOMUS TUMOR (glomangioma): fingers. Some are found in viscera (stomach, lung)

...HEMANGIOPERICYTOMA: lower extremity and retroperitoneal space

...HEMORRHAGE, intracerebral: putamen, cerebral white matter, thalamus, pons, cerebellum

...HEMORRHOIDS: in the left lateral, right anterior, and right posterior anal canal

External: beneath the dentate line

416

The Most Common
SITE OF:

...HERNIAS: the vast majority of hernias occur in the inguinal region, with approximately 50% of these being indirect and 25 per cent being direct inguinal hernias. Incisional hernias (including ventral hernias) make up about 10 per cent of all hernias, femoral hernias approximately 5 per cent, and umbilical hernias 3 per cent; rare hernias account for the remainder

Abdominal: inguinal (75-80%). Then incisional ventral hernias (8-10%), and umbilical hernias (3-8%)

Dorsal (Lumbar):
the most common sites are the superior and inferior lumbar triangles. The superior triangle (Grynfelt's) is the larger and more frequently involved, whereas the inferior triangle (Petit's) is less involved

Inguinal: right side > left side

in Children:
on the right (about 60%), on the left about 30%, and bilateral between 10% and 15% of the time

Lumbar (Dorsal):
the most common sites are the superior and inferior lumbar triangles. The superior triangle (Grynfelt's) is the larger and more frequently involved, whereas the inferior triangle (Petit's) is less involved

Spigelian: through the Spigelian fascia inferior to the semicircular line of Douglas

...HERNIATED MUCOSAL POUCHES OF DIVERTICULOSIS:
in the left colon

...HOUSE FIRES IN THE UNITED STATES:
in the East and Southeast

The Most Common
SITE OF:

...HYPERPLASTIC POLYPS OF THE COLON:
> in the rectosigmoid (60-80%) > the ascending colon (20%). The remainder are in other colonic locations

...HYPERTENSIVE HEMORRHAGE OF THE BRAIN:
> basal ganglia-thalamus, pons, cerebellum

...HYDROPIC SWELLING:
> highly metabolic cells (e.g. epithelial cells, proximal tubular cells, liver, and heart)

...INFARCTION FROM ARTERIAL EMBOLI:
> brain, retina, heart (left ventricle), spleen, kidney, small intestine, lower leg

...INFECTION:
> in Aspergillosis:
>> the lung, but any organ may be invaded, as well as virtually any orifice or surface, including the ear, nose, nasal sinuses, eye, skin, and intestine
>
> in Blastomycosis:
>> Disseminated:
>>> the skin, bone, urogenital organs, and less commonly, the brain
>>
>> Local: the lung
>
> in Cryptosporidiosis:
>> the terminal ileum and cecum
>
> with Diphtheria:
>> the membranes of the pharynx, but the nasal fossae, tonsils, lower respiratory tract, gut, conjunctiva, umbilical stump, and skin are other sites
>
> in Rhinosporidiosis:
>> hyperplastic polypoid lesions of the nasal mucosa. Less frequently the infection involves the conjunctiva and mouth, and in rare in-

418

stances it involves the skin and viscera

with Trichomonas vaginalis:
: the vagina in females, but also near the urethra of both sexes

...INGUINAL HERNIAS:
: right side > left side

in Children:
: on the right (about 60%), on the left about
30%, and bilateral between 10% and 15% of
the time

...INSULINOMAS:
: insulinomas occur with equal frequency in the
head, body, and tail of the pancreas; less than
1% develop outside the pancreas

...INTESTINAL LYMPHOMA, primary:
: the stomach

...INTESTINAL OBSTRUCTION:
: about 85% of mechanical obstructions occur
in the small intestine and 15% in the large intestine

in Gallstone Ileus:
: the terminal ileum

of the Large Bowel:
: the left colon, followed by the cecum

in Tuberculous Peritonitis:
: obstruction due to constriction by a tuberculous lesion usually develops in the distal ileum and cecum, although multiple skip areas
along the small bowel may exist

...INTESTINAL PERFORATION IN AMEBIASIS:
: the cecum

...INTIMAL THICKENING OF ARTERIES:
: coronary arteries, abdominal aorta

...INTRA-ABDOMINAL (PERITONEAL) ABSCESSES:
: subphrenic space, subhepatic space, lateral

The Most Common
SITE OF:

> gutters along the posterior peritoneal cavity, pelvic area, periappendiceal or pericolonic areas

...INTRADUCTAL PAPILLOMA OF THE BREAST:
> within the principal lactiferous ducts

...INTUSSUSCEPTION:
> ileocecal valve

Postoperative: unlike idiopathic ileocolic intussusception, most postoperative intussusceptions are ileoileal or jejunojejunal

...INVOLVEMENT:
in Acute Staphylococcal Osteomyelitis:
in Adults over 50 years of age:
> the vertebrae

in Young patients:
> the bones of the legs

in Adhesions, postoperative abdominal:
> the omentum, small bowel, colon, and rectum

of Amebic Abscess:
> the right lobe of the liver

of Chemodectoma (paraganglioma):
> the carotid body (neck mass) or glomus jugulare (petrous bone)

in Crohn's Disease:
> the distal ileum (most frequent) and proximal right colon

in Diphtheria: the membranes of the pharynx, but the nasal fossae, tonsils, lower respiratory tract, gut, conjunctiva, umbilical stump, and skin are other sites

in Diverticulosis:
> the sigmoid colon, with other portions of the large bowel involved to a greater or lesser extent

in Endocarditis, Rheumatic:

420

the mitral valve

in Gonorrhea:

    in Men: the urethra

    in Women:

        the endocervix

of Heart Valves in Nonbacterial Thrombotic Endocarditis (marantic endocardiosis):

    mitral, aortic, tricuspid, pulmonic

in Hirschsprung's disease:

    the rectosigmoid colon, but the entire colon may be involved

in Lymphadenitis, toxoplasmic:

    the posterior cervical lymph nodes, although nodes at other sites may also be affected

of Lymphangitis and Lymphadenitis:

    an extremity

in Mallory-Weiss Syndrome:

    about 75% of these lesions are confined to the stomach; 20% straddle the esophagogastric junction; and 5% are entirely within the distal esophagus. The disruption extends through the mucosa and submucosa but not usually into the muscularis mucosae

in Miliary tuberculosis:

    the lung, lymph nodes, kidneys, adrenals, bone marrow, spleen, liver, meninges, brain, eye grounds, and genitalia. Miliary tubercles rarely develop in the pancreas, thyroid, striated muscle, or heart

of Mucoid (basophilic) Degeneration of the heart:

    the left ventricle

in Multiple myeloma:

    skull, spine, ribs, pelvis, and femur

in Nocardiosis of the lung which has spread systemically:

    the brain and skin and, less commonly, the

421

The Most Common
SITE OF:

thyroid, liver, or other organs

in Noma:
soft tissues and bones of the mouth and face, and, less commonly, other sites, such as chest, limbs, or genitalia

in Osteomyelitis, acute Staphylococcal:
in Adults over 50 years of age:
the vertebrae
in Young patients:
the bones of the legs

of Paraganglioma (chemodectoma):
the carotid body (neck mass) or glomus jugulare (petrous bone)

of Peripheral Arterial Disease:
the vessels of the lower extremities and the extracranial cerebral circulation

in Postoperative Adhesions, abdominal:
the omentum, small bowel, colon, and rectum

in Pseudomembranous Colitis:
the colon

in Rhinoscleroma:
the nasal mucosa (less commonly, the nasopharynx, larynx, and trachea)

in Septic arthritis:
the knee, hip, ankle, elbow, wrist, and shoulder

in Staphylococcal Osteomyelitis, acute:
in Adults over 50 years of age:
the vertebrae
in Young patients:
the bones of the legs

in Syphilitic Cardiovascular Disease:
ascending portion and arch of the aorta

in Systemic Lupus Erythematosus:
joints, kidney, heart, serosal membranes

in Toxoplasmic lymphadenitis:

422

the posterior cervical lymph nodes, although nodes at other sites may also be affected

in Tuberculosis, miliary:

the lung, lymph nodes, kidneys, adrenals, bone marrow, spleen, liver, meninges, brain, eye grounds, and genitalia. Miliary tubercles rarely develop in the pancreas, thyroid, striated muscle, or heart

in Werdnig-Hoffmann disease:

the anterior horn cells of the spinal cord

...JUVENILE RETENTION POLYPS:

in the rectum

...*KLEBSIELLA* PNEUMONIA:

Superior segment of lower lobes or posterior segments of upper lobes, the areas most often affected by aspiration

...LARGE BOWEL OBSTRUCTION:

the left colon, followed by the cecum

...LEG PAIN CAUSED BY PERIPHERAL ARTERIAL OCCLUSIVE DISEASE AT ANY LOCATION IN THE EXTREMITY:

calf claudication

...LEIOMYOMA, uterine:

intramural, in corpus of uterus

...LESIONS:

in Chronic obstructive emphysema:

in the lower lobes of the lung

due to Herpes simplex virus:

lips and mouth (e.g., primary gingivostomatitis leading to recurrent herpes labialis) and on the genitals, primary or recurrent keratoconjunctivitis, and occasionally encephalitis

in Mallory-Weiss Syndrome:

about 75% of these lesions are confined to the stomach; 20% straddle the esophagogastric

423

The Most Common
SITE OF:

junction; and 5% are entirely within the distal esophagus. The disruption extends through the mucosa and submucosa but not usually into the muscularis mucosae

Miliary, in miliary tuberculosis:

the lung, lymph nodes, kidneys, adrenals, bone marrow, spleen, liver, meninges, brain, eye grounds, and genitalia. Miliary tubercles rarely develop in the pancreas, thyroid, striated muscle, or heart

in Tuberculosis, miliary:

the lung, lymph nodes, kidneys, adrenals, bone marrow, spleen, liver, meninges, brain, eye grounds, and genitalia. Miliary tubercles rarely develop in the pancreas, thyroid, striated muscle, or heart

...LUNG CYSTS, Congenital:

these may occur anywhere in the lungs but involve the lower lobes twice as often as other sites

...LYMPHADENITIS:

in Children with *Mycobacterium scrofulaceum*:

cervical

Toxoplasmic: the posterior cervical lymph nodes, although nodes at other sites may also be affected

...LYMPHADENOPATHY IN PATIENTS WITH INFECTIOUS MONONUCLEOSIS:

the posterior cervical nodes; other anatomic sites may also be affected

...LYMPHANGIOMA:

the tongue (macroglossia), often combined with soft tissue of neck (cystic hygroma colli)

...LYMPHOMAS OF THE GASTROINTESTINAL TRACT:

the stomach and small intestine. The next

424

most favored sites are the ileum, large intestine, and appendix

...MALLORY-WEISS SYNDROME TEARS:

about 75% of these lesions are confined to the stomach; 20% straddle the esophagogastric junction; and 5% are entirely within the distal esophagus. The disruption extends through the mucosa and submucosa but not usually into the muscularis mucosae

...MELANOMA: skin, eyes, anal canal

...MENINGIOMA: parasagittal, lateral convexity, parasagittal arising from the falx, olfactory groove, sphenoid ridge, clivus

...MESOTHELIOMA in asbestos workers:

pleura. Then peritoneum

...METASTASIS FROM:

Ewing's sarcoma:

the lung. Metastases to other bones or lymph nodes rarely develop. Central nervous system metastases, particularly meningeal, have been reported but are very rare

Neuroblastoma:

bone, bone marrow, liver, skin, and lymph nodes

Sarcomas (all):

the lung (almost always bilateral and multiple). Other structures, such as the liver, bone, and subcutaneous tissue, are affected by hematogenous dissemination much less frequently than are the lungs. Regional lymph node metastases are relatively infrequent in most types of sarcomas but do occur with greater frequency in certain types

Wilm's Tumor:

The Most Common
SITE OF:

lung. Liver and lymph nodes are the next most common sites. Bone is rarely, if ever, involved. Bone marrow metastases are extremely rare and tend to be associated with clear cell subtypes of sarcomatous Wilms' tumor. Central nervous system metastases are extremely rare

...MILIARY LESIONS IN MILIARY TUBERCULOSIS:

the lung, lymph nodes, kidneys, adrenals, bone marrow, spleen, liver, meninges, brain, eye grounds, and genitalia. Miliary tubercles rarely develop in the pancreas, thyroid, striated muscle, or heart

...MINOR SALIVARY GLAND TUMORS:

the palate

...MONOMORPHIC ADENOMAS OF THE SALIVARY
         GLANDS:

the minor salivary glands of the lip

...MUCOEPIDERMOID TUMORS OF THE LUNG:

centrally located > peripherally

...MUMPS INFECTION:

the parotid salivary glands. Less often the virus attacks the pancreas, ovaries, testes, and other organs

...MYELOMENINGOCELE:

thoracolumbar or lumbar spinal cord, although lesions may be anywhere along the spine

...MYOCARDIAL INFARCTION:

the left anterior descending coronary artery in its extramural portion; the left ventricular subendocardium

...MYOCARDITIS IN RHEUMATIC HEART DISEASE:

the interventricular septum or posterior wall

426

of the left ventricle

...NEUROFIBROMA:

skin, major nerve plexuses, large deep nerve trunks, retroperitoneum, GI tract

...OAT CELL CARCINOMA OF THE LUNG:

centrally located (80%) > peripherally located (20%)

...OBSTRUCTION, Intestinal:

about 85% of mechanical obstructions occur in the small intestine and 15% in the large intestine

in Gallstone Ileus:

the terminal ileum

of the Large Bowel:

the left colon, followed by the cecum

in Tuberculous Peritonitis:

obstruction due to constriction by a tuberculous lesion usually develops in the distal ileum and cecum, although multiple skip areas along the small bowel may exist

...OCCULT TUMOR WHICH METASTASIZES TO THE HEAD AND NECK:

Primary in the Head and Neck:

the nasopharynx, hypopharynx (piriform sinus), and oropharynx (tonsillar fossa), but lung and esophagus occasionally are implicated

Primary outside the Head and Neck:

the lung. Other sites include the pancreas, esophagus, stomach, breast, ovary, and prostate

...OLIGODENDROGLIOMAS in:

Adults: cerebrum

...OSTEOGENIC SARCOMA:

The Most Common
SITE OF:

> distal femur, proximal tibia, proximal humerus, proximal femur

...OSTEOMYELITIS:
  in Children: in the long bones of the lower extremities and, to a lesser extent, in the upper extremities

...PAGET'S DISEASE:
> nipple

...PANCREATIC ADENOCARCINOMA:
> the head of the pancreas

...PAPILLOMAS OF THE BREAST:
> within the principal lactiferous ducts

...PARAGANGLIOMA (CHEMODECTOMA):
> carotid body (neck mass) or glomus jugulare (petrous bone)

...PAROTID GLAND TUMOR:
> superficial and caudal part of the gland

...PEDIATRIC INGUINAL HERNIAS:
> on the right side

...PEPTIC ULCER DISEASE:
  in Children older than 6 years of age:
> duodenum > stomach

  in Children younger than 6 years of age:
> duodenum = stomach

  Duodenal ulcer:
> about 95% are situated within 2 cm of the pylorus, in the duodenal bulb

  Gastric ulcers: 95% of gastric ulcers are located on the lesser curvature, and 60% of these are within 6 cm of the pylorus

    Type I ulcers:
> 95% are on the lesser curvature, usually near the incisure angularis. They are usually located within 2 cm of the boundary between parietal cell and pyloric mucosa, but always in the latter

428

Type II ulcers:

    these are usually located close to the pylorus

Type III ulcers:

    these occur in the antrum

Perforation: most perforated ulcers are located anteriorly on the duodenum, although occasionally gastric ulcers perforate into the lesser sac

...PERFORATION OF THE INTESTINE IN AMEBIASIS:

    the cecum

...PERFORATION OF THE COLON IN ULCERATIVE COLITIS:

    the sigmoid colon and the splenic flexure

...PERFORATION OF A PEPTIC ULCER:

    most perforated ulcers are located anteriorly on the duodenum, although occasionally gastric ulcers perforate into the lesser sac

...PERFORATION WHEN THE COLON IS OBSTRUCTED:

    the cecum

...PERITONEAL (INTRA-ABDOMINAL) ABSCESSES:

    subphrenic space, subhepatic space, lateral gutters along the posterior peritoneal cavity, pelvic area, periappendiceal or pericolonic areas

...PHEOCHROMOCYTOMA:

    the adrenal medulla (about 90% - approximately 10-20% of these are bilateral). Of the extra-adrenal 10%, most are found in the organs of Zuckerkandl, the sympathetic ganglia, the extra-adrenal paraganglia, the urinary bladder, and the mediastinum. Extra-abdominal locations are rare (1-2%)

...PHLEBOTHROMBOSIS:

    deep leg veins

...PHLEGMASIA CERULEA DOLENS:

    it is more common in the left leg

The Most Common
SITE OF:

...PLEURAL EFFUSIONS in severe pancreatitis:

> left > right

...POLYPS OF THE LARGE BOWEL:

Adenomatous: rectosigmoid colon

Tubular adenomas:
> in the left colon, including the rectum (75%). About 50 to 60% arise in the rectosigmoid

Villous adenomas:
> rectum (50-55%), sigmoid (30%), descending colon (10%). The remainder are distributed throughout the more proximal levels of the large bowel

Hereditary/Familial:
> scattered

Hyperplastic: in the rectosigmoid (60-80%) > the ascending colon (20%). The remainder are in other colonic locations

Juvenile: rectum

Puetz-Jeghers: chiefly small (intestine) (Sabiston)

Villous: rectosigmoid

...POSTTRAUMATIC ANEURYSM OF THE THORACIC AORTA:
> the descending thoracic aorta, just distal to the origin of the left subclavian artery. The arch and ascending aorta are next in frequency

...PRIMARY INTESTINAL LYMPHOMA:
> the stomach

...PRIMARY MALIGNANT NEOPLASM:
> lung, colorectum

...PRIMARY NEOPLASM WHICH METASTASIZES TO THE:

Heart: lung, breast, lymphoma, leukemia, melanoma

...PRIMARY ORGAN SYSTEM INVOLVEMENT IN SYSTEMIC LUPUS ERYTHEMATOSUS:
> joints, kidney, heart, serosal membranes

...PRIMARY SMALL BOWEL LYMPHOMA:

430

ileum

...PULMONARY SEQUESTRATIONS:

within the left lower lobe. At times this cyst-like mass of nonfunctioning lung tissue some-times develops entirely outside the lungs

...PURULENT TENOSYNOVITIS OF THE HAND:

occurs from penetrating injury to the flexion creases of the fingers, most commonly the in-dex, middle, and ring fingers

...PYOMYOSITIS: the quadriceps, gluteus, shoulder, and upper arm muscles, with multiple areas of involve-ment in about 40% of patients

...RAYNAUD'S PHENOMENON:

in the upper extremities

...REACTIVATION TUBERCULOSIS:

subapical area of the upper lobes of the lungs

...RECURRENCE:

in children with relapse of Acute lymphocytic leukemia:
bone marrow, CNS (used to be the most com-mon site of recurrence prior to CNS prophy-laxis), testes (are becoming the most common site of extramedullary relapse)

of Carcinoma of the hypopharynx:
at the primary site or neck

...RHABDOMYOSARCOMA:

the head and neck (35%), the trunk and ex-tremities (35%), and the genitourinary tract (30%)

...RHINOSPORIDIOSIS:

hyperplastic polypoid lesions of the nasal mu-cosa. Less frequently the infection involves the conjunctiva and mouth, and in rare in-stances it involves the skin and viscera

...RUPTURE OF THE COLON:

the cecum

431

The Most Common
SITE OF:
...SACCULAR (BERRY) ANEURYSMS:

branch points in the Circle of Willis: 1) the internal carotid complex (the internal carotid, posterior communicating, anterior cerebral, and anterior choroidal arteries); 2) union of the anterior cerebral and anterior communicating arteries; 3) the trifurcation of the middle cerebral artery; 4) other sites

...SCABIES (Sarcoptes scabiei) infection:

hands, wrists, breasts, and buttocks

...SCHWANNOMA:

intracranial (most commonly cranial nerve VIII), intraspinal (most commonly from the dorsal [sensory] spinal roots, peripheral nerves)

...SINUSITIS, ACUTE:

in Children: the ethmoid sinuses. The maxillary sinuses may also be involved but are not clinically important until after 18 months of age. Frontal sinusitis and sphenoidal sinusitis are rare before 10 years of age

...SMALL BOWEL LYMPHOMA, primary:

ileum

...SOLID TUMOR FORMATION in childhood:

the intra-abdominal tissues

...SPONTANEOUS CHOLECYSTOENTERIC FISTULA:

duodenum or colon

...SPREAD OF ANGIOSARCOMA (MALIGNANT HEMANGIOENDOTHELIOMA) OF THE LIVER:

locally to the spleen, and distantly to the lungs

...SQUAMOUS CELL CARCINOMA OF THE:

Esophagus: in the middle third (50%) > in the lower third (30%) > in the upper third of the esophagus (20%)

Lung: centrally near the hilum (two-thirds) > periph-

432

erally (one-third)

Nasal cavity and paranasal sinuses:

the maxillary antrum; primary malignant neoplasms of the nasal cavity are rare

...STOMACH TUMORS:

pylorus and antrum (50-60%) > cardia (10%) > whole organ (10%) > other areas. The lesser curvature is involved in about 40%, the greater curvature in 12%, and the entire circumference in about 25% of instances; the remainder are found on the anterior or posterior walls. Thus, a favored location is the lesser curvature of the pyloroantrum

...SUBADVENTITIAL FIBROPLASIA of the renal arteries:

right > left

...SUICIDES BY HOSPITAL INPATIENTS:

the bathroom

...SYNOVIAL SARCOMAS:

around the knee joint

...SYPHILITIC ANEURYSM:

the arch and ascending aorta, especially about the right innominate artery

...SYRINGOMYELIA:

in the cervical or thoracic spinal cord

...SYSTEMIC CANDIDIASIS:

the urinary tract

...the TIP OF THE APPENDIX:

pelvic, but it may be subcecal, retrocecal, retrocolic, ileocecal, or, rarely, subhepatic.

...TOXOPLASMIC LYMPHADENITIS:

the posterior cervical lymph nodes, although nodes at other sites may also be affected

...TRANSITIONAL CELL CARCINOMA:

trigone of the bladder

433

The Most Common
SITE OF:
of the Ureter: more than 60% of these tumors occur in the lower ureter

...TUBERCULOSIS infection:

the lung

Miliary: the lung, lymph nodes, kidneys, adrenals, bone marrow, spleen, liver, meninges, brain, eye grounds, and genitalia. Miliary tubercles rarely develop in the pancreas, thyroid, striated muscle, or heart

...TUBULAR ADENOMAS OF THE COLON:

in the left colon, including the rectum (75%). About 50 to 60% arise in the rectosigmoid

...TUMORS OF THE STOMACH:

pylorus and antrum (50-60%) > cardia (10%) > whole organ (10%) > other areas. The lesser curvature is involved in about 40%, the greater curvature in 12%, and the entire circumference in about 25% of instances; the remainder are found on the anterior or posterior walls. Thus, a favored location is the lesser curvature of the pyloroantrum

...TYPHOID NODULES:

the intestine, mesenteric lymph nodes, spleen, liver, and bone marrow. Less commonly, the kidney, testes, and parotid gland are affected

...ULNAR NERVE INJURY, compressive:

cubital tunnel, Guyon's canal

...URETHRAL STRICTURE:

Postinflammatory:

in Males: the membranous segment of the urethra

...VALVULAR INVOLVEMENT IN NONBACTERIAL THROMBOTIC ENDOCARDITIS (marantic endocardiosis):

mitral, aortic, tricuspid, pulmonic

...VARICOCELE OF THE SPERMATIC CORD:

434

on the left side of the scrotum

...VENTRICULAR SEPTAL DEFECT:

subaortic, in the membranomuscular portion

...VILLOUS ADENOMAS OF THE COLON:

rectum (50-55%), sigmoid (30%), descending colon (10%). The remainder are distributed throughout the more proximal levels of the large bowel

...VISCERAL INJURY ASSOCIATED WITH TRAUMA TO THE GALLBLADDER:

the liver

...VOLVULUS:

the sigmoid colon. Also occasionally in the cecum. It almost never occurs in the transverse colon

...WORMS IN *ENTEROBIUS VERMICULARIS* (pinworm) INFECTION:

the cecum, appendix, and adjacent large intestine

...X-RAY CHANGES IN BRONCHIECTASIS:

in the lower lobes of the lungs

The Most Common
SITE OF:

References

Beck, WW: *Obstetrics and Gynecology*. (The National Medical Series for Independent Study). New York, John Wiley & Sons, Inc., 1989.

Braunstein, H: *Outlines and Review of Pathology*. St. Louis, C.V. Mosby Company, 1987.

Casciato, DA, ed: *Manual of Clinical Oncology*, 2nd ed. Boston, Little, Brown and Company, 1988.

Chandrasoma, P: *Key Facts in Pathology*. New York, Churchill Livingstone, Inc., 1986.

Creighton University Lecture Series, Introduction to Clinical Medicine course, Pathology course, Microbiology Course, 1988-89.

Day, AL, MD. Subarachnoid hemorrhage. *AFP*. 1989;40:95.

Dworkin, PH: *Pediatrics* (The National Medical Series for Independent Study). New York, John Wiley & Sons, Inc., 1987.

Hsu, B: *Physiology*. Boston, Little, Brown and Company, 1987.

Jarrell, BE: *Surgery* (The National Medical Series for Independent Study). Media, Harwal Publishing Company, 1986.

Kingsbury, DT, ed: *Microbiology* (The National Medical Series for Independent Study). Media, Harwal Publishing Company, 1985.

LiVolsi, VA, ed: *Pathology* (The National Medical Series for Independent Study). Media, Harwal Publishing Company, 1984.

The Merck Manual of Diagnosis and Therapy. Rahway, Merck Sharp & Dohme Research Laboratories, 1987.

Robbins, SL: *Pathologic Basis of Disease*. Philadelphia, W.B. Saunders Company, 1984.

Rubin, E, ed.: *Pathology*. Philadelphia, J.B. Lippincott Compa-

436

ny, 1988.

Sabiston, DC: *Sabiston's Essentials of Surgery*. Philadelphia, W.B. Saunders Company, 1987.

Schrock, TR, ed.: *Handbook of Surgery*, 9th ed. Greenbrae, Jones Medical Publications, 1989.

Scialabba, FA, MD. Saccular Aneurysms of the Thoracic Aorta. *AFP*. 1990;41:1475.

Sierles, FS: *Behavioral Science for the Boreds*. Miami, MedMaster, Inc., 1987.

Stillman, RM: *Surgery Diagnosis and Therapy*. East Norwalk, Appleton and Lange, 1989.

Straub, WH, ed.: *Manual of Diagnostic Imaging*, 2nd ed. Boston, Little, Brown and Company, 1989.

Way, LW: *Current Surgical Diagnosis and Treatment*. Norwalk, Appleton and Lange, 1988.

Woods, SM, ed.: *Psychiatry*, 5th ed. (Pre-Test Series). New York, McGraw Hill Inc., 1989.

The Most Common

Site Of Origin Of...

The Most Common
SITE OF
ORIGIN OF:

...AORTIC DISSECTION ("Dissecting Aneurysm"):
> over 60% of dissections arise in the ascending aorta, roughly 20% in the transverse or distal arch, and the remainder in the descending thoracic or abdominal aorta

...APPENDIX:
> most often arises at the convergence of the teniae coli on the cecum

...ARTERIAL EMBOLI TO THE MESENTERIC ARTERIES:
> the heart

...ARTERIAL VASCULAR THROMBOSIS TO THE MESENTERIC ARTERIES:
> the superior mesenteric artery

...BRAIN TUMORS IN CHILDREN:
> below the tentorium (two-thirds), above the tentorium (one-third)

...BRONCHOGENIC CARCINOMA:
> parenchyma - peripheral zone comprising the minute bronchi and bronchioles. Then major bronchus - mainstem or segmental bronchus in zone extending to the smallest visible bronchiole

...CEREBRAL HEMORRHAGE:
> the region of the external capsule

...CHONDROBLASTOMAS:
> almost always located in the epiphyseal ends of long bones

...CORONARY EMBOLISM:
> endocarditis and endocardiosis. Also atherosclerotic plaques; coronary arterial thrombus; thrombi in the left atrium or appendage

...DEEP VENOUS THROMBOSIS:
> The condition usually originates in the lower extremity venous system, starting at the calf vein level and progressing proximally to involve the popliteal, femoral, or iliac system.

The Most Common SITE OF ORIGIN OF:

Some 80-90% of pulmonary emboli originate here

...DISSECTING ANEURYSM OF THE AORTA (Aortic Dissection):
over 60% of dissections arise in the ascending aorta, roughly 20% in the transverse or distal arch, and the remainder in the descending thoracic or abdominal aorta

...DYSPLASIA: in hyperplastic squamous epithelium, and in areas of squamous metaplasia, sites other than squamous epithelium such as dysplastic changes in the mucosal cells

...ECTOPIC PACEMAKERS of the heart:
these develop most commonly in the AV node, the bundle of His, or the Purkinje system; however, modified cells of the atria or ventricles may become aberrant pacemakers

...GIANT CELL TUMORS OF BONE:
almost always located in the epiphyseal ends of long bones

...HEMANGIOENDOTHELIOMA:
the skin and subcutaneous tissue of children
Malignant (hemangiosarcoma):
bones, muscle, liver, and spleen

...HEMANGIOSARCOMA (malignant hemangioendothelioma):
bones, muscle, liver, and spleen
associated with Vinyl chloride exposure:
liver

...HEPATOBLASTOMAS:
right > left lobe of the liver

...LOCALIZED MESOTHELIOMAS (of the pleura):
usually arise from the visceral pleura

...LUNG METASTASES, diffuse lymphangitic type:
breast, prostate

...MESOTHELIOMAS (of the pleura):

442

Localized: usually arise from the visceral pleura

...METASTASES OF UNKNOWN ORIGIN:

(Determined antemortem in only 15% of cases. When a primary site *is* determined, the sites of origin are:) pancreas (25%); lung (20%); stomach, colorectum, hepatobiliary tract (8 to 12% each); kidney (5%); breast, ovary, prostate (2 to 3% each), other sites (< 1% each)

...NOSEBLEEDS: an estimated 90% of nosebleeds originate in Kiesselbach's plexus (also called Little's area), a junction of blood vessels located in the anterior nasal septum

...OAT CELL (undifferentiated small cell) CARCINOMA OF THE LUNG:

centrally

...OSTEOGENIC SARCOMA (osteosarcoma):

over half of all osteosarcomas occur about the knee, most often in the distal femoral metaphysis, or less frequently in the proximal tibial metaphysis. The metaphysis of any long bone may be affected. The hands, feet, skull, and jaw are less common sites for this disease, but they are affected more frequently in patients older than 24 years of age

...OSTEOID OSTEOMAS:

most commonly located in the diaphyses of the tibia and femur, but nearly every other bone in the body has been involved at one time or another, with the possible exceptions of the skull, sternum, and clavicles

...OSTEOSARCOMA (osteogenic sarcoma):

over half of all osteosarcomas occur about the knee, most often in the distal femoral metaphysis, or less frequently in the proximal tibial

443

The Most Common
SITE OF
ORIGIN OF:

metaphysis. The metaphysis of any long bone may be affected. The hands, feet, skull, and jaw are less common sites for this disease, but they are affected more frequently in patients older than 24 years of age

...PROSTATE ADENOCARCINOMA:

in the subcapsular zone. Rarely in the median zone. Almost always in the posterior or lateral lobes. Many reference sources state that almost all are posterior. This is undoubtedly incorrect; in many publications, frequency at least equal in lateral lobes is indicated

...RENAL CELL CARCINOMA:

proximal tubules

...RENAL CORTICAL ADENOMAS:

in proximal tubules

...RHABDOMYOSARCOMAS:

in Childhood: head and neck (38%: orbit tumors, nasopharyngeal and middle ear tumors, neck tumors); genitourinary tract (21%: bladder and prostate tumors, vaginal and uterine tumors); extremity tumors (18%: solid masses on the upper or lower extremities); miscellaneous presentations (a mass or obstructing lesion in the following locations: trunk, retroperitoneum, paratesticular region, perianal region, gastrointestinal and biliary tracts)

...SQUAMOUS CELL CARCINOMA:

of the Anus: in the anterior or posterior anal quadrants

of the Larynx: on the (anterior half of the) true vocal cords . Also in the laryngeal ventricles, false cords, aryepiglottic folds, epiglottis, arytenoid, and subglottic areas.

of the Lung: centrally

...THROMBOEMBOLI:

444

The Most Common
SITE OF
ORIGIN OF:

deep veins of the leg

References

Braunstein, H: ·*Outlines and Review of Pathology*. St. Louis, C.V. Mosby Company, 1987.

Casciato, DA, ed: *Manual of Clinical Oncology*, 2nd ed. Boston, Little, Brown and Company, 1988.

Creighton University Lecture Series, Pathology course, 1988-89.

Dworkin, PH: *Pediatrics* (The National Medical Series for Independent Study). New York, John Wiley & Sons, Inc., 1987.

Jarrell, BE: *Surgery* (The National Medical Series for Independent Study). Media, Harwal Publishing Company, 1986.

Medical Student. Epistaxis: Diagnosis and Treatment. *Medical Student*. November/December, 1990, p. 20.

Purdy, RE.: *Handbook of Cardiac Drugs.* Boston, Little, Brown and Company, 1988.

Robbins, SL: *Pathologic Basis of Disease.* Philadelphia, W.B. Saunders Company, 1984.

Rubin, E, ed.: *Pathology.* Philadelphia, J.B. Lippincott Company, 1988.

Sabiston, DC: *Sabiston's Essentials of Surgery.* Philadelphia, W.B. Saunders Company, 1987.

Schrock, TR: *Handbook of Surgery.* Chicago, Jones Medical Publications, 1989.

Way, LW: *Current Surgical Diagnosis and Treatment.* Norwalk, Appleton and Lange, 1988.

The Most Common

Symptoms Of...

The Most Common
SYMPTOMS OF:

...ABDOMINAL IRRADIATION:
> decreased appetite

...ACUTE DIVERTICULITIS:
> left lower quadrant pain and a change in normal bowel habits, either constipation or diarrhea. Nausea and vomiting may also be present

...ANAL FISSURES:
> excruciating pain during and after defecation

...BRAIN TUMOR:
> headaches, irritability, vomiting, and gait abnormalities. Morning headaches are most characteristic, but drowsiness and abnormal behavior are also quite common. Symptoms may be intermittent, particularly in very young children, who have open fontanelles

...CANCER OF THE PANCREAS:
> pain

...CARCINOMA OF THE CERVIX, invasive:
> postcoital or irregular bleeding

...CELIAC DISEASE, in children:
> diarrhea. Failure to thrive is frequently seen. Vomiting is more common in younger patients. There may be abdominal distention and irritability. Short-stature, iron-resistant anemia, and rickets may be seen in older children

...COLITIS CYSTICA PROFUNDA:
> rectal bleeding, mucus stools, diarrhea, pain, tenesmus, weight loss

...CONGESTIVE HEART FAILURE:
> dyspnea

...COW'S MILK AND SOY PROTEIN INTOLERANCE IN

The Most Common
SYMPTOMS OF:

CHILDREN:

vomiting and diarrhea. Rectal bleeding may be seen if colitis is present. Edema secondary to excessive enteric protein loss may be dramatic and is often associated with anemia. Rhinorrhea, wheezing, and eczema may occasionally be seen and are frequently accompanied by eosinophilia and an elevated serum immunoglobulin E (IgE) level. Anaphylaxis rarely is observed but may be life threatening

...DEPRESSION:

Cognitive features:

self-criticism, <u>sense of worthlessness</u>, guilt, pessimism, <u>hopelessness</u>, despair, distractible, <u>poor concentration</u>, uncertain and indecisive, variable obsessions, somatic complaints (<u>particularly in the elderly</u>), memory impairment, delusions and hallucinations

Emotional features:

<u>depressed</u> mood,"blue", <u>irritability</u>, anxiety, <u>anhedonia</u>, <u>loss of interest</u>, loss of zest, diminished emotional bonds, interpersonal withdrawal, preoccupation with death

Vegetative features:

<u>fatigability</u>, no energy, <u>insomnia</u> or hypersomnia, anorexia or hyperrexia, weight loss or gain, psychomotor retardation, psychomotor agitation, impaired libido, frequent diurnal variation

...DIVERTICULITIS, acute:

left lower quadrant pain and a change in normal bowel habits, either constipation or diarrhea. Nausea and vomiting may also be present

450

The Most Common
SYMPTOMS OF:

...ECTOPIC PREGNANCY:

abnormal uterine bleeding or spotting, which usually begins 7-14 days after the missed menstrual period. Then unilateral pelvic pain, which may be knife-like and stabbing or dull and less well-defined

...ENDOMETRIAL CARCINOMA:

irregular menses or postmenopausal bleeding

...ENTEROBIASIS:

pruritus ani

...GASTROESOPHAGEAL REFLUX IN CHILDREN:

vomiting

...GRAVE'S DISEASE:

emotional lability, increased appetite, heat intolerance, weight loss, frequent loose stools, deterioration of behavior and school performance, and poor sleeping. Weakness and inability to participate in sports are sometimes noted

...HEMATOMA, Subdural, chronic:

headache

...HEMORRHOIDS:

protrusion, bleeding, dull pain, and pruritus

...HERPES SIMPLEX VIRUS (HSV):

recurrent vesiculoulcerative genital lesions

...INVASIVE CARCINOMA OF THE CERVIX:

postcoital or irregular bleeding

...LUNG TUMORS, Benign:

bronchial obstruction by the lesion, pneumonitis, and hemoptysis. Clubbing or hypertrophic osteoarthropathy does not occur in benign tumors except in fibrous mesotheliomas

...MANIA:

Cognitive features:

elevated self-esteem, <u>grandiosity</u>, speech dis-

451

The Most Common
SYMPTOMS OF:

turbances (loud, word rhyming [clanging], pressure of speech, flight of ideas, progression to incoherence), <u>poor judgement</u>, disorganization, paranoia, delusions and hallucinations

Emotional features:

excited, elevated mood, euphoria, emotional <u>lability</u>, rapid temporary shifts to acute depression, <u>irritability</u>, low frustration tolerance, demanding, egocentric

Physiological features:

boundless energy, insomnia, <u>little need for sleep</u>, decreased appetite

...MOOD DISORDERS:

Depression:

Cognitive features:

self-criticism, <u>sense of worthlessness</u>, guilt, pessimism, <u>hopelessness</u>, despair, distractible, <u>poor concentration</u>, uncertain and indecisive, variable obsessions, somatic complaints (<u>particularly in the elderly</u>), memory impairment, delusions and hallucinations

Emotional features:

<u>depressed</u> mood,"blue", <u>irritability</u>, anxiety, <u>anhedonia</u>, <u>loss of interest</u>, loss of zest, diminished emotional bonds, interpersonal withdrawal, preoccupation with death

Vegetative features:

<u>fatigability</u>, no energy, <u>insomnia</u> or hypersomnia, anorexia or hyperrexia, weight loss or gain, psychomotor retardation, psychomotor agitation, impaired libido, frequent diurnal variation

Mania:

Cognitive features:

452

The Most Common
SYMPTOMS OF:

elevated self-esteem, <u>grandiosity</u>, speech disturbances (loud, word rhyming [clanging], pressure of speech, flight of ideas, progression to incoherence), <u>poor judgement</u>, disorganization, paranoia, delusions and hallucinations

Emotional features:

excited, elevated mood, euphoria, emotional <u>lability</u>, rapid temporary shifts to acute depression, <u>irritability</u>, low frustration tolerance, demanding, egocentric

Physiological features:

boundless energy, insomnia, <u>little need for sleep</u>, decreased appetite

...MYASTHENIA GRAVIS:

ptosis, double vision, dysarthria, dysphagia, nasal speech, and weakness of the arms and legs

...OSTEOMYELITIS IN OLDER CHILDREN:

fever and localized bone tenderness. Local swelling, redness, warmth, and suppuration may occur subsequently

...OVARIAN CANCER:

abdominal pain and distention, urinary and gastrointestinal tract symptoms due to compression by tumor or cancer invasion, and abdominal and vaginal bleeding are the most common symptoms

...PANCREATIC CANCER:

pain

...PERICARDITIS: inspiratory chest pain

...PMS (PREMENSTRUAL SYNDROME):

Emotional: irritability, tension, depression, anxiety, crying spells and fatigue are among the most common

453

The Most Common
SYMPTOMS OF:

Physical: breast tenderness, abdominal bloating, swelling of the ankles, and weight gain

...PREMENSTRUAL SYNDROME (PMS):

Emotional: irritability, tension, depression, anxiety, crying spells and fatigue are among the most common

Physical: breast tenderness, abdominal bloating, swelling of the ankles, and weight gain

...PYELONEPHRITIS:

Xanthogranulomatous pyelonephritis:
fever and flank or abdominal pain

...REFLUX IN CHILDREN:

Gastroesophageal:
vomiting

...SINUSITIS IN YOUNGER CHILDREN:
fever, purulent nasal discharge, and daytime cough that persists longer than 10 days. Suggestive signs of acute sinusitis include periorbital swelling, localized tenderness to pressure, and malodorous breath

...SQUAMOUS CELL CARCINOMA OF THE VAGINA:
vaginal discharge, which is often bloody

... SUBDURAL HEMATOMA, Chronic:

headache

...TESTICULAR CANCER:
a painless enlargement usually noticed during bathing or after a minor trauma. Painful enlargement of the testis occurs in 30 to 50% of patients and may be the result of bleeding or infarction in the tumor.

...related to the THYROID GLAND IN PEOPLE WITH A GOITER:
an awareness of increasing size of the neck or the presence of a mass

454

...TRICHINOSIS: fever, weakness, and muscle pain. Also eyelid edema, a maculopapular rash, and petechial hemorrhages in the conjunctiva and beneath the nails. Serious complications include congestive heart failure, delirium, psychosis, paresis, and coma. Hemoptysis and pulmonary consolidation are common.

...ULCERATIVE COLITIS:
rectal bleeding, diarrhea, abdominal pain, weight loss, and fever

...URINARY CALCULI (acute symptom):
Upper urinary calculi:
pain. Other symptoms include hematuria, nausea and vomiting, irritative bladder symptoms, general abdominal discomfort mimicking gastrointestinal disease

...VULVAR HYPERPLASTIC DYSTROPHY:
constant pruritus

...VULVAR LICHEN SCLEROSUS:
chronic soreness associated with "vulvar dysuria", pruritus

...VULVOVAGINITIS:
Vulvar symptoms:
burning, inching, odor

...WILMS' TUMOR:
enlarged abdomen, abdominal pain, and painless hematuria

...XANTHOGRANULOMATOUS PYELONEPHRITIS:
fever and flank or abdominal pain

The Most Common
SYMPTOMS OF:
References

Barcia, PJ, MD, FACS, COL, USA, MC. Colitis Cystica Profunda: An Unusual Surgical Problem. *The American Surgeon*. 1979;45:61.

Beck, WW: *Obstetrics and Gynecology*. (The National Medical Series for Independent Study). New York, John Wiley & Sons, Inc., 1989.

Casciato, DA, ed: *Manual of Clinical Oncology*, 2nd ed. Boston, Little, Brown and Company, 1988.

Dworkin, PH: *Pediatrics* (The National Medical Series for Independent Study). New York, John Wiley & Sons, Inc., 1987.

Jarrell, BE: *Surgery* (The National Medical Series for Independent Study). Media, Harwal Publishing Company, 1986.

Kingsbury, DT, ed.: *Microbiology* (The National Medical Series for Independent Study). Media, Harwal Publishing Company, 1985.

Myers, AR, ed.: *Medicine* (The National Medical Series for Independent Study). Media, Harwal Publishing Company, 1986.

Robbins, SL: *Pathologic Basis of Disease*. Philadelphia, W.B. Saunders Company, 1984.

Sabiston, DC: *Sabiston's Essentials of Surgery*. Philadelphia, W.B. Saunders Company, 1987.

Schwartz, SI: *Principles of Surgery*. New York, McGraw-Hill Book Company, 1989.

Stillman, RM: *Surgery Diagnosis and Therapy*. East Norwalk, Appleton and Lange, 1989.

Tomb, DA: *Psychiatry for the House Officer*. Baltimore, Williams & Wilkins, 1988.

Way, LW: *Current Surgical Diagnosis and Treatment*. Norwalk, Appleton and Lange, 1988.

Woods, SM, ed.: *Psychiatry*, 5th ed. (Pre-Test Series). New York, McGraw Hill Inc., 1989.

The Most Common

Time...

...that AIR EMBOLISM OCCURS:

Arterial:	occurs as a consequence of tears in pulmonary parenchyma, opening venous channels
Venous:	during the course of brain or head and neck surgery performed with patient in a sitting position

...that AKATHISIA APPEARS DURING ANTIPSYCHOTIC THERAPY:

between the second and tenth weeks of therapy

...of ANOVULATION:

during the 2 years after menarche (i.e., the first menses) and the 3 years before menopause

...that BILIARY COLIC OCCURS:

1 to 2 hours postprandially, usually in the evening and almost never in the morning

...that BONE MARROW CHROMOSOME STUDIES ARE USED:

in the evaluation of leukemias

...during which BRAIN DYSFUNCTION/HYPERACTIVITY/ ATTENTION DEFICIT DISORDER USUALLY PRESENTS:

the school aged child (age 7-10)

...that CARNEOUS DEGENERATION OF UTERINE LEIOMYOMAS OCCURS:

during pregnancy

...of DIAGNOSIS OF AORTIC ANEURYSM:

routine physical examination

...of DIAGNOSIS OF GALLBLADDER TRAUMA:

at laparotomy

...of infestation with HEAD LICE IN CHILDREN:

during the winter

...that HOUSE FIRES OCCUR:

at night; in December through March

The Most Common

TIME:

...during which INVERSION OF THE UTERUS OCCURS:
> immediately following delivery

...that JAUNDICE SECONDARY TO ANTIPSYCHOTICS AND NON-MAO INHIBITOR ANTI-DEPRESSANTS OCCURS:
> between the second and fourth weeks of therapy

...for MISCARRIAGE:
> first trimester pregnancy

...that MECKEL'S DIVERTICULA IS DETECTED:
> incidental finding at laparotomy, then as a result of a significant complication

...that MYOCARDIAL INFARCTION, Perioperative, OCCURS:
> during the first 3 postoperative days. The remainder occur during the next 3 days.

...that NAUSEA AND VOMITING, DISTASTE FOR FOOD, AND QUEASINESS OCCUR DURING THE FIRST 3 MONTHS OF PREGNANCY:
> most often noted upon rising (therefore called "morning sickness")

...that PERIOPERATIVE MYOCARDIAL INFARCTION OCCURS:
> during the first 3 postoperative days. The remainder occur during the next 3 days.

...of PRESENTATION OF:
> severe, Abdominal Pain in acute occlusion of the superior mesenteric artery:
>> early in the course of the disease
>
> Insulin-dependent diabetes mellitus (IDDM) in children:
>> in early adolescence
>
> Necrotizing enterocolitis in preterm infants:
>> within the first week of feeding
>
> adult Polycystic Kidney:
>> in the fifth decade

460

...that PSEUDOPARKINSONISM APPEARS DURING ANTI-
PSYCHOTIC THERAPY:
between the second and tenth weeks of therapy
...of infection with ROTAVIRUS:
during the cooler months of the year
...of RUPTURE OF THE HEART AFTER AN MI:
within the first few days
...that UMBILICAL HERNIAS CLOSE BY:

closure by the age of 2 years

References

Beck, WW: *Obstetrics and Gynecology*. (The National Medical
Series for Independent Study). New York, John Wiley &
Sons, Inc., 1989.

Benson, RC: *Handbook of Obstetrics and Gynecology*. Los Altos, Lange Medical Publications, 1983.

Braunstein, H: *Outlines and Review of Pathology*. St. Louis,
C.V. Mosby Company, 1987.

Creighton University Lecture Series, Introduction to Clinical
Medicine course, 1988-89.

Creighton University Lecture Series, Department of OB/Gyn,
1989.

Dworkin, PH: *Pediatrics* (The National Medical Series for Independent Study). New York, John Wiley & Sons, Inc., 1987.

Gregory, I: *Psychiatry*. Boston, Little, Brown and Company,
Inc., 1983.

Jarrell, BE: *Surgery* (The National Medical Series for Independent Study). Media, Harwal Publishing Company, 1986.

The Most Common

TIME:

Sabiston, DC: *Sabiston's Essentials of Surgery*. Philadelphia, W.B. Saunders Company, 1987.

Sierles, FS: *Behavioral Science for the Boreds*. Miami, MedMaster, Inc., 1987.

The Most Common

Type Of...

The Most Common
TYPE OF:

...ABNORMALITY IN DOWN'S SYNDROME:

presence of an extra chromosome > unbalanced translocations > mosaics

...ACUTE CYSTITIS:

hemorrhagic. Other varieties are sometimes seen (bullous, fibrinous, gangrenous, suppurative)

...ACUTE LEUKEMIA IN CHILDREN:

acute lymphocytic leukemia (ALL) (accounts for 80% of all childhood acute leukemia); acute nonlymphocytic leukemia (ANLL) (accounts for the remaining 20% of cases of acute leukemia in children)

...ADENOCARCINOMA OF THE:

Gallbladder: scirrhous (60%), papillary (25%), or mucoid (15%)

Stomach: ulcerative (~75%), polypoid (10%), scirrhous (localized or linitis plastica) (10%), superficial spreading (5%)

...ADENOMATOUS POLYP OF THE COLON:

tubular adenomas (~75%)

...AMENORRHEA:

hypogonadotropic, or secondary amenorrhea

...ANEURYSM: berry aneurysm

Intra-abdominal:

aneurysms of the aorto-iliac system, splenic artery aneurysms

Intracranial: most are saccular and arise from a bifurcation of vessels that form the Circle of Willis

Splanchnic: aneurysms of the splenic artery (>60%), hepatic artery aneurysms (20%)

Superior mesenteric:

mycotic (60%), and most of the rest are atherosclerotic

The Most Common
TYPE OF:
Thoracic aorta:

Caused by:

Atherosclerosis:
fusiform aneurysm. Up to 20% may be saccular

Cystic medial necrosis:
dissecting aneurysm

Mycotic:
saccular aneurysm

Posttraumatic:
saccular aneurysm

Syphilitic:
saccular aneurysm (~75%)

Non-dissecting:
atherosclerotic (~70%), posttraumatic (15-25%), syphilitic (< 5%; this represents a considerable reduction from the 30 percent of earlier times), nonsyphilitic mycotic aneurysms (2%; found with a higher frequency in intravenous drug abusers), congenital. A small mixed group of other aneurysms occurs with Marfan's syndrome, Turner's syndrome, giant-cell arteritis, and congenital subaortic stenosis

seen in the United States today:
atherosclerotic

...ANGIOMA OF THE BRAIN:
arteriovenous malformations (AVMs)

...AORTIC STENOSIS, congenital:
the valve is bicuspid, with a single fused commissure and an eccentric orifice

...AORTOILIAC OCCLUSIVE DISEASE:
atherosclerosis extends from the aorta to include femoral and distal vessel; then atherosclerosis extends from the aorta to the level of the inguinal ligament, but there is little or no

466

disease more distally; fewest with atherosclerosis limited to the aortic bifurcation and common iliac arteries

...ARTERIOSCLEROSIS:

atherosclerosis

...ASTHMA IN CHILDREN:

extrinsic (IgE mediated) > others. Mixed extrinsic- and infection-induced is also common. Others include intrinsic (no IgE mechanism demonstrated, often triggered by infection), solely exercise-induced, or aspirin-induced - these are rare during infancy or childhood

...ATRIAL SEPTAL DEFECT:

ostium secundum defects account for the majority of atrial septal defects. Sinus venosus defects and ostium primum defects occur less commonly. A patent foramen ovale is not considered an atrial septal defect

...ATYPICAL MYCOBACTERIA WHICH CAUSE CERVICAL ADENITIS IN CHILDREN:

Mycobacterium scrofulaceum and *Mycobacterium avium-intracellulare*

...BASAL CELL CARCINOMA OF THE SKIN:

nodular-ulcerated BCC

...BILIARY DISEASE in Hong Kong:

recurrent pyogenic cholangitis (oriental cholangiohepatitis)

...BIOPSY MADE:

excisional biopsy

...BLADDER CALCULI:

primary, about foreign body

...BLADDER CANCER:

single papillary cancers

...BLADDER INFLAMMATION:

The Most Common
TYPE OF:

acute inflammatory process with much erythrocyte extravasation (hemorrhagic cystitis). Other varieties are sometimes seen (bullous, fibrinous, gangrenous, suppurative)

...BRAIN ANGIOMA:

arteriovenous malformations (AVMs)

...BRAIN HERNIATION seen clinically:

transtentorial (uncal) herniation

...BRAIN TUMOR:

primary (60%) > metastatic (40%)

in Children: medulloblastoma

...BREAST TUMOR, malignant:

infiltrating duct carcinoma

...BRONCHIAL ADENOMA OF THE RESPIRATORY TRACT:

bronchial carcinoid (85%). Also adenoid cystic (10-15%), mucoepidermoid (rare)

...BURN, Severe: thermal injury from fire, steam, or scalding liquids

...CALCULI of the urinary tract (urolithiasis):

calcium oxalate, phosphate, uric acid

...CANCER in:

Adenoma of the colon:

well differentiated

Childhood:

Black children:

leukemia, central nervous system, lymphoma including Hodgkin's, soft tissue sarcoma, Wilms' tumor, neuroblastoma, eye and germ cell

White children:

leukemia, central nervous system, lymphoma including Hodgkin's, neuroblastoma, soft tissue sarcoma, Wilms' tumor, bone, eye, germ

468

cell, liver

...CARCINOID TUMOR OF THE APPENDIX:

benign

...CARCINOMA:

of the Biliary tract:

carcinoma of the gallbladder

of the Esophagus:

poorly or well-differentiated squamous cell
carcinomas (60-70%), adenocarcinomas that
originate either from the esophageal mucous
glands or from changes previously referred to
as Barrett esophagus (5-10%), and the remainder are undifferentiated tumors. Some of
these undifferentiated neoplasms are composed of large, pleomorphic anaplastic cells.
A few are so-called "oat-cell" carcinomas,
composed of small uniform cells that have
deeply chromatic nuclei. These oat cell lesions are probably derived from endocrine
cells and so belong to the family of APUDo-
mas capable of secreting a variety of amine
and polypeptide hormones

of the Gallbladder:

adenocarcinoma

Adenocarcinomas:

scirrhous (60%), papillary (25%), or mucoid
(15%)

of the Thyroid:

well-differentiated papillary carcinoma

of the Vulva: squamous carcinoma. Fewer are adenosquamous carcinoma, adenocarcinoma, malignant
melanoma, verrucous carcinoma, and sarcomas

...CATARACT: senile cataract

...CELL INJURY: ischemic

469

The Most Common
TYPE OF:

...*CLOSTRIDIUM NOVYI* CAUSING GAS GANGRENE, ISO-
LATED:
type A

...*CLOSTRIDIUM PERFRINGENS* IN ENVIRONMENTAL ISO-
LATES:
type A

...CELLS
in children with Acute lymphocytic leukemia (ALL):
L1 lymphoblasts (small lymphoblasts with
scant cytoplasm and absent or inconspicuous
nucleoli); L2 lymphoblasts are less common
than L1 cells (these are larger, with more
abundant cytoplasm and one or more prominent nucleoli, and are sometimes mistaken for
myeloblasts); L3 lymphoblasts are rare (these
are large, with deeply basophilic and vacuolat-
ed cytoplasm and prominent nucleoli, and
usually indicative of the equally rare B-cell
ALL)
in children with Non-Hodgkin's Lymphomas:
T-cell origin (almost half of the cases); B-cell
origin (most other cases); non-T, non-B cell
origin (uncommon); true histiocytic or non-
lymphoid origin (rare)

...CHILDHOOD LEUKEMIA:
acute lymphocytic leukemia

...CHRONIC MYELOGENOUS LEUKEMIA IN CHILDHOOD:
adult CML > juvenile CML (2 times)
Blastic CML: myeloid > lymphoid

...COCCIDIOIDOMYCOSIS:
primary pulmonary and disseminated

...COLLAGEN IN:
Bone: Type I collagen
Cartilage: Type II collagen
Mature scars: Type I collagen

470

Pliable organs, such as blood vessels, the uterus, and the gastrointestinal tract:
Type III collagen

Skin: Type I collagen

Tendon: Type I collagen

...COMMON BILE DUCT STONES:
secondary, then primary

...CONGENITAL AORTIC STENOSIS:
a bicuspid valve with a single fused commissure and an eccentric orifice

...CONGENITAL NEPHROSIS:
"Finnish" (characterized by widespread foot process fusion, microcystic change in proximal tubules, nephrotic picture and early death from renal failure)

...CRITICAL AORTIC STENOSIS ASSOCIATED WITH PATENT DUCTUS ARTERIOSUS (PDA):
the valve most often is bicuspid but may be unicuspid with an eccentric small opening. Annular hypoplasia almost always is present in the neonatal period; often, left ventricular hypoplasia and endocardial fibroelastosis also are found

...CROUP: acute laryngotracheobronchitis

...CYST, renal: solitary

...CYSTITIS, acute:
hemorrhagic. Other varieties are sometimes seen (bullous, fibrinous, gangrenous, suppurative)

...DEGENERATIVE CHANGE of uterine leiomyomas:
hyaline degeneration. Others include cystic degeneration, necrosis, carneous degeneration, mucoid degeneration, rarely sarcomatous degeneration

...DEVELOPMENTAL LANGUAGE DISORDER:

471

The Most Common
TYPE OF:

receptive type > expressive type

...DIAPHRAGMATIC HERNIA IN THE NEWBORN:
hernias through the foramen of Bochdalek.
Hernias through the foramen of Morgani are
somewhat rare

...DISEASE: inherited, congenital, toxic, infectious, traumatic, degenerative, allergic, autoimmune, neoplastic, nutritional, metabolic, molecular,
psychosomatic, factitious, iatrogenic

...DUODENAL ULCER PERFORATION:
ulcers on the anterior surface of the duodenum. Occasionally, ulcers can perforate pos-
teriorly into the lesser sac

...EDEMA seen clinically:
vasogenic edema

...EMBOLUS: venous thromboembolus

...EMPHYSEMA: centrilobular emphysema is the form of the
disease most frequently encountered and the
one usually associated with clinical symptoms. It is most common and most severe in
the upper zones of the lung (upper lobe and
superior segment of lower lobe)

...ENDOMETRIAL CARCINOMA:
adenocarcinoma, adenocanthoma. The remaining types are papillary serous carcinoma,
clear cell adenocarcinoma, and adenosquamous carcinoma

...ERYTHROBLASTOSIS FETALIS:
mild hemolytic disease > moderate hemolytic
disease > severe hemolytic disease

...ESOPHAGEAL ATRESIA:
esophageal atresia with distal tracheoesopha-
geal fistula

...ESOPHAGITIS: reflux esophagitis
Viral: herpetic

472

Fungal: *Candida albicans*

...FISTULAS:

Vesical: vesicovaginal, vesicointestinal, and vesicocutaneous

...FLUID AND ELECTROLYTE IMBALANCE IN SURGICAL PATIENTS:

isotonic hypohydration (dehydration)

...GALLSTONE:

in the Western World:

bile supersaturated with cholesterol. Small percentage is pure cholesterol stones

Pigment stones:

pure pigment stones > calcium bilirubinate stones

in the Orient: calcium bilirubinate stones

...GANGLIOSIDOSE:

Tay-Sachs disease

...GASTRIC ULCERS:

Type I ulcers > Type II or Type III ulcers.

...GASTROINTESTINAL LYMPHOMA:

diffuse histiocytic lymphoma (60%); lymphocytic lymphoma, nodular or diffuse, well or poorly differentiated, were the next most common type. The remainder of cases in one series included rare instances of primary Hodgkin's disease of the gastrointestinal tract

...GENETIC HYPERLIPIDEMIA IN CHILDHOOD:

familial hypercholesterolemia

...GERM CELL TUMOR:

in Children: sacrococcygeal germ cell tumors

...GINGIVOSTOMATITIS:

in Children: herpetic gingivostomatitis. Most cases are due to herpes simplex virus type 1 rather than type 2

...HSMN (Hereditary Sensory and Motor Neuropathy):

The Most Common
TYPE OF:

Charcot-Marie-Tooth disease (peroneal muscular atrophy)

...HAMARTOMA of the lung:

localized type (cartilaginous) - tumors composed of islands of cartilage and cleft spaces lined by ciliated epithelium.

...HAMARTOMATOUS COLONIC POLYPS:

juvenile polyps

...HEAD-RELATED INJURY:

contusion

...HEMORRHAGE, intracranial:

in Newborn infants:

periventricular/subependymal hemorrhage

Post-traumatic:

subarachnoid hemorrhage

...HERNIAS: the vast majority of hernias occur in the inguinal region, with approximately 50% of these being indirect and 25 per cent being direct inguinal hernias. Incisional hernias (including ventral hernias) make up about 10 per cent of all hernias, femoral hernias approximately 5 per cent, and umbilical hernias 3 per cent; rare hernias account for the remainder

Inguinal: indirect > direct

Pediatric, Inguinal:

indirect hernia > direct hernia

Strangulated: in a review of a series of patients with strangulated hernias, 40 to 50 per cent of the hernias were inguinal. 30 to 35 per cent were femoral, 10 to 15 per cent were umbilical, and the remainder were incisional or epigastric. Ten per cent of all inguinal hernias presented as incarcerated hernias, whereas 20 to 25 per cent of femoral hernias presented as incarcerations (Andrews, NJ, in Sabiston)

474

Ventral: incisional hernias
in Women: indirect inguinal hernias

...HERPES GENITALIS:

herpesvirus (*Herpesvirus hominis*) type 2
(HSV-2). Remainder is herpesvirus type 1
(HSV-1)

...HERPES SIMPLEX VIRUS WHICH CAUSES GINGIVOS-
TOMATITIS IN CHILDREN:

type 1 > type 2

...HISTOLOGY IN RHABDOMYOSARCOMA OF CHILD-
HOOD:

favorable histology, which is predominantly
embryonal (80%) > unfavorable histology, of
various subtypes (20%)

...HYPERLIPIDEMIA IN CHILDHOOD:

Genetic: familial hypercholesterolemia

...IMPERFORATE ANUS:

in Males: the supralevator (high) type (the rectum does
not pass through the puborectalis sling)
in Females: the infralevator (low) type (the rectum passes
through the puborectalis sling)

...INFARCTION: myocardial infarction, pulmonary infarction,
cerebral infarction, intestinal infarction, renal
infarction

...INFECTION:

in Humans: #1 not available. Urinary tract infection is the
second most common

in the Newborn:

perinatally acquired bacterial infections. Infections that are acquired in utero remain an
important source of long-term disability

...INGUINAL HERNIA IN CHILDHOOD:

indirect inguinal hernia > direct inguinal hernia

...INJURY:

The Most Common
TYPE OF:

    associated with Abuse in children:
        burns
    that requires an Emergency room visit by children:
        falls

...INSULINOMA: benign (80%) > malignant (10%) > multifocal (10%)

...INTRA-THORACIC MASS IN CHILDHOOD:
        mediastinal masses

...KIDNEY STONES:
        calcium salts (70%) (calcium oxalate, calcium oxalate and hydroxyapatite [67%], brushite and hydroxyapatite [3%]); struvite (20%); uric acid (5%); cystine (3%); insoluble organic compounds (2%)

...LEUKEMIA:
    in Children: acute lymphocytic leukemia (ALL)
    Acute: acute lymphocytic leukemia (ALL) (accounts for 80% of all childhood acute leukemia); acute nonlymphocytic leukemia (ANLL) (accounts for the remaining 20% of cases of acute leukemia in children)

    in Western countries:
        chronic lymphocytic leukemia (CLL) (accounts for one-third of cases)

...LIVER TUMOR:
    in Children: hepatoblastoma
    in Men: malignant
    in Women: benign

...LUNG CANCER:
        metastatic
    Primary: squamous cell (epidermoid) carcinoma (about 35%-40%), adenocarcinomas (mucinous type) (30%), small cell undifferentiated (oat cell) carcinomas (25%), large cell undifferentiated carcinomas (5%)

476

The Most Common
TYPE OF:

Cured by Radiotherapy:
> radiotherapy cures lung cancer in only 1-2% of cases, most often undifferentiated tumors

...LUNG LESIONS IN HISTOPLASMOSIS:
> lesions like caseocavitary tuberculosis and peripheral coin lesions

...LUNG MALFORMATION:
> cartilaginous hamartoma

...LYMPHATIC SPREAD OF RECTAL CANCER:
> upward displacement

...LYMPHEDEMA, primary:
> lymphedema praecox

...LYMPHOMA:
Gastrointestinal:
> diffuse histiocytic lymphoma (60%); lymphocytic lymphoma, nodular or diffuse, well or poorly differentiated, were the next most common type. The remainder of cases in one series included rare instances of primary Hodgkin's disease of the gastrointestinal tract

Malignant:
in the Pediatric patient:
> lymphoblastic lymphoma

...MALFORMATION OF THE LUNG:
> cartilaginous hamartoma

...MALIGNANT SALIVARY GLAND TUMOR following salivary gland irradiation:
> mucoepidermoid carcinoma

...MALNUTRITION:
in Surgical Patients:
> protein-calorie malnutrition
in the World: Kwashiorkor, which is caused by a severe deficiency of protein

...MECHANICAL INTESTINAL OBSTRUCTION:
> extrinsic lesions > intrinsic lesions > obtura-

The Most Common
TYPE OF:

tion obstruction

    Extrinsic: adhesions

...MEDIASTINAL TUMOR:

benign (75%) > malignant

...MEDULLARY CYSTIC DISEASE (nephronophthisis):

juvenile nephronophthisis (50% of cases), sporadic nephronophthisis (about 20%), renal-retinal dysplasia (about 15%), adult-onset medullary cystic disease (about 15%)

...MELANOMA: superficial spreading (70%), nodular melanoma (15%), lentigo maligna melanoma (10-15%), acral lentiginous

...MENTAL RETARDATION:

mild retardation > moderate retardation > severe retardation > profound retardation

    Moderate and severe types:

Down's syndrome

...MESOTHELIOMA:

pleural malignant mesotheliomas outnumber peritoneal ones by a ratio of 3:1

...METASTASES OF UNKNOWN ORIGIN:

adenocarcinomas and undifferentiated carcinomas (> 75%)

...MUSCULAR DYSTROPHY:

Duchenne (pseudohypertrophic) muscular dystrophy. Other genetic muscular dystrophies include Becker's dystrophy (a later-appearing, more benign form that otherwise resembles Duchenne muscular dystrophy), Landouzy-Dejerine dystrophy (facioscapulohumeral), Leyden-Moebius dystrophy (limb-girdle, or scapulohumeral), and the myotonic muscular dystrophies

...MYCOBACTERIUM, atypical, which cause cervical adenitis in children:

478

Mycobacterium scrofulaceum and *Mycobacterium avium-intracellulare*

...MYOMATA UTERI:

> intramural myomas. Others include submucous and subserous

...NEPHRONOPHTHISIS (medullary cystic disease):

> juvenile nephronophthisis (50% of cases), sporadic nephronophthisis (about 20%), renal-retinal dysplasia (about 15%), adult-onset medullary cystic disease (about 15%)

...NEPHROSIS, congenital:

> "Finnish" (characterized by widespread foot process fusion, microcystic change in proximal tubules, nephrotic picture and early death from renal failure)

...NEUROPATHY, SENSORY AND MOTOR:

Hereditary (HSMN):

> Charcot-Marie-Tooth disease (peroneal muscular atrophy)

...ORGANIC BRAIN SYNDROMES:

> delirium, dementia, and intoxication and withdrawal

...OSTEOCHONDRITIS DISSECANS:

> unilateral

...OVARIAN CANCER:

> serous cystadenoma carcinoma

Malignant: epithelial malignancies

Epithelial: Serous > mucinous > endometroid

...POLYPS:

Colorectal: hyperplastic polyps

Adenomatous:

> tubular adenomas (~75%)

...PAROTID TUMOR:

> benign

...PEDIATRIC INGUINAL HERNIAS:

The Most Common
TYPE OF:

indirect hernia

...PEMPHIGUS seen in North America:

pemphigus vulgaris

...PEPTIC ULCERS:

duodenal ulcers are 10 times more common than gastric ulcers in young patients, but in the older age groups the frequency is about equal

...PERSISTENT TRUNCUS ARTERIOSUS:

a short main pulmonary artery segment originates from the trunk.

...PHEOCHROMOCYTOMA:

benign (90%) > malignant (10%)

...PIGMENT STONES:

in the USA: pure pigment stones > calcium bilirubinate stones

in the Orient: calcium bilirubinate stones

...PITUITARY ADENOMA:

Hypersecretory:

prolactin-secreting adenoma and growth hormone-secreting adenoma

...PLEURAL NODULAR LESION:

fibrous plaque composed of poorly cellular laminated collagen bundles of non-neoplastic origin

...POLYP OF THE LARGE BOWEL (in adults):

adenomatous (60-75%), villoglandular (15-20%), villous adenoma (10-15%). Rarely hereditary familial or Puetz-Jeghers

...PRIMARY LYMPHEDEMA:

Lymphedema praecox

...PROSTATE ADENOCARCINOMA:

well differentiated, small acinar adenocarcinomas

...PSYCHOTHERAPY:
    Group therapy:
                interpersonal exploration groups
    Individual therapy:
                supportive therapy, psychoanalytic psycho-
                therapy, and cognitive therapy

...PULMONARY TUMOR associated with endocrine effects:
                oat cell carcinoma

...REFLUX, Vesicoureteral:
                primary reflux is by far the most common
                type. Secondary reflux is relatively rare

...RENAL CYST: solitary

...RESPIRATORY VIRUS WHICH CAUSES ACUTE LARYN-
                GOTRACHEOBRONCHITIS:
                parainfluenza virus

...RICKETTSIAL INFECTION in the United States:
                Rocky Mountain spotted fever

...SARCOMA:
    Bone: osteosarcoma (45%), chondrosarcoma (20%),
                Ewing's sarcoma (15%), chordoma (9%), fi-
                brosarcoma of bone (7%), parosteal sarcoma
                (<2%), and adamantinoma, malignant giant
                cell tumor, and polyhistiocytoma (each < 1%)
    Small bowel: leiomyosarcoma
    Soft tissue: Fibrosarcoma (10-20%) and fibrous histiocy-
                toma, malignant (10-20%); liposarcoma and
                rhabdomyosarcoma (each 15%); synovial sar-
                coma (10%); neurofibrosarcoma (malignant
                schwannoma, malignant neurilemmoma)
                (5%), angiosarcoma (3%), hemangiopericyto-
                ma (1%)

...SCHIZOPHRENIC OR SCHIZOPHRENIFORM DISORDER
                AMONG PATIENTS RECENTLY ADMIT-
                TED FOR INPATIENT CARE:
    in the United States:

The Most Common
TYPE OF:

paranoid

in many South American and African countries:

catatonic

...SEIZURE:

in Children:

Acute, non-recurring:

febrile convulsions. Other causes of acute seizures include toxic substances (e.g., drugs,
household poisons), metabolic disturbances
(e.g., hypoglycemia, tetany), and intracranial
disorders (e.g., brain tumors, meningitis)

Chronic, recurring (epilepsy):

in most cases, no specific cause can be found
(idiopathic, cryptogenic, primary, or essential
epilepsy); in about 20% of cases, a specific
cause is identified (symptomatic, organic, secondary, or acquired epilepsy)

...SEQUESTRATIONS OF THE LUNG:

intralobar (85%) > extralobar (15%)

...SHOCK: neurogenic

...SKELETAL DYSPLASIA, generalized:

achondroplasia

...SMALL BOWEL SARCOMA:

leiomyosarcoma

...SYMPTOMATIC BOWEL WALL TUMOR:

malignant tumors

...TERATOMA OF THE TESTICLE:

malignant > benign. Most common types are
intermediate, multigerminal (nonmalignant
mixtures with foci of malignant tissue); teratocarcinoma; differentiated multigerminal
(many types of tissue, nonmalignant); undifferentiated malignant (various varieties of malignant tissue in mixtures); malignant trophoblastic (choriocarcinoma)

...TETRALOGY OF FALLOT:
        cyanotic type (right to left shunt) > acyanotic
        type (left to right shunt)

...THYMOMA: benign (70%). 30% are locally invasive

...THYROID CARCINOMA:
        well-differentiated papillary carcinoma

...TRACHEOESOPHAGEAL MALFORMATION pattern:
        esophageal atresia (the proximal segment of
        the esophagus ends as a blind pouch in the
        midthorax [proximal pouch]) with a distal tra-
        cheo-esophageal fistula (distal segment of
        esophagus [connected to stomach] forms a
        connection to the bronchus near the carina)
        (86% of cases); the next two occur almost
        equally (in 6% of cases) and are pure esopha-
        geal atresia (proximal and distal blind pouch-
        es) without fistula, and tracheoesophageal fis-
        tula without atresia (H fistula); the most
        uncommon type (in 2% of cases) combines
        both a proximal and a distal tracheo-
        esophageal fistula with a proximal atresia

...TRANSFUSION REACTION:
        allergic reaction (i.e. fever, chills, urticaria,
        and itching)

...TRICUSPID ATRESIA:
        atresia with normally related great arteries and
        with or without VSD (70% of cases), atresia
        with D-transposition of the great arteries and
        VSD (23%), atresia with L-transposition of
        the great arteries (7%)

...TUMOR:
    in Men: lung, prostate, colon and rectum, urinary, leu-
        kemia and lymphoma, oral, skin, pancreas
    in Women: lung, breast, colon and rectum, uterus, leuke-
        mia and lymphoma, ovary, urinary, pancreas,

The Most Common
TYPE OF:
skin, oral

...TUMOR CAUSING INTESTINAL OBSTRUCTION:
    adenocarcinoma of the colon or rectum. Other malignant tumors include carcinoid or lymphoma

...TUMOR, vaginal:
    malignant

...ULCERS:
    duodenal > gastric

  Duodenal, that perforate:
    ulcers on the anterior surface of the duodenum. Occasionally, ulcers can perforate posteriorly into the lesser sac

...URACHAL CANCER:
    adenocarcinoma

...UTERINE INVERSION:
    acute > chronic; complete > incomplete inversion

...VAGINAL TUMOR:
    malignant

...VALVE IN CONGENITAL AORTIC STENOSIS:
    bicuspid valve with a single fused commissure and an eccentric orifice

...VENOUS RETURN IN CONGENITAL ABNORMALITY OF THE PULMONARY VEINS:

  Partial anomalous venous return:
    The right upper pulmonary vein drains into the superior vena cava

  Total anomalous venous return:
    supracardiac (50% of cases) - blood drains into the innominate vein and thence to the superior vena cave; cardiac (20% of cases) - blood drains into the coronary sinus or directly into the right atrium; infracardiac, also known as infradiaphragmatic (20% of cases) - blood drains into the portal or hepatic vein

and thence into the inferior vena cava; mixed (10% of cases) - blood returns to the heart via a combination of the above routes

...VENTRAL HERNIAS:

incisional

...VENTRICULAR SEPTAL DEFECT:

infracristal (membranous). Others include supracristal, in the atrioventricular canal, muscular

...VESICOURETERAL REFLUX:

primary reflux is by far the most common type. Secondary reflux is relatively rare

...VIRUS, respiratory, which causes acute laryngotracheobronchitis:

parainfluenza virus

...VULVAR CARCINOMA:

squamous carcinoma. Fewer are adenosquamous carcinoma, adenocarcinoma, malignant melanoma, verrucous carcinoma, and sarcomas

The Most Common
TYPE OF:

References

Andrews, NJ: Presentation and outcome of strangulated external hernia in a district general hospital. *Br. J. Surg.*, 68:329, 1981 in Sabiston, DC: *Sabiston's Essentials of Surgery*. Philadelphia, W.B. Saunders Company, 1987.

Beck, WW: *Obstetrics and Gynecology*. (The National Medical Series for Independent Study). New York, John Wiley & Sons, Inc., 1989.

Braunstein, H: *Outlines and Review of Pathology*. St. Louis, C.V. Mosby Company, 1987.

Casciato, DA, ed: *Manual of Clinical Oncology*, 2nd ed. Boston, Little, Brown and Company, 1988.

Chandrasoma, P: *Key Facts in Pathology*. New York, Churchill Livingstone, Inc., 1986.

Creighton University Lecture Series, Pathology course, 1988-89.

Creighton University Lecture Series, Department of OB/Gyn, 1989.

Day, AL, MD. Subarachnoid hemorrhage. *AFP*. 1989;40:95.

Dworkin, PH: *Pediatrics* (The National Medical Series for Independent Study). New York, John Wiley & Sons, Inc., 1987.

Evans, MI: *Obstetrics and Gynecology* (Pre-Test Series). New York, McGraw Hill, Inc., 1989.

Gregory, I: *Psychiatry*. Boston, Little, Brown and Company, Inc., 1983.

Jarrell, BE: *Surgery* (The National Medical Series for Independent Study). Media, Harwal Publishing Company, 1986.

Kingsbury, DT, ed: *Microbiology* (The National Medical Series for Independent Study). Media, Harwal Publishing Company, 1985.

Kravath, RE, ed.: *Pediatrics* (Pre-Test Series). New York, McGraw Hill Book Company, 1987.

LiVolsi, VA, ed: *Pathology* (The National Medical Series for Independent Study). Media, Harwal Publishing Company, 1984.

Myers, AR, ed.: *Medicine* (The National Medical Series for Independent Study). Media, Harwal Publishing Company, 1986.

Robbins, SL: *Pathologic Basis of Disease.* Philadelphia, W.B. Saunders Company, 1984.

Rubin, E, ed.: *Pathology.* Philadelphia, J.B. Lippincott Company, 1988.

Rudolph, AM, ed.: *Pediatrics*, 18th ed. Norwalk, Appleton & Lange, 1987.

Sabiston, DC: *Sabiston's Essentials of Surgery.* Philadelphia, W.B. Saunders Company, 1987.

Schrock, TR, ed.: *Handbook of Surgery*, 9th ed. Greenbrae, Jones Medical Publications, 1989.

Scialabba, FA, MD. Saccular Aneurysms of the Thoracic Aorta. *AFP.* 1990;41:1475.

Straub, WH, ed.: *Manual of Diagnostic Imaging*, 2nd ed. Boston, Little, Brown and Company, 1989.

Tisher, CC, ed.: *Nephrology for the House Officer.* Baltimore, Williams & Wilkins, 1989.

Tomb, DA: *Psychiatry for the House Officer.* Baltimore, Williams & Wilkins, 1988.

Vaughan, D: *General Ophthalmology.* 9th ed. Los Altos, Lange Medical Publications, 1980.

Way, LW: *Current Surgical Diagnosis and Treatment.* Norwalk, Appleton and Lange, 1988.